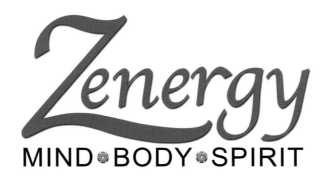

Cover Artwork: Christine Brisley, Brownwood, Texas
Photography, Graphics and Cover Design: Tad Browning, Georgetown, Texas
Book Design: The Oh Group, LLC, Dallas, Texas
Printed in USA by Buzz Print, Dallas, Texas
ISBN: 978-1-7333706-0-8
LCCN: 20290173

This book is dedicated to elevating spiritual consciousness and the health of humankind. May those who read it receive a blessing.

ACKNOWLEDGEMENTS

I offer special thanks to my amazing husband, Tad Browning, for all the quality images and graphics presented throughout the entire book. Without his professional eye for perfection and consistent loving support, this book would not be possible. Tad's mother, Helen Widener, has been a wonderful source of inspiration and encouragement over the course of completion. Helen's joy, wisdom, experience in writing four books and genuine friendship over the years has motivated me immensely. I am very grateful to be a part of their family!

Tad worked as a MediArtist, Photographer, Videographer and Graphics Illustrator since 1990. He began his career as a US Army Combat Photographer, worked with the Texas Rangers as a Forensic Photographer and currently oversees the Audiovisual Support for Operational Testing for the US Army. He also served as a Broadcast Journalist for 16 years in the Texas National Guard, completed two tours to Iraq, and retired as a First Sergeant in 2012 after 22 years of military service. Besides military imagery, Tad earned his FAA drone license for aerial photography and videography, enjoys underwater photography and recently discovered an interest in VR 360 video. As a MediArtist, Tad continues to find his passion for all things visual. For more information view his videos on YouTube, visit *GeorgetownMultimedia.com*, or call 512-GT-Media.

FRONT COVER ARTWORK BY CHRISTINE BRISLEY

I give a special thanks to my good friend Christine Brisley for the cover artwork. Christine is an internationally known artist who exhibited her art since age 15 and was one of the first Europeans invited to attend the Nam Yang Academy of Fine Art in Singapore. This early exposure to Oriental culture can still be seen in her watercolors today. Since then she has had over 60 one-woman exhibitions in England, America, Cyprus, Singapore and the Channel Islands, and she has shown her art in numerous galleries including the famous Grosvenor Park Gallery in Mayfair, London and the Spencer Coleman Galleries throughout England. She now resides in Brownwood, Texas. To see more of Christine's artwork visit *BrisleyArt.com*.

THANK YOU!

This book would not have been possible without the support and assistance from Renee Curtis, Rosa Oh, Laura Steelman, Sue Arney, Cathy Battle, Sue Angle, Helena Ovington, Eileen Pennington, Chris McKee, Dr. Jagit Khalsa, Dr. James Miles, Dr. Scot Knight, Tammy Holstrom, Dr. Jeanine Wade, Kathy Herring, LoAnne Mayer, Ray Stafford, Doug Willoughby, Keith Adelstein, and my parents, Joe and Peggy Steelman. My parents supported me in numerous ways over the years through education, travel and their own personal practices. Although "Wellness and Life Coach" were not words when I first started my quest, my parents gave me space to find my own path, and I thank them for my independence.

ENDORSEMENTS

Karen Lee Loenser, Director of Operations, Discovery Digital Media
Zenergy offers a spiritual buffet for seekers searching for nourishment for their souls. This work is like the masterpiece of a seasoned artist, who has carefully gone out into the world and studied and simplified some of its best practices. Ki assembled it for the reader as a personal offering for them to nibble, sample and savor it in bite-sized pieces for themselves.

This work offers an incredible portfolio of experience for both new and seasoned seekers who rely on authentic teachers like Ki Browning who have ventured out into the world with no roadmap, have re-discovered these ancient, magical (and much needed) practices and wrapped it with a loving ribbon of clarity and simplicity.

John Van Auken, Director of the Edgar Cayce Foundation
The vast breadth of information in Ki Browning's mind is matched by the depth and detail that she brings to us in this book. I've spent 50+ years researching and reporting on the many ways toward human wellness, now I have it all in one book. What she has gathered together for us is impressive; it's a resource for our physical, mental, and spiritual wellness. I can feel a genuine understanding in her teachings about being well despite all of our daily challenges. Zenergy is not in my book case, it's on my desk!

Ron Miller, 4 Time Ironman Finisher, All World Athlete, Proud Husband and Father, and Corporate Executive
Zenergy is food for my soul. Ki lays out foundational practices that have lead me to a happy healthy life. I've suffered from anxiety, stress and depression and only through my faithful practices have I learned that my mind, body and soul all need nourishment.

Carol Ritberger, PhD, Author of Healing Happens with Your Help...Understanding the Hidden Meanings Behind Illness
Ki's book a must-read for those who want to heal themselves, and it's a must-read for those who want to learn how to manage the daily challenges of life. Ki has gifted us with a great reference book that's rich with suggestions and techniques that can teach us how to live a happy, healthy, and peaceful life.

Chris McKee, Certified Nutritionist, The Nomadic Nutritionist

I had the privilege of being one of the first to preview Ki Browning's new book Zenergy. As a nutritionist and natural health enthusiast for over thirty years I found this book to be very comprehensive. Ki covers all aspects of health, nutrition, physical, emotional and spiritual. To lead a healthy and productive life we must address all of these areas, and Ki does it in an easy to understand yet far reaching manner. I would highly recommend this book be your guide to a long, healthy and active life!

Peter Woodbury, MSW, Harvard University Graduate and Past Life Regression Teacher

Ki does a wonderful job in her chapter on reincarnation. She makes a complicated subject very accessible, drawing parallels from multiple sources. The field of reincarnation studies is just in its fledgling state, and Ki has added a valuable resource to the field. A must-read for anyone even remotely interested in reincarnation.

INTRODUCTION

Are you happy? If you don't feel joyful right now, what are you going to do about it before sundown? Zenergy offers a multitude of ways that help you feel better quickly. I've designed this book so you can read it cover-to-cover or open it to just about any page and glean a nugget of wisdom to apply immediately. Read the Table of Contents and select a topic of your choosing. This book is full of many time tested scientifically proven methods that you can implement today. You will get the maximum benefit from this book when you practice the Zenergy Boosts. They are short mental and physical activities, when applied, can transform your outlook and understanding much more than just reading a few pages. Practice at least one suggested technique each day for the next 90 days for maximum benefit.

In the past decade employers increased spending on health and wellness, boosting participation in corporate wellness programs, biometric screenings, yoga and fitness classes and even incentives to walk more in attempts of achieving a healthier workforce. Whether at work or home, the day you incorporate wellness practices into your life, you will feel better instantly.

Consider the following signs that you're well, healthy, healed and whole.
1. You appreciate yourself and others.
2. You're height-weight proportional.
3. You're flexible physically and mentally.
4. You set healthy boundaries when needed.
5. You're in touch with your emotions and share authentic expression.
6. Your life has meaning.
7. You value experiences more than possessions.
8. You offer natural sincerity and convey reverence for all life.
9. Your supportive disposition allows others to trust you.
10. You exercise regularly and meditate daily.
11. You live inside your financial means.

Appreciation is a key factor to enjoying life. Do you take time to acknowledge yourself for your efforts day-after-day? Spending just one minute to prepare for the day and set your intentions can improve your overall outlook. Take measures into your own hands so that you feel fantastic and achieve your daily goals. Waiting for others to recognize you may lead to feeling undervalued, resentful or even angry. Knowing what's important to you can breathe new life into common activities and interactions. Many times when doing a favorite thing, like eating, we rush through the experience to complete the task. Don't miss the enjoyment and benefits of your favorite activity just to check it off your to-do list. Learning to be present will enrich your life and give you a sense of complete health and wellness. Let's get *Zenergized*!

TABLE OF CONTENTS

MIND SECTION

I. THE INNER YOU 2
    A. What is Wellness 2
    B. Healing the Mind 4
    C. Obtain Your Highest Frequency 7
    D. Managing Anxiety 11
    E. Sadness is a Part of Life 13
    F. Living and Coping with Trauma 16
    G. Changing a Habit 19
    H. Under-Thoughts and Thought-Storms 22
    I. Compassion, The Ultimate Love 29

II. SETTING HEALTHY BOUNDARIES 31
    A. Conscious Communication 31
    B. Brain-Drains 36
    C. Slicers 38
    D. Adult Adolescents 41
    E. Punctuality Matters 42
    F. Win/Win Negotiations 44
    G. Forgiveness Relaxes Your Guard 46

III. PEACE PROVOKING APTITUDE 52
    A. Stress Management Skills 52
    B. Meditation 101 56
    C. Meditation Practices 61
    D. Breathing Techniques for Relaxation 63
    E. Meditation Frustration 68
    F. Resolving Scatter Chatter 69

IV. CHARTING YOUR FUTURE 71
    A. Magnetize Your Heartsong 71
    B. Magnetizing Your Heartsong Worksheet 78
    C. Taking Action 88

BODY SECTION

V. NUTRITIONALLY STARVED & PHYSICALLY FAT 92
  A. Genetically Modified Organisms/Foods (GMOs) 93
  B. Strains, Grains and Brain Fog 96
  C. Sugar Shocker 97
  D. Kicking the Can 98
  E. Fast Food Frenzie 99

VI. HOW TO READ NUTRITION LABELS 102
  A. Grocery Shopping 102
  B. Reading Labels 104
  C. Food Journal 106

VII. INTRODUCTION TO AYURVEDA 107
  A. Dosha Quiz 111
  B. Balancing Techniques for Each Mind Dosha 115
  C. Enjoying All 6-Tastes Pacifies the Body Doshas 117
  D. Balance Your Body Through Suitable Nutrition 120
  E. 6-Tastes Shopping List 123
  F. Components of an Ayurvedic Daily Routine 125
  G. Healthful Hints 126

VIII. THE GOODNESS OF FOOD 127
  A. Cinnamon Oatmeal with Apples 128
  B. 6-Tastes Magic Muffins 130
  C. Quick 6 Breakfast: Eggs & Spinach 132
  D. Hearty or Lite Turkey and Cheese Delight 134
  E. Robust Lentil Soup Crockpot 136
  F. Fresh Flounder and Cabbage Flower 138
  G. Veggie Stir Fry with Tricolor Quinoa 140
  H. Grass-Fed Beef Spaghetti and Roasted Vegetables 142
  I. Fresh Salmon and Zestful Zucchini Boat 144
  J. 6-Tastes Munchie Mix 146
  K. Beverages 148
  L. Spiritualizing Your Food 152

IX. DETOXING 154
    A. Do You Need to Detox? 154
    B. Castor Oil Packs for Detoxing 157
    C. Detoxifying the Skin 158
    D. Top Digestion Stressors 160
    E. Dirty Dozen and Clean Fifteen 160
    F. Nutritional Tips 162
    G. How to Lose 10 Pounds Fast 163

X. INTEGRATIVE AND NATURAL THERAPIES 164
    A. Mind-Body Integration 164
    B. Placebo Effect 166
    C. East Meets West 170
    D. Chiropratic Care 170
    E. Acupuncture 172
    F. Dry Needling 173
    G. Massage Therapy 174
    H. Hypnosis Works! 176
    I. Essential Oils 177
    J. Benefits of CBD, Cannabidiol 179
    K. Natural Remedies 180

XI. LET'S TALK ABOUT SEX 183

XII. YOGA 189
    A. Exercise with Mindful Awareness 192
    B. Keep Moving 192
    C. Benefits of Yoga and Exercise 195
    D. Reframing Exercise 195
    E. Sun Salutation 196
    F. Spinal Health Yoga Sequence 201
    G. Sciatica Release Yoga Sequence 211
    H. Yoga for Weight Management and Strength 215
    I. Yoga for Digestion 220
    J. Postures for Balance & Poise 223
    K. Advanced Yoga Asanas 229
    L. Yoga on a Peg ~
        A Yogi recounts her harrowing motorcycle adventure through the Andes............ 232

SPIRIT SECTION

A. What is Spiritual Wellness 238

B. Contacting Your Angels & The Power of Prayer 243

C. Becoming Zen 245

D. Equinoxes and Solstices 246

E. Spirit Animals 248

F. Oracle Cards 251

G. Numerology 253

H. Astrology 257

I. The Power of Your Dreams 263

J. What's Your Superpower? 269

K. Chakras & Their Influence 277

L. Reiki Healing Energy 288

M. Near Death Experiences 291

N. Reincarnation 294

O. Past Life Recall 302

P. Heavenly Stargate 309

Glossary 311

Bibliography 317

Biography 327

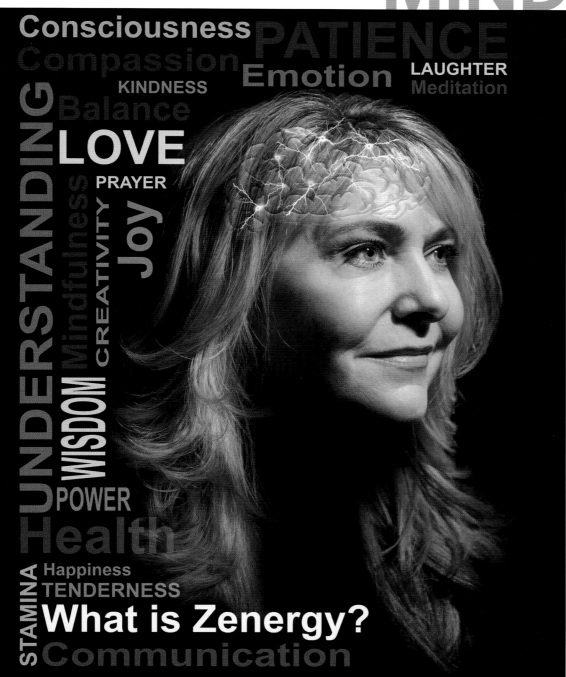

THE INNER YOU

WHAT IS WELLNESS?

Wellness is more than just diet and exercise. Wellness includes many aspects of our lives— family, work, society, even the part of you who grocery shops, repairs the vehicle or mows the lawn. How mindful are you in the different areas in your life? What type of person are you in your community? What is your communication style? What is your spouse's communication style? Are you friendly, serious, resentful, shy? Identifying your personality traits gives great wisdom into your personal wellness. Finding many ways to keep yourself happy and healthy is important along your temporary journey on Earth. Remember, no one gets out alive. So take the next 40, 50 or 70 years to explore this vast planet. Take note of the five people that you spend the majority of your time with because they influence you the most. Knowing them intimately will certainly help you along your path to staying well and happy.

Implementing a wellness routine into your daily activities can positively transform your life. Be mindful during the large and small tasks you do today. Change can be awkward at the beginning and many won't even take the first step; however, when the fecal matter hits the ventilator, there is high motivation to do something, anything, to create a new way of living. Why wait until you're in complete crisis? Acknowledge yourself for the efforts you've already made and add a simple wellness practice today.

 ZENERGY BOOST FOR DEFINING YOUR WELLNESS PROGRAM
Make a list of the positive things you're doing already and a list of 3-5 things you would like to improve in your life. Be looking for new strategies in these pages.

Accessing memories fires the brain in a different way than when you're reading. Shifting back and forth between the creative-emotional-spiritual side (right brain) and the analytical-scientific-logical side (left brain) is a skill that improves brain functioning. Noticing your body periodically (like how the clothes rest on your skin or the quality of your breath) makes you more present. Your body is talking to you and, more importantly, it's listening to you. Every thought you have is being registered by your cellular structure. Identify what you're thinking which leads to lifestyle choices that are healthy or toxic. The hidden self, or subconscious, makes decisions behind the scenes. For instance, many people say they want to lose 30 pounds, and then eat a pizza. This incongruent behavior creates confusion and confliction. That's the hidden self we will uncover over the course of this book, and the suggested Zenergy Boosts will, over time, uncover that decision maker.

The Value of Wellness

Many Human Resource Directors are looking for new ways to enhance company culture by incorporating wellness. Stressful situations at work and home can lead to high blood pressure, anxiety, sadness, depression, or insomnia which, in turn, can lead to tardiness, lack of accountability, excessive sick leave, presentism (the employee should be absent but they are physically present) or employee disengagement. When stress levels are high, cortisol increases and IGA goes down. IGA, immunoglobulin A, naturally rebuilds cells creating the primary defense against bacteria and viruses. Better than a flu shot, your body has an innate pharmacy and making wellness a natural part of a company culture is comparable to choosing the right benefits package for staff.

Today, we frequently hear about the positive impact corporate wellness programs have to train and retain quality staff members. According to the 10th Annual Health and Wellbeing Survey from Fidelity Investments and the National Business Group on Health, "the average per employee incentive of $762 for 2019 is nearly three times the average employee incentive of $260 reported in 2009. Wellness programs include emotional and mental health, financial health [education], community involvement, social connectedness and job satisfaction. As employers recognize the relationship between employee wellbeing and productivity, wellbeing programs have taken on an increasingly meaningful role in employers' business strategies" (April 2019).

Many employees will rarely admit to the stress associated with just one person in the office. If employees were better equipped with quality coping and communication skills they might overcome those difficulties, and the corporation retain their skill set. Employee disengagement or changeover is challenging for both the employee and the company, especially after the one-year marker.

The worst thing for an organization is to have a senior staff member suddenly die from a heart attack or stroke. Equally challenging is living with the issues after a stroke. According to the American Heart Association, about 30% die from strokes annually; 70% recover and live with disabilities. That can also takes its toll on a company and its leadership, not to mention the family but mostly the survivor. Which may mean you. Are you at risk for a stroke? Adopting health and wellness practices, whether mind, body or spirit, provides a process for self-care and work-life balance that brings a higher level of workplace productivity and a deeper level of contentment.

HEALING THE MIND

Each day there is an onslaught of information to process—news, emails, relationships, workflow, traffic jams, home repairs, financial planning, IRAs, medical care, family health. The brain is like a computer organizing events, storing memories and defragging the mainframe. It can be overwhelming to process the mass of data day after day. Some days we like it, other days not-so-much. Information overload is common and many people become ill due to mental and emotional strain. However, like professional athletes, victory awaits those who recharge before returning to the game. I counseled many high achievers over the years whose demanding schedules crippled their health and who eventually ended up on their knees with cancer or another disease.

Executives focusing on the big corporate picture and profits frequently lose sight of their own wellbeing. They forget the collaboration of a healthy mind-body-spirit to achieve their professional goals. Moms can undermine their own happiness concentrating on their child's accomplishments. Moms are the glue to most families and if Mom gets sick the familial conveyor belt can come to a screeching halt. Even recreational athletes push to the edge and can over-train only to injure themselves a few days prior to the event. Working or training 12-hour days is unhealthy, and can even cause permanent damage to your physique, immune and endocrine system. Finding balance is the key.

Karen (names have been changed) came to me after she had been diagnosed with breast cancer. She chose not to have chemotherapy as it would only have a 50/50 affect on her type of cancer. She decided on radiation and a lumpectomy. Upon awakening she learned the doctor also removed 14 lymph nodes. During our counseling sessions we uncovered her hidden emotions spurring her exemplary career achievements. She devoted 15 years to building a clinic, being an integral part of the management team and taking the company to the top in their region. She caught the brass ring, but didn't realize it until she was in my office dealing with the aftermath of cancer treatment. It never occurred to her that she had actually earned the title and respect she craved from that company. She enjoyed her career but underneath her desire for high achievement she wanted acceptance from others. Fearful thoughts can have us do all kinds of things at the expense of ourselves. Regretfully, she passed up a few marital offers in lieu of corporate achievement hoping to gain further admiration from her employer by working nights and weekends. She compromised her health along the way due to her narrow vision toward work and was devastated when she realized the missed opportunities. After our sessions she began taking steps to lessen her workload and dedicate more time for wellness strategies. Accepting the decisions she made that directed her life path away from marriage and children, she restored her mental and physical health. Repetitive feelings of gratitude toward the positive decisions made (toward her career, home ownership or other endeavors) allowed her to understand her choices better.

I can't tell you how many times I've counseled clients on this topic. Yes, the details are different but, generally speaking, high achievers can give all that they have at the cost of their health. Don't give it all away, Folks! Save some for yourself and your family. Accepting certain career decisions doesn't mean one cannot make time for other joys, like pursuing outside interests. Plus, think about professional athletes, and how they sit on the bench for a round or two and regain energy before jumping back into the game. Periodically, reflect on the life you're living. Is it your destiny or have you fallen into some bad habits? Stress and inflammation are the main causes of disease and working non-stop definitely precipitates physiological imbalance.

Set realistic goals to reduce your stress and improve your health. (Goal setting is discussed in later chapters.) You're in charge. Stress is a choice. You invite most, if not all, of the stress that comes your way. What? You might think, "How can that be true?" Let's look at the typical choices of how you prefer to live. Do you live in a clean environment? Cluttered messy homes attract germs, mold and potential illness. Organizing and cleaning your home can help you manage your mental obligations. What food are you choosing? The wrong nutritional choices can cause inflammation; stress and inflammation are the foremost causes of disease. Do you choose to meditate and relax for a few minutes each day? The intensity of the days and weeks and years adds up, and your choices today may cause imbalances in your mind, body and spirit tomorrow.

Healing the mind is one of the best ways to overcome the anxiety of a fast-paced life, or the potential onset of depression and negativity after the diagnosis of a disease. Sometimes we can overcome hardship alone, but frequently we need someone positive to walk with us. We need a healthy, compassionate friend to bounce ideas off of and who can share an objective observation. Don't underestimate the power of talking to a friend, support group or even a stranger. Sometimes sitting on an airplane you can strike up a conversation with a complete stranger and disclose personal things about yourself since they don't really know you or your circle. You can exchange ideas and even intimate details without the concern of gossip; however, don't fail to recognize the benefits of a professional therapist. The brain that created the problem is not the brain that will solve it. Think outside your own box and welcome new ideas to expand your outlook. Consider new wellness ideas to incorporate into your day-to-day activities, and this will help you maintain healthy brain-body functioning. Curiosity will keep you youthful and expand your personal evolvement.

Begin to notice how much time you watch TV and consider reducing it by one hour each week. Use that time doing your favorite healthy hobby or learn a new skill. Some people get emotionally charged from watching the 6 o'clock news. Be particular about what you watch as memories stay in your mind for a very long time. It is the same with social media. Who's on your feed? Are those people actually feeding you? Be choosy. You don't have to watch all the negativity TV shows broadcast. It's called "programming" for a reason. You are getting programmed. Don't watch highly charged, opinionated or negative TV for a day or a week and notice how much better you feel. Your friends will tell you about the major disasters (for which typically you can do little). One objective of mainstream media is to sell pharmaceuticals. Reporters discuss the tragedies all over the planet, followed by an anti-depressant pharmaceutical ad. News anchors can deliver a narrative on mud-slinging politicians, corruption and even tragic earth changes, and then an anti-anxiety pharmaceutical ad airs.

Release the stress by taking a few minutes each day to defrag, relax and contemplate the day's activities. Unrecognized stress due to information overload can cause frustration or even sideways anger. Yelling at a colleague because you couldn't find a parking place and consequently were late for the meeting is a common example of sideways anger. Emotions like irritation, anger, hatred, sadness or suicidal thoughts frequently go unheard. Men especially may not discuss their feelings of fear, dread or depression as it could appear weak or show vulnerability. Women may talk incessantly, but rarely disclose deep concerns, leaving many to feel isolated or misunderstood. Taking time to explore your feelings could save your career and marriage. A lot of marital stress is due to incompatible communication styles and can be resolved with a little bit of self-discovery. If your marriage causes you undue stress then get to a counselor or a marital retreat and learn new communication strategies. One visit could change your life for the better.

Healing the mind starts with excavating your authentic self and uncovering what is truly important to you. Notice how often you are doing things that are essential to you versus doing what others expect of you. Finding authentic self-expression is one of the keys to inner peace and contentment. With a little observation you may find you're already on the right path. It just takes a little awareness, patience and commitment. As you find new ways to openly express yourself, mental health and emotional freedom are obtainable.

 ZENERGY BOOSTS FOR MENTAL & EMOTIONAL HEALING
1. Create a gratitude journal.
2. Upon awakening, log your dreams each morning & interpret them.
3. Wear a different style of clothing for a day or two; document how you felt about it and what was the response from your friends and co-workers.
4. Walk 15 minutes twice a week.
5. Bat a phone book or pillow to released pent-up emotions.
6. Write your resignation speech (don't deliver it, just write it) and identify where you're going from here.
7. Yell at the wall instead of a coworker or child.
8. Get a hot oil massage or spa treatment.
9. Take a drama, acting, modeling or comedic improv class.

OBTAIN YOUR HIGHEST FREQUENCY

We all emit a frequency ~ upbeat, offbeat, flat, dissonant, andante, or allegro. Brainwaves are measureable yet invisible. We recognize frequency on an intuitive level, but we don't have a common language for it yet. The electromagnetic spectrum is the range of frequency from radio waves to microwaves to ultraviolet and even gamma rays. Some we can see; most we cannot. Vibration is all around us. Plants, animals, humans, everything, all emit a vibrational frequency. The world is one big vibration.

Animals acknowledge the frequency with transparency; they either like you or they don't. They can sense risk or danger based on frequency and odors well before humans can. Maybe you've heard your dog bark at a pedestrian through the front windows of your home well before you could see that person walking on the sidewalk. This is a good example of their abilities. There are sounds that humans cannot hear but dogs can, like the dog whistle. Dogs pick up on your vibrations quickly. As the good adage goes, "if my dog likes you, I like you."

Remember a time when you met someone that you instantly didn't like. No real reason, you just didn't resonant with them. So, you avoided them in the future. In the 1960s they said, "Bad vibes, Man." Your collaborative frequency was dissonant so you circumvented your time together. We're always looking for harmony whether you register it like that or not.

Those who are positive or optimistic emanate a higher harmonious frequency. They are upbeat, buoyant, constructive, joyful and/or encouraging. When you are negative, gloomy thoughts can preoccupy your outlook and this lowers your frequency. Negative, or negativity, is a number, a frequency, a low tempo. Like a symphony, each phase of our life can create a different movement or mood, and each has its own beginning and end. Are you stuck in a mood?

Emotions like fear, negativity, anger, and hopelessness can create an inner dialogue which block you from experiencing day-to-day happiness. Your body generates a vibration just from your bones and tissue, but also with every act, thought, encounter and each meal you ingest. You're giving off vibrations with everything you do. Negativity is just as contagious as positivity. When you complain about the weather or traffic usually someone will chime in with an equally downbeat story. When you smile at a stranger, frequently they will catch your vibe and smile back recharging both of you. "Good vibes, Man." Our moods can be contagious.

Emotions like guilt, shame and apathy vibrate at a slower rate. You feel slow and sluggish when you're down in the dumps, and you feel upbeat, high and inspired when you experience joy, peace and love. You are sending out a signal, or a vibe, with your thoughts and feelings. Each thought you have creates energy in you and around you. If you're joyful, you smile more or are more patient. If you're angry, you honk your horn or offer finger gestures while driving. Your vibrations are generated from repetitive thoughts and actions throughout each day and decade. If you think angry thoughts day after day, that moves from a mood to a disposition to a personality or even a personality disorder. Others are picking up on these vibes from you and responding whether you realize it or not.

Was there a time when you used to be more cheerful and felt fairly healthy? Where did that go? Did you become prideful, fearful or apathetic? Maybe joy disappeared behind the responsibilities of adulthood, child rearing, paying the mortgage and the daily grind. Pleasure disappears due to the stress response, and this lowers your internal frequency. If we reflect on the past, frequently we access some fun memories of riding the roller coaster at an amusement park, dancing until the wee hours or laughing loudly. As we mature, decisions are made and our life changes. We move from one phase to the next and life has its ups and downs. These crescendos and decrescendos allow us to appreciate the fluctuations in life. Otherwise, it would all be quite flat and boring. Take a few minutes to enjoy some of your playful past times to increase your frequency, your optimism and resiliency.

Listening to music or attending a concert could be just the answer too. Facilitating emotional wellbeing through music has been understood since before recorded time. Sadly today, many people miss the joyous experience when attending a concert because they are so intent on recording it on their cell phones. They spend most of the concert adjusting their technology and staring at a small screen even though they are standing near the stage in the middle of the action. Enjoy the concert and if you want to see it again, visit the band's website. They will have a higher quality recording than your cell phone, and visiting their website is another way to support your favorite bands. The benefits of music include improving memory, reducing pain and stress and lowering anxiety, sometimes within the first few notes. Hearing your favorite song can shift your mood almost instantaneously. It has been proven that babies enjoy listening to music even in the womb. Music lifts your spirits in a profound nonverbal way. Learn to vibrate at your highest possible frequency through uplifting harmonies.

Music is the bridge between heaven and earth.
Chinese Proverb

ZENERGY BOOST FOR UPLIFTING YOUR FREQUENCY

1. Listen to upbeat or classical music with eyes closed. Truly listen to it, don't multitask, and notice how your mood shifts with the notes.
2. Look at a mandala or attractive scenic photo for 2-5 minutes.
3. Tap into the joy of your childhood again with the new adult coloring books. Coloring mandalas and/or looking at them is nourishing for the mind-body-spirit connection.
4. Hold a mineral or crystal in your hand or leave in your pants pocket; it's most effective to wear it on your neck over the heart chakra (Chakras discussed in Spirit Section).
5. Watch a comedy or attend a comedy show.
6. Politely step away from the gossip table. Gossip hurts everyone. Stop listening.
7. Visit a museum or look at illusionist art. Enjoying art and surreal images help you think outside your box.

Mentally positive people have staying power. They typically don't get sick (or as sick) as their contemporaries. Raising your frequency allows you to rebound quickly after an emotional or financial setback, or to take the high road in conversations and conflict. Seeing the bright side of life improves your overall immunity. Negativity opens the door for injury, illness and disease.

We are an electromagnetic vibration emanating a pulse. When you're overwhelmed, resentful or dejected you generate static about you, and those around you notice it. Your family, friends and colleagues might tolerate it, but they certainly would prefer that you're kind, optimistic or at least pleasant. In one way you're sucking the life out of a situation; in the other, you are energizing it. You can transform an average or unpleasant day just by planning ahead. Having a date for dancing or billiards can increase your optimism after an offbeat day. Prepare!

If you find that emotions are building up or spilling over, find your imaginary helicopter and fly away. You already know what's down that path. Don't take it. When dark emotions arise and try to get the best of you, stand up, and change your environment. Stop entertaining those negative notions and physically change what you're doing immediately. Go for a walk or watch a funny video. Later you can factually evaluate your circumstances and transcend your emotions through logic. Don't sit and dwell. Dwelling extends karma.

We all have a rhythm in life. Women's cycles are generally 28-days and for men it's approximately 32-days. Determine yours as soon as possible. During the month we have both a crest of the wave and then a time when we plunge deeply into a well. Women, discover your PMS time–are you pre-menstrual, during-menstrual or post-menstrual? Generally speaking, identify the time when you just don't feel good for two or three days per month. Your hormones are shifting or maybe even imbalanced. Find a calendar and start charting your rhythm. Which days are high (usually during ovulation) and which are low? Don't try to fight it, flow with it. Understanding your cycle can save you years of unexpected turbulent times. Men, you can do the same thing. Of course, you don't have a menstruation to guide you but begin to chart your feelings. Notice when you're on the crest of the wave, high fiving your pals and singing in the shower. And, document when you're out of rhythm, needing more cave time. Record your highs and lows throughout the month.

Take time to pamper yourself when your energy or frequency is low. This is the time to keep yourself mentally and emotionally balanced. Generally speaking, women generate oxytocin (the happy hormone) by getting a massage, mani/pedi or enjoying quality aromatherapy. Men generate it by being alone, driving fast, or watching a sporting event or action film. Both sexes become much happier after an orgasm. Think of it as a reset button. Whatever floats your boat, set time aside just for yourself on those down days. Many arguments can be alleviated with a little forethought. Don't lash out at your friends and family because you need some self-time. Schedule your self-time into your calendar in advance. Doing that is not a selfish act; yelling at your family because you need more space is selfish. If possible, avoid interviews or signing contracts when you're in the depths of your well. Sometimes we just don't have a choice, as life keeps moving fast; however, if you can, circumvent important meetings and first dates until you're on the crest of your wave again.

Like a symphony, your frequency rises and falls throughout the day. Avoid getting stuck in any one beat or mood. Go with the flow and allow the rhythm to uplift you. Don't enable the cacophony of a demanding day to steal your inner peace. Choose harmony and reap the rewards immediately.

 ZENERGY BOOST FOR FINDING THE CREST OF YOUR WAVE
1. Find a calendar and begin rating your emotional state daily from 1 to 10.
    1—sad, bitchy, asshole, road rage day; 10—generous, joyful, easily humored day.
2. Look for the trend in your monthly cycle and increase your frequency by staying prepared.
3. Plan something nurturing when you're in the well next time.
4. Use your phone calendar for privacy

MANAGING ANXIETY

Driving on Interstate-35 where construction continues between Dallas and Austin, I've had more than one harrowing experience. It's been ongoing for years and many people have died on I-35. The drive used to be easy and mostly straight. Texas is so big and highways seem to go on forever. Long distance travel can turn into a leisurely drive with the handy use of cruise control. Then, the main artery to the state capitol went under construction for years, the speed limit changed constantly, 18-wheelers hauled past on two narrow lanes while watchful police officers sat on the sidelines with their radar detectors hoping to make their quota.

One time, I was driving between a cement road divider and an 18-wheeler, which can be a little daunting, especially at night. The lanes began to zigzag as I entered the most technical part of the drive. It was hard not to imagine slamming into the cement wall or gliding under the nearby truck. I noticed the rubber tire marks on the road and the cement divider from others who may not have made it. My shoulders inched toward my ears as my hands gripped the steering wheel tighter. I took a deep breath and tried to relax my shoulders. I opened my fingers one at a time while my sweaty palms pressed firmly to the column to maintain control of the vehicle. My shoulders edged upward toward my tight jaw and my achy neck while the cycle continued for another 90 minutes until I safely arrived home.

Driving tension is common. It's easy to get overwhelmed in traffic or construction. Sometimes you might not even notice you're stressed, but if you get angry and offer an unfavorable hand gesture, don't pretend that it's the other person's fault. You're the one who shot the dove, even if the other person cut you off. Yes, they too are stressed, but don't blame them for your flying finger. The mind-body can maintain high levels of adrenaline and cortisol hormones even though we're not in any eminent danger. Worrying can elevate adrenaline. So, don't let your brain fly off your neck during times of construction or traffic jams. Feel the clothes on your skin and feel your feet on the floorboard. Anxiety is a legitimate feeling and acknowledging it is the beginning of the healing process. You can't heal something you haven't noticed.

Identify sources of your anxiety ~ driving, work, finances, relationships, society, health. What is the worst-case scenario that can happen in any of these situations? Exploring this subject with many clients over the years I've come to find that underneath all the tension for most people is really the fear of dying or worse, dying in a Maytag box or even worse, in a box alone. Now, I understand that this is extreme, but if you will ask yourself the question, "what if the worst happens?" and keep asking yourself about the worst, you will uncover what motivates your anxiety.

Death and dying are often taboo topics yet they dominate our lives. Fear of dying is illogical because you are going to die. Fear of being unfinished when you die is common because you cannot possibly do everything in one lifetime. You must know there is a limit to what you can do and how long you get to do it. So think deeply about your ultimate goal and start moving toward that. Acquiring the goal isn't as important as moving toward it. Being on the path toward your vision is the primary function of life and deep down many people feel anxious because they aren't moving toward their dreams at all. Are you? Are you living your dreams or someone else's? Is it bringing you happiness, despair or anxiety? Successful people know that there will be victories and failures throughout life. You are not going to win at every thing you ever try, but if you never try then you've not lived fully. And, many won't try to reach their dreams because of anxiety. So again I ask, what is the worst-case scenario that gives you so much anxiety?

Sometimes anxiety can come from hanging onto what is ineffective or obsolete just because it's familiar. Are you hanging onto the past? If a part of you longs for the past, yearning for the way things used to be, spend a few minutes each day to reminisce and memorialize the past. Have a ceremony for it. Spend 5-10 minutes each day paying homage to the past you lost and then 5-10 minutes creating the future you truly want, possibly with some of the same elements. Remember, nothing stays the same. Acknowledge the past and step into the present audaciously. You don't drive forward looking in your rearview mirror, do you? Of course not. So, don't live today by focusing on yesterday (or yester-year or yester-decade). If you're on autopilot you cannot correct or improve your outlook. First, you have to decide to take charge of your personal choices. Waking up anxious is a bad habit. The day hasn't even started yet. Give it a chance to be better than yesterday. Becoming conscious is a choice.

Proper nutrition, exercise and positive thinking are powerful tools for staying grounded and managing anxiety. Exercise and nutrition can make a huge difference in your mental-emotional state. Blood draws indicate lower cortisol and higher dopamine and serotonin after subjects exercise and eat quality food. Walking is free and making better nutritional choices just requires a little knowledge and, of course, the desire to be healthier. If you know that particular foods make you more anxious or moody, consider eliminating them, at least during stressful times like end-of-month accounting, annual reviews or holidays with the in-laws. Even premenstrual syndrome (PMS) can be reduced significantly by adding exercise and making smarter nutritional choices. Fried foods, heavy carbohydrates and high fructose corn syrup irritate the body and hormones; fruits, vegetables and salmon balance the body. If you awaken and you're already a little anxious, don't drink coffee. That will only irritate your body more. Start with a shower. If that's not enough then drink a cup of tea, but limit it to only one cup. Many people, especially those with anxiety, do not need caffeine at all. They're zooming naturally.

ZENERGY BOOST TO ALLEVIATE ANXIETY FAST
1. Sit in a chair, place your hands on your heart and navel and breath slowly for five minutes. Intend that your heart beat slow and steady.
2. Take a deep breath and retain the breath for 3-5 seconds. Do this for 3-30 breaths.
3. Rescue Remedy contains five flower essences. You can ingest it sublingually (under the tongue) for immediate relief. Found at health food stores.
4. Exercise for 30-60 minutes.
5. Take a hot shower and wash your hair.
6. Luxuriate in a hot Epsom salt bath for 15-30 minutes (2-3 cups per tub).
7. Laugh. Watch a comedy, adorable kid or funny pet videos. It's refreshing.
8. Contribute to another when you feel low. Volunteerism takes the focus off you and is very helpful in moving past personal problems.

SADNESS IS PART OF LIFE

Many people have sad thoughts and feelings, which are different from depression. We use the word depression to casually describe a gloomy mood; however, depression is a clinical term that refers to a chemical imbalance frequently managed by pharmaceutical drugs. Depression is not the same as thinking sad thoughts, although, if you think enough sad thoughts, eventually you're going to get depressed. Thoughts that are fired get hard-wired in the neurology. Sad thoughts can lead to depression because every thought you have delivers a chemical throughout your body. Pessimism keeps the focus on what is wrong, broken or missing from your environment. Complaining and lamenting or even commiserating with your friends drives you down a bumpy road, solidifies poor behavior and reduces resiliency. Sad people focus on what's missing day after day. They concentrate on bad things in their environment, rarely noticing the good. They could be standing in the middle of a joyous celebration and still feel miserable. Repetitive thoughts, or looped thinking, eventually get hard-wired into the brain.

Sometimes you need medication, and anti-depressants can be useful at different times. It's helpful to have many alternatives to deal with stress. Sometimes medication is a part of the answer, but you still have to deal with what you're thinking. Wherever you go, there you are! Whatever you ingest, you're still there. The problem didn't leave because you took a pill. You still need to find the solution, and for many people the drugs just aren't enough.

Resiliency can help you cope with trauma and move on after a distressing event. Characteristics of resilient people include self-confidence, positive outlook, sense of humor and flexibility. Moving toward a new goal and developing a positive view of yourself can be useful behaviors to reorientate. Avoid seeing the crisis as insurmountable and reach out to loved ones for support. You can learn from your mistakes and choose more wisely in the future. Just because you made a mistake doesn't mean you ARE a mistake.

The 2015 Disney movie, *Inside Out*, had a sweet way of identifying emotions. The movie portrays a visually inventive viewpoint toward emotional expression encouraging children to be emotionally authentic. The movie starts from a daring intangible premise within the psyche of a girl named Riley. The film's characters are her feelings ~ Joy, Sadness, Fear, Disgust and Anger. Stay with me here, I'm not rabbit trailing. When do we learn about authentic self-expression? Childhood. It can be an insufferably challenging time and that outlook can move into adulthood. I like the movie because it portrays the secret life of feelings in an abstract way, but which can ultimately become the bedrock of your personality. Those who are generally sad consistently remember what went wrong on any particular day, instead of what went right.

The narrative continues during a birthday celebration. Joy (one of the characters) remembered her fun birthday party and was enthusiastic about the celebration. Then, Sadness (another character) remembered that the sprinkler system went off inadvertently, and she lamented on how cold she was at her birthday party. The character Sadness focused on how unfortunate it was that the party wasn't perfect. Joy tried to bring Sadness out of those dark feelings by reminiscing on the delight experienced at the party. Take a moment to reflect now. Do you focus on what went wrong in any given situation or how you were offended or embarrassed, or can you refocus on the thrill of it all? When you express sadness or even anger is it a momentary emotional expression or is it your personality? Sadness and happiness are choices.

Your thoughts and your outlook determine your unhappiness. Unfortunately, the mind can dwell on disappointments or fears even though there is nothing you can do about that circumstance. For instance, remember a time when you didn't get a date with the new girl in the office. Thinking about the unfulfilled wish is only natural, but longing for that one person could lead to an obsession. Those obsessive thoughts alter your blood chemistry and discourage positive action. Focus on the *qualities* of the person you desire instead of one person specifically (since that new girl is unavailable).

Sadness can weasel its way into our hearts and yet so many people don't take time to cry. When was the last time you had a good cry? Why so long? Frequently, we don't feel safe to share our vulnerabilities with anyone, even our spouse. We may find ourselves standing among friends and family but no familiar shoulder to lean upon. Find a good tearjerker movie and settle in for a couple hours. Bring the tissues to the couch, and be intentional about your desire to release stagnant emotions. Initially, you may cry about the content of the movie, but after a minute or two you might find that you're crying about your own discord. Embrace it. You're not weak because you cry; you're repressed and stressed because you don't. Being pent-up can lead to hopelessness, loss of self-worth or even despair. Journal a few pages about your sorrow, and let your stream of consciousness flow. Don't edit or use grammatical phrases. Just spew. Then, back to the movie. Back and forth for an hour or two might be just what your tender heart ordered.

Remember most people, your spouse and friends included, are likely not formally trained communicators. They probably haven't attended the university or learned how to communicate effectively. Keep that in mind when sharing your sensitive side. Don't expect a friend or family member to be your personal coach or therapist. Albeit, they may have compassion and even be a good listener, but they may not have the words of wisdom required for your specific situation. Frequently, well-meaning friends say the wrong thing just from a lack of understanding. So, when crying on a friend's shoulder, keep in mind that they care, but they are not your counselor.

After a good cry and journaling, think about how you want the future to be. Imagine a positive scenario coming to pass very soon and put aside unhappy or worrisome thoughts. Over time your inner peace (and faith) will prevail. Meditation is a useful tool for transforming heavy emotions and cultivating your spirituality. Relaxation techniques quiet the mind so that you can regain awareness of what you're thinking and manage your emotions (Meditation Methods discussed in future chapters). When negative thoughts arise, flip them off. Give 'em a flip, turn them upside down. Affirm the opposite. If you don't want to be single, then focus on the qualities of an appropriate partner. If you don't want a car wreck then drive safely. If you don't want to get fired, then appreciate the job you have, and give your best effort. If you don't want to be fat, then think about being healthy. Affirm the positive and flip those dark thoughts. And remember, why worry when you can pray!

 ZENERGY BOOST TO REDUCE SADNESS FAST
1. Eat or drink St. John's Wort. Found at most grocery stores.
2. Make a list of what you lost and a detailed list of what you want now.
3. Stop watching the news for one week and notice how much better you feel.
4. Go for a walk. Any type of exercise is very helpful~dance, skateboard, ski, tai chi.
5. Listen to upbeat music and sing along.
6. Make amends to someone you've upset.
7. Get involved in a co-op (community opportunity), church group or volunteer project.
8. Write a list of 5 people whom you've helped over the years and think about all the good that you created for them.
9. Cry it out. Get a tear-jerker movie to get the tear ducts moving. Then, journal afterwards.

LIVING & COPING WITH TRAUMA

You can create a new life after a Significant Emotional Event (SEE) and learn to see life with a new perspective. Significant emotional events and post traumatic stress can be serious and disruptive. According to the Mayo Clinic approximately 70% of adults have experienced a traumatic event at least once in their lives. Events like the loss of a loved one, getting fired from a job, childhood trauma, natural disasters, disease diagnosis, witnessing violence, combat, and more can produce serious stress. Emotional and physical responses to trauma vary. Nightmares, flashbacks, loss of connection to loved ones, loss of concentration, excessive defensiveness, or insomnia name a few symptoms which may be experienced from post-traumatic stress disorder (PTSD).

Each time the traumatic memory arises, your brain responds the same way as when the original event occurred. The hypothalamus gland in the brain produces hormones and biochemicals like during the original experience; therefore, the body lives in a constant state of pure anxiety making it very difficult to sleep, think, laugh or enjoy life. Recurring memories are uncontrollable initially; it's almost as if they have a life of their own. It is not a sign of weakness to experience difficulties from stressful events. It's only human. When someone is lost in trauma, the memories just flood in over and again. Many people have traumatic experiences in their lives, but they still are able to work and manage daily tasks. Resiliency can be easier for some. They might see a therapist once a week or once a month and that gives them coping skills; however, for someone who has PTSD the pain just remains.

Signs of PTSD
• Self-harm & risky behavior
• Reckless driving
• Suicide attempt
• Excessive use of sick leave
• Withdrawal and isolation
• Lack of empathy
• Unwillingness to trust
• Excessive drinking, binge eating or gorging

Disease feeds off toxic biochemicals generated from the trauma. Inflammation in the body comes from eating poorly, or a sedentary lifestyle and/or consistent fearful or negative thoughts. Diseases are born in a toxic, acidic, inflamed body. Small health concerns can turn big when the body is out of balance.

Common Health Symptoms Can Include
• Mood swings or angry outbursts
• Regular insomnia, nightmares or fitful sleep
• Constipation
• Belching, gas or gastrointestinal problems
• Indecisiveness or powerlessness feelings
• Numbness, disconnection or despair
• Survivor guilt

It is well-documented that women and men who experienced a significant emotional event have a difficult time with their feelings as they are frequently lost in a memory of the ordeal. Understanding anger-related disorders can alleviate uninhibited anger, anger turned inward or even low-grade frustration. Self-awareness skills, like interpersonal relationship knowledge, learning to set healthy boundaries and postponing thoughts that sustain anger can accelerate the healing process. Investigating the health risks resulting from constant irritation and persistent negative feelings can lessen the stress.

When coping with traumatic events, continue moving toward your goals, develop a positive image of yourself and look for opportunities for self-discovery. Developing ways to stay resilient is an empowering life-long skill. Remember, talking about trauma with untrained people can be detrimental because they don't know what to say. Even with well-meaning intentions, our friends and family can make things worse. Don't expect compassionate family members to be your professional counselor. An objective listener and professionally trained therapist can offer guidance that family members just don't know how to give.

 ZENERGY BOOST FOR DEVELOPING RESILIENCY
1. Think about a problem you recently resolved and apply that skill in other areas.
2. Be mindful of what you're eating and drinking by logging your intake.
3. Reduce compulsive activities like gambling or looking at porn.
4. Choose to eliminate ONE unhealthy behavior each month.
5. Avoid seeing the predicament as insurmountable.
6. Avoid triggers which stimulate anxiety.
7. Help someone who is less fortunate than you.
8. Avoid negative people, TV and violence.

When you are listening to someone who has had a traumatic event happen to them, check-in and make sure they're still attentive to your conversation. Sometimes it's useful to touch them on the shoulder or hand. Periodically you can adjust your body position, alternating from standing to sitting occasionally through your conversation. The movement will maintain awareness of the conversation at hand, but too much can be perceived as threatening. Continue engaging the person to bring them back to the present moment. Resolving PTSD is a more advanced skill, but recognizing the symptoms is beneficial for friends and family. You might be able to help a loved one today.

Recognized as an effective form of treatment for trauma by the American Psychiatric Association, the World Health Organization and the Department of Defense, Eye Movement Desensitization Reprogramming (EMDR) offers comprehensive recovery in as few as 1-12 sessions. What, in the past, might have taken years of therapy, this new technique provides faster results. The EMDR website states, "Studies show that 84%-90% of single-trauma victims no longer have PTSD after only three 90-minute sessions. Another study funded by HMO Kaiser Permanente, found that 100% of single-trauma victims and 77% of multiple trauma victims no longer were diagnosed with PTSD after only six 50-minute sessions. In another study, 77% of combat veterans were free of PTSD in 12 sessions." EMDR uses visual, audio and tactile cues to encourage the patient to move out of the amygdala. When a person is lost in shock, disbelief or denial, the brain is stuck in the flight or fight mechanism. The amygdala hosts the primary role in processing memory, judgment and determination of situations, as well as emotional wellbeing. EMDR techniques move patients out of this portion of the brain (amygdala) and restore whole-brain coherence. Many insurance companies cover this type of therapy.

If you're frustrated with the Western medical approach to trauma, you might consider Hypnosis and Regression Therapy. If a part of you lives in that disturbing scene and you just can't get it out of your mind, I would assert that your soul fragmented at the point of impact. Swinging between traumatic memories of the past and apprehension of potential threats in the future make it difficult to find a place in the present. A portion of you remains back there. Reclaiming your life after trauma can be difficult, and a regression can restore the fragmented soul. Regression Therapy gently takes you back in time to the origination of the trauma with a trained professional so that you can effectively unblock repressed memories, remove negative emotions, reframe the event and create a new approach to life. You can learn not only new coping skills but a fresh way to reframe-and-contain the trauma. Many people experience great results in one to four visits.

Start on your own with the simple wellness methods discussed in this book. After a few days or weeks, locate a nearby Counselor, Psychiatrist, Board Certified Hypnotherapist or Regression Therapist to assist you on your path. Don't sit alone in isolation. Open up and let someone help you.

ZENERGY BOOST FOR MOOD ENHANCEMENT
1. Stand outside and feel the sunshine on your head. Breathe in the solar rays.
2. Be gentle with yourself when you have an unexpected emotional reaction. Remember feelings are always changing ~ joy, sadness, fear, disgust and anger. Don't make long-term decisions based only upon your feelings. Definitely include some logic in there too.
3. Journal 1-3 pages about your discordant emotions each morning for 15 minutes. Journaling is an intimate conversation with yourself.
4. Cry alone or with someone for 10 minutes.
5. Add salmon, turmeric, yogurt or dark chocolate to your weekly diet.
6. Avoid sodas, fried foods and caffeine as much as possible.
7. Try herbal supplements like rhodiola rosea to rebalance stressed adrenal glands from the flight or fight response.
8. Consider St. John's Wort, Valerian Root or Ashwaghanda herbal supplements and tea formulas. If you're currently taking medication, confirm with your doctor in advance that their pharmaceuticals won't have a negative side effect with plants and other natural therapies.
9. Dilute rose or lavender oil with filtered water and spray on your pillow at night or add 5-10 drops to your next bath.

CHANGING A HABIT

When you decide to change a habit, please set a realistic goal. Don't set a goal doing something you know darn well you're never going to fulfill. That just generates more disappointment. You're probably not going to exercise daily or never eat another candy bar or drink another cocktail. You might overcome a sedentary lifestyle or consuming excess sugar (which includes alcohol), but I encourage you to focus on a reasonable goal, not the obstacle. The end result may be that you "never" or "always" but don't start there. The goal is to be healthy or healthier.

Set your intention for how you want to *feel* in the future. How is that feeling different from how you're feeling now? Typically, it means a bit less self-loathing, maybe a lot. Ah, wouldn't that be nice if some of the day weren't over-wrought with negative self-talk? What if you spent that same time (even just half of it) complimenting yourself and noticing all the good around you? Increasing self-confidence occurs in many ways; sometimes we just start with less apprehension and build self-assurance.

Keeping your word to yourself is a great way to build self-esteem. Do you show up for work daily and timely? Do you care for your body through food and water and bathing? Are you available for your children most of the time? Do you provide for them food, water and shelter? Do you follow the driving rules relatively speaking? Do you care for any pets? These little and large accomplishments virtually go unnoticed as the days and years pass with very little acknowledgement to yourself at how well you're currently performing. When trying to change an undesired habit, begin first by realizing all the wonderful things you're doing already.

According to the 12-step program, the best way to change a habit is to begin one-day-at-a-time. Only think about the next 24-hours (or even less, if necessary). Remind yourself, "I am postponing eating sugar/drinking alcohol/being sedentary today. Just for the next hour I will refrain from ingesting unhealthy food or alcoholic beverages." If you're approaching the end of the day and you haven't reached your exercise goals yet, then walk around the block, dance in your living room or march in place for ten minutes.

Keep your goals reachable. Weight Watchers has helped millions since 1963. The crux of that program is to count points, be mindful of what you're ingesting and enjoy a supportive group. There are many ways to change a habit, and it's best to break it down into small segments, first with refraining, then rewarding your results.

Refraining
Drug and alcohol addiction are generally more complex than other undesired habits; however, hypnosis can be a powerful tool for most addiction recovery. You can reduce triggers, decrease the appetite for your drug of choice, as well as reframe the underlying emotional shock, suffering and sorrow. Hypnosis can make you feel better naturally without side effects while creating a sense of wholeness. During a session you may recall the first time you had certain emotions that led to the addictive behavior. When you recognize them with a therapist, you can gain more clarity and release the shackles those emotions had on you in the past. After several sessions, old behaviors disappear and new ones are formed regaining a more optimistic outlook. It doesn't feel like refraining, you simply choose healthier behaviors. Hypnosis is not about surrendering power; it is an interactive process giving you the ability to take charge of your life proactively. Hypnosis can help reduce cravings, develop willpower, and produce rational responses to daily challenges. You can effectively restore peace in your life and establish new ways of living.

Many people who just binge at night can be relieved to know you only have to apply your willpower (or won't power) after work. Knowing that at 6pm you won't be able to do what you normally do (which might mean hitting happy hour with friends or being a couch potato snacking for a few hours) requires you to handle stress differently through the day. The standard stress relief (drinking or binging) won't be waiting for you when you finish working, so set the tone for the week in advance. Be prepared to exchange old habits with new curiosities. Certainly at the beginning of habit breaking behavior it's good to be prepared and get to bed early for the first week or month. Avoid bars, parties or the candy aisle where you know you'll be tempted.

When you decide that you're going to abstain for one month, break it into four one-week segments. Set a task for each week trying a new interest in the place of the old routine.

ZENERGY BOOST TO CHANGE YOUR ROUTINE
1. Attend an exercise, dance or painting class.
2. Listen to different lecturers (whether in person or on YouTube).
3. Learn a new language, skill or talent (whether in person or on YouTube).
4. Volunteer your time and talents to a cause that interests you (local theater, food bank, animal rescue, hospital, park rangers, etc.)
5. Be a pet sitter or a foster-care pet parent.
6. Remodel your home, start with organizing or painting a closet.
7. Clean your garage or attic.
8. Be a scribe. Help an elderly person write their life story.
9. Locate a soldier or veteran and assist them as you can.
10. Teach a class at a school, park, local YMCA or assisted living facility.
11. Become a mentor.
12. Join the Boys & Girls Club.
13. Find a Sponsor or Life Coach.

Pick an activity that is of keen interest to you that will take you out of your typical life to reduce thoughts about indulging. For instance, when you're attending a new fitness class like Yoga, Zumba or QiGong, you have to be alert and follow directions. It's ideal for quieting the scatter chatter. Same with attending a woodshop course and learning how to use power tools, you need to be sober and attentive to the instructor and machinery.

Eliminating a bad habit for the rest of your life sounds daunting, but if you just give it up for today, then one day at a time leads to a week. Usually, if you can get to hump day (3-day marker), then you're halfway there. Little by little you'll get to one month (by counting three days at a time). Be sure not to have a lot of "down time" at the beginning. Make a point to interrupt yourself with some of the above suggestions when familiar patterns arise, and congratulate yourself for the big changes you're making. Have a reward system for each week and each month.

When you're changing a big habit you're requesting yourself to step into a different you. How do you not be you? Quantum Physicist, Dr. Joe Dispenza, author of *Breaking the Habit of Being Yourself* (2012) teaches on this exact subject. "Emotions are a record of the past. If you're stuck thinking about the past, you cannot move into the future. Unfortunately, the body cannot tell the difference between what's actually happening and a memory. So the longer you hang onto shame, blame or guilt (or other self-loathing emotions) your body will continue to crave food, beverages and behaviors from the past. Uneasy emotions keep you stuck in an experience that you'd rather forget anyway." You can't drive forward looking in your rear view mirror.

Create, generate and pontificate (silently) the new you. Think about who you will be in the future when XYZ occurs. Fall in love with your new future. Convince your body so that you feel a new reality, chemically speaking. The brain doesn't know the difference between reality and a thought. So begin to think about your new life and imagine yourself in your new reality. See it, feel it, hear it and experience it! Your brain will begin to create new bio-chemicals that complement what you're thinking instead of the common chemistry that matches self-limiting emotions. Remember to reward yourself with something healthy on a regular basis.

ZENERGY BOOST TO REWARD YOUR PROGRESS
1. Shoot for 100%, celebrate at 90%
2. Buy a new outfit.
3. Enjoy a day at the park.
4. Attend a concert, show or theater.
5. Receive a massage or spa treatment.
6. Take a mini-vacation.
7. Go to the museum.
8. Add a plant to your garden.

UNDER-THOUGHTS & THOUGHT-STORMS

The four scientifically measured brainwaves are beta, alpha, theta and delta. We have customary cognitive thoughts that guide us through daily life. This established form of thinking is found in the beta brainwave. When engaged in an activity, conversation, dancing or working on a project, you are in the beta brain. The frequency of beta waves ranges from 15 to 40 cycles a second. Very active. We use the alpha brainwave for things like contemplating the future or daydreaming in an elevator. When you are chillin', zoned out or resting on the couch watching TV you are in the alpha brainwave. The frequency ranges from 9 to 14 cycles per second. We experience theta brainwaves while in deeper meditation, like when you access the gap, and during hypnosis. Athletic runners rave about "runner's high" when they get into the zone and just fly over the pavement. This high is associated with alpha. We experience theta when the images appear prior to falling asleep. This frequency range is normally between 5 and 8 cycles per second. Sleeping generates the slowest brainwave of delta at 1.5 to 4 cycles per second. Of course, it's never at zero because then the brain would be dead, but dreamless sleeping is the slowest brainwave (ScientificAmerican.com). Generally speaking, most people are either thinking in beta or on autopilot sleeping in delta, and a huge portion of the brain is not optimized during the alpha-theta brainwave.

The alpha-theta brainwave is the mental state when you consciously create your reality. I link these two together because in restful awareness, deep meditation or hypnosis, the brain cycles slower receiving new messages without the critical mind evaluating all the content. Unfortunately, unless you're a regular meditator, most people waste this precious resource on TV. If you plunk yourself down in front of the TV when you are most creative (in alpha and theta) then you allow the TV to direct your creative mind with their mainstream programming. For instance, subliminal (silent) messages are received on the alpha-theta brainwave. When a person listens to subliminal audio tracks, say for smoking cessation or anxiety reduction, cognitive recognition doesn't occur. You wouldn't hear or even remember the exact suggestions but the subconscious does. Ultimately, behavior changes because these recommendations are made subliminally (or silently) on the alpha-theta brainwave. The subconscious monitors the environment constantly and responds with 'fight or flight' or 'rest and relax.' I strongly discourage you from falling asleep in front of mainstream TV because the suggestions from commercials move directly into the subconscious mind encouraging you to think or behave similarly to the commercials recommendation.

The subconscious mind processes life behind the scenes and your *under-thoughts* guide your actions even when you are unaware of your behavior. Autopilot or knee-jerk reactions are indications of *under-thoughts*. They are under your common or normal thoughts. Identifying the motive behind behavior can frequently be a surprise. These *under-thoughts* are steering your behavior whether you want it or not. For instance, if you felt you got the short end of the stick in a divorce, you might not trust new relationships that are forming. Even though cognitively you long for love again, underneath that desire is a fear of intimacy or a fear of being taken advantage of again. If your previous employer dismissed you and forced you out unfairly, there could be a residue of that memory which impacts your behavior at your next job. You show up for work late because secretly you fear being discharged. If you were mocked as a child, you might be self-conscious as an adult due to these *under-thoughts*. These thoughts are typically about the past imbalances and in one way you're attempting not to recreate them; yet in another way, the *under-thought* draws to you a repeat performance. When you watch a lot of TV, you are receiving suggestions from the programming and the commercials and that information moves directly into the subconscious mind because you are in the alpha brainwave while watching TV. Consequently your behavior will correspond to these recommendations, whether you actually need that merchandise or not. You might not recognize your newfound interest in a certain athletic shoe or pharmaceutical drug until you link the fact that you've seen 30 commercials (or 300) for that product. (If you can sing along or recite the commercial then it is stored in your subconscious mind.) You may even begin adopting certain opinions from TV because when you hear a certain narrative repeatedly, you begin to believe it. With thousands of radio stations, YouTube channels, cable, internet TV, streaming videos, podcasts and more, why limit yourself to the same TV station with basically the same programming everyday?

Accurate interpretation or not, *under-thoughts* mysteriously weave the storyline to our behavior. For example, when you reflect on the previous year's holidays, you will have a certain feeling. Take one minute right now and reflect on what happened last year. If you did that exercise, then only certain memories returned. You don't remember everything that happened, just the major events, like the travel, hugs, food, religious services, and what presents were exchanged. When you consider what happened 10 holidays past, the memories might be faded, but some situations regardless of how long ago they occurred may linger. They can float through the mind and direct the behavior on a certain path, whether your interpretation was accurate or not. Opinions, judgments and resentments generate certain behavior in the future. Some behavior you may intend and some you may not (passive behavior or passive-aggressive behavior). You might not even understand why you don't like the holidays or another festive experience that others enjoy because of these suppressed *under-thoughts*.

Indications that *under-thoughts* are interfering with your mental-emotional state:
• A surge of sadness, loneliness or feeling lost overwhelms you.
• Unhealthy or negative feelings overcome you from out of the blue.
• Resentments you can't seem to shake.
• Random waves of anxiety occur for no reason.
• You avoid certain situations at all cost.
• You avoid certain conversations at all cost.
• You purchase products you don't really need.

If in some way you felt harmed by someone, society, a former lover, previous employer or your parents, you may have learned to cope with that discomfort, yet replay it continually as a suppressed *under-thought*. Albeit an unhealthy choice, suppression is a common tool for handling these big and small losses, and can lead to questionable behavior or even addiction. Suppressing disturbing feelings may cause unfamiliar behavior to take you down unfortunate roads. I counseled some who cheated on their spouses because they didn't know how to communicate effectively resulting in habitual arguments. Sweeping miscommunications under the rug is a common trait in marriage and can lead to regrettable choices.

If you have a pessimistic outlook, even when good things come your way, you will most likely miss these gifts because you're drawn to focus on the negative. For instance, if you've been trying to get a date with that cute guy in the office, and he finally looks your way, you might not even notice. Even if he asks you out, you may hear it as a joke or something worse, so you decline. Let's say your boss offers you an opportunity to give a presentation at work that ultimately can help your career, but you don't prepare properly because you don't think anything can help at this point and you deliver a slipshod performance sabotaging yourself. This unconscious behavior occurs in the alpha-theta brainwave. It's stored there, and we can transform it there.

We each think negative thoughts from time-to-time, even daily, but there is a level. Let's use a scale of 1-10 measuring your emotions~1 being good/happy and 10 being awful/depression. Let's say you have sad thoughts and they linger on low end of the scale at 2 or 3. Occasionally, you have some, but they don't really bother you. Then one day they escalate to a 7, 8, or 9, and you can't shake them. They not only linger, they begin to have a life of their own. They are loud and distracting and cause intense self-loathing. I call that a thought-storm. You had sad thoughts before (some recognized, some unconscious), and even these exact ones but never on this scale. It's overwhelming. That's when *under-thoughts* become a *thought-storm*.

Parasitic thoughts, negativity, fear, blame or hate can sneak up and the next thing you know it's overpowering. You feel awful all day, and it's hard to do good things for yourself (and maybe even others). You start to take an emotional nosedive. You might even be able to hide it from others initially, but inside you feel dreadful. I see *thought-storms* like a cloud or emotional parasite, and they can cause a lot of unnecessary psychological damage. *Thought-storms* leave you with a murky outlook, more imbalanced than ever before. Negative thoughts, statements, feelings, or words start flowing from your mouth. Statements like, "I'm not good enough. I blew it again. I'll never get ahead in life." Or blaming remarks toward others like, "You're not good enough. You blew it again. You're holding me back." These "I am not" statements or "You are not" statements affirm the negative and influence behavior. These thoughts have power to attract what you don't want. This is self-hypnosis of the worst kind because frequently you don't even realize what you're saying or doing, consequently drawing to you exactly what you fear the most.

Here's an example of self-hypnotic semantics. Don't think of a purple tree. Don't think of a luxurious bathtub. Now, don't think of a sacred garden. You can't stop thinking those things. Your subconscious mind is your dutiful servant or your masterful manipulator. So if you're saying to yourself all day, "I don't want to be fat" or "I'm so broke" then you're setting yourself up for sad thoughts about your body or financial status. Neither of those are static situations anyway; in fact, nothing is static on this planet. Affirm encouraging statements throughout the day like, "I am healthy" or "I live inside my means" or "Money comes to me." Constructive statements influence you positively. Positive reinforcement works.

Listening to a recording of my own voice saying positive things changed my common daily thinking. Years ago, I created and recorded a list of 75 inspirational statements, looped it to play continuously, and listened to them almost daily for several years. Every other year I re-recorded myself affirming many of the same statements and adding new ones. When you do this exercise and hear your inspired declarations repeated throughout the day, your behavior changes because of your belief in the affirmations. You start to live and act like the person you wish you could be. Ultimately, your vibrational frequency elevates with your new beliefs, and next time you record your voice the sound will be slightly altered. It may be undectable, but your subconscious mind will recognize it. Quietly play the recording in the background, like a subliminal. It's very effective.

Remember, the beta-brain is the problem-solving mind. It's handling the day-to-day activities. The alpha-theta brainwave is the creative mind. Discarding the self-sabotaging negativity, and identifying what you want are basic steps to creating a meaningful harmonious future. This practice of imagining your ideal life in your mind's eye and fueling it with emotion and energy, while in the alpha-theta brainwave, can transform your life.

Usually a *thought-storm* hovers around the head or to one side of the brain. You'll notice this more by where your eyes "look" when the lids are closed. While contemplating what is bothering you, the eyes will dart from one side to the other, indicating different parts of the brain being accessed during the *thought-storms* ~ mental disturbances in the left brain, emotional disturbances in the right brain. You may feel your eyes darting to see a past love or hearing your boss dismiss you. Just notice your eyes move around following sights, sounds and memories in the mind's eye while in restful awareness.

ZENERGY BOOST & GUIDED MEDITATION TO CLEAR NEGATIVE ENERGY
Find a comfortable chair, close your eyes and become aware of your breathing. Spend 2-5 minutes deliberating smoothing out the breath, balancing the inhale with the exhale. Bring your awareness to the center of your brain, and breathe slowly with your attention at the pineal gland, located at the midbrain. Focus on what's bothering you. Think about that problem, the sadness, the failure, the anger or whatever is occupying your mind's time. Now, center the eyes on the point between the eyebrows at the Third Eye. Become single focused. Keep the ocular muscle relaxed while noticing your inner dialogue. Regardless of the thoughts or feelings, notice your breath flowing through your nostrils and stay restfully aware. Don't fall asleep. Envision a sphere of indigo light with a golden rim for protection surrounding your body. Imagine the light in you and around you. Silently affirm, "Only that which is for my highest and greatest good can stay with me now. Any negativity, anxiety, sadness, tension, anything which does not hold a positive vibration must leave NOW." Continue this affirmation (or a similar statement), and imagine a violet flame transmuting all negativity. Freely release any suffering into the flame. Maintain the feeling that you are being cleaned and cleared of negativity by discarding those emotions outside the indigo light of protection and into the violet flame. Finish the process by affirming I AM statements.

First release the negativity, and then declare the positivity. Consider one or two of the affirmations from the list below. Memorize it and say it 100 times each day. You know how to think positively and at times you have to be extremely disciplined to dissolve an under-thought or a thought-storm. You are creating a new habit of transforming yourself at the alpha-theta level.

Suggested Affirmations
I am safe and secure.
I am loved and protected.
I am financially secure.
I am joyously abundant.
I am filled with vibrant vitality.
I am happily married to my Soulmate.
We have a dynamic romantic marriage.
I am healthy, wealthy and wise.
I am peaceful and joyous.
I am on my path and I trust my pace.
God is my Source!

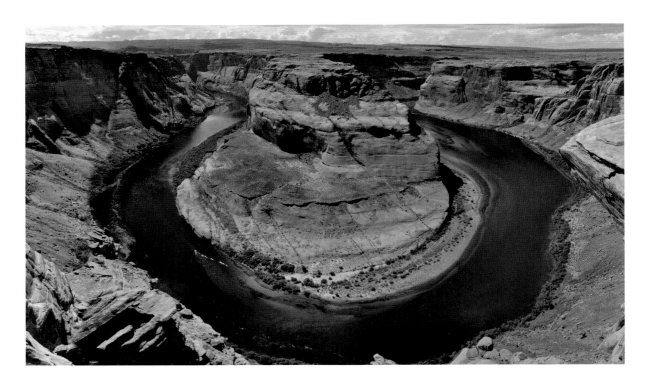

 ZENERGY BOOST TO SHIFT YOUR UNDER-THOUGHTS FAST
1. Wash your face with clean water.
2. Take a shower and wash your hair.
3. Listen to soothing ambient music or nature noises.
4. Visualize or look at a gorgeous scenic photo.
5. List and memorize 10 affirmations; recite them daily or hourly.
6. Focus your attention on a new project ~ woodworking, painting, singing, planning a party.
7. Exercise ~ walking around the block is free.
8. Get a hug, give a hug (even a handshake will suffice).
9. Pray ~ God is Always Ready to Assist!

COMPASSION, THE ULTIMATE LOVE

Where does one learn compassion? How can you tell when someone is compassionate? Compassion is a gift, skill and talent. Being trustworthy of someone's vulnerability is an honor.

One time while at the grocery store a woman stopped me. I'm not sure if she thought I was someone else, but she proceeded to share a tender story with me. Through her details she began to sob. I reached out to hold her hand and allowed her sharing to continue. I didn't bother to look around to notice who was watching. It really didn't matter. She was so scattered and distressed, and I knew that I should just look at her with a neutral gaze and witness her pain. I did not indicate with my facial expressions whether I agreed or disagreed. Agreeing with someone's distress can sometimes encourage them to stay in a victim mentality and delay healing. Witnessing someone's pain can be very healing for both of you. You may not even need to respond. Just don't discourage it. Maintain a kind, unbiased facial expression. Let them cry and share what's heavy on their heart. They need to release in that moment and your ability to invite authentic expression could be the miracle you both need.

Compassion is likened to altruism. Recognizing that another human being is grieving and reaching out for love can aide in immediate healing. Put yourself in their shoes. Don't squelch the sharing of their misfortune. We live in an emotionless-capitalistic society where our primary focus is acquiring more–more goods, services, sex, money, respect, attention. When someone is in pain, they too need to acquire something at that time–more love.

According to the University of California at Berkley, "cynics may dismiss compassion as touchy-feely or irrational; however, scientists have started to map the biological basis of compassion, suggesting its deep evolutionary purpose. This research has shown that when we feel compassion, our heart rate slows down and we secrete the 'bonding hormone' oxytocin. Regions of the brain linked to empathy, caregiving and feelings of pleasure light up, which often results in our wanting to care for other people." Next time someone reaches out for you, lower your cell phone and offer your ear or shoulder.

Connecting to others ignites feelings of selfless behavior that deepens the bond between us, not to mention diminishes the notion of isolation. Advancing technologies and even addiction to technology is leading us away from one another. In the past, we lived in tribes; we belonged to a group. Today, we grow up quickly and frequently move away from our parents, migrating for work and various other reasons. Or just stay glued to our tech (resulting in the new word called "tech neck"). That disengagement can lead to a loss of belonging and connection in the real world.

Visiting an acquaintance at work or in your neighborhood builds bridges that can keep you grounded and feeling stable. Volunteerism is a positive way to build compassion and there are numerous ways to contribute to countless organizations. Many hospitals have a Neonatal Intensive Care Unit (NICU) that need support in cuddling babies. Simply hugging a newborn is greatly needed in some regions, and it boosts bountiful feelings of love, connection, belonging, importance, compassion, sense of purpose and more. Even just imagining hugging an infant can generate constructive and magnificent feelings.

According to Researcher, Author and Storyteller Brené Brown, compassion is linked with vulnerability and setting healthy boundaries. Frequently, when we hear the word vulnerability, we think of weakness, but it takes a lot of courage to be vulnerable. Remember the last time you risked with someone and felt vulnerable? You had to be courageous first. It is very brave to be vulnerable. I find it emotionally heroic when someone shares authentically. Taking your mask off to reveal the real you takes a lot of self-compassion, openness and audacity.

Additionally, compassion goes hand-in-hand with setting healthy boundaries. If you give at the expense of yourself that sacrifice comes at a huge price, and it is unsustainable. Eventually, you are going to avoid that person or organization or just burnout. Given your current schedule and responsibilities, consider what is reasonable for you to give ~ of time, talent, energy and finances. Brown recommends being generous in your assumptions of others; anticipate that they have good intentions. When you set healthy boundaries its easy to give freely with eyes wide open. When you assume the best about others and give when you can, you expand your ability to love. Compassion brings us closer to each other. Emotional resonance and connectivity build love and belonging, and the world definitely needs more love today!

 ZENERGY BOOST FOR DEVELOPING COMPASSION
1. Be a Hero or a Shero. You decide how.
2. Be a first responder and contribute to those in a natural disaster.
3. Envision your loving arms around the globe and give love to humanity.
4. Buy a stranger's groceries.
5. Plant a tree for a deceased relative or friend.
6. Tell a musician, celebrity or another person in your life how their amazing works of art or community contribution impacts you.
7. Send wisdom to world leaders.

SETTING HEALTHY BOUNDARIES

CONSCIOUS COMMUNICATION

If I ask you to read an email or watch a documentary that takes 20-minutes, do you think that's a long time? Today, many people do. Next time when you talk with your friends, observe yourself. Be mindful if you hog all the airtime and jammer on and on about yourself. Learn to listen to your spouse, friends and children. You can really learn a lot by listening and asking questions. Plus, you might be able to reduce some of your inner scatter chatter by focusing on someone else's issues for 15-minutes. Conversely, if you're an introvert, stop hiding. Step out and speak up, "I've got something to say." You'll be surprised at how many of your friends are waiting for you to share. You might need to jump in there, interrupt and start talking about your point of view. It feels awkward the first few times, but keep trying.

Communication relays a clear vision of what you're thinking. Are you able to share your message concisely? Convey your point while staying connected to your audience, whether it's a family member, employer or even a stranger. Speaking succinctly shows your confidence in the message you are relaying. Think before you speak and be your authentic self. Maintain your poise and observe the reaction of others to your statements. Exhibiting some animation with hands and facial expressions conveys a dynamic presence. Maintain consistent nonverbal communication.

Body language, eye contact, hand gestures and the tone of your voice all play a meaningful role in self-expression. Whether talking or listening, while engaged in a conversation establish eye contact without staring. If you are seated avoid slouching and slightly lean forward indicating your interest in the topic. Listen carefully. Don't interrupt and try not to multitask (i.e. don't use your cell phone unless you are specifically taking notes from the discussion). Nodding periodically demonstrates you're keeping up with the dialogue. Try to maintain open arms which is a neutral stance; folded arms can convey defensiveness. So, if you are closed to the topic or the request, then crossing your arms maintains a congruent expression. Avoid laughing or smiling when you don't agree. I remember laughing at many off-color, even sexist, jokes when I was younger because I thought I was required to express amusement. If you're insulted by a joke or just don't find it funny, don't laugh. Keep it real.

Typically at work, colleagues listen with an edge. They're trying to one-up each other and compete for the boss' attention or the boss' position. Sitting at company meetings initiates the competitor in many team players. It's good to have your agenda when you arrive for a meeting, and if you don't get your points addressed, follow up with a concise email. Prepare for the next meeting in advance. Be proactive about your role at work and don't be a wallflower. Wallflowers rarely get the promotions, raises or awards, and sometimes even get dismissed because they appear not to contribute very much. Rotate your eye contact to various people in the group. Your style of communication (or lack thereof) can brand you as pushy or as a pushover.

Take longer deeper breaths when you're nervous. Clasp your hands together to avoid fidgeting but don't grip until your knuckles are white. Concentrate on the ideas you want to convey, and use your vocal speed and volume to set the tone for your message. I like the aphorism, "Fake it until you make it." In these types of situations, when you pretend that you're confident, you gain experience and eventually you won't be nervous. Psychologist Amy Cuddy discusses her research findings on how "faking it actually leads to becoming it" (Ted Talks, 2016).

Toastmasters is an excellent organization for learning public speaking skills in social and professional circles. Small groups gather weekly at restaurants and business complexes around the globe providing a structure to learn graceful public speaking skills. Participants grow steadily in their confidence and communication abilities. You would be pleased at how comfortable you can become communicating with strangers, and even from a podium, in just a few weeks. Many people have social anxiety now because they spend so much time with computers. Toastmasters is a great way to meet new friends, and the singles group is a good way to find a date. Visit *Toastmasters.org* to find a group near you.

The Secrets of Exceptional Speaking Course is a California-based internationally recognized company educating executives and staff alike. They provide an excellent one-day course that offers proven techniques to help you gain the edge as an exemplary public speaker. It's perfect for one-on-one training or corporate departmental improvement. I attended the online classes and quickly improved my overall communication abilities. Visit *ExceptionalSpeaking.com* to learn more.

Whether you are shy or talk too much, find a podium. Locate an audience that you can teach for one hour per week or per month. If you're not comfortable talking, then this activity will give you an opportunity to see how much you have to contribute, and how valuable your sharing can be to others. If you're used to hogging the show then you'll have an audience. Consequently, it will be easier for you to listen after your attention needs are fulfilled. Generally speaking, people who talk too much need more attention than they are currently receiving. Find healthy ways to get that attention without wearing down your family, friends and spouse.

Better Speaking Skills
• Think Before You Speak
• Read Your Audience
• Maintain Rapport
• Connect & Convey
• Build Trust
• Listen Actively
• Keep Practicing

Communication is about relaying a story. Are you able to share your story successfully? My father was a trial attorney in Houston for 25 years. He practiced his opening and closing arguments in the garage and in the mirror prior to trial to gain comfort when speaking before the judge and jury. I found practice performances to be very useful in my professional speaking engagements too. Listen to yourself speaking aloud in your home. Watch yourself in the mirror as you practice giving a brief presentation or even a casual talk. You will feel more comfortable with consistent effort. Practice makes permanent.

Learning to communicate consciously takes attention. Many times people are just spewing words without even thinking about their intent to speak. It's easy to miscommunicate because so many people are multitasking all day long. If you miscommunicated with someone, identify the facts of the situation and label the feelings arising inside you. Labeling feelings is a powerful tool as most people are happy, angry, sad or fine (which isn't a feeling at all). Acquire new words to describe how you feel. Joyful, elated, relaxed, comforted, remorseful, sensitive, irritated, enraged, belittled, sorrowful, forgiving, tolerant, compassionate. Expand your vocabulary.

When you recognize your feelings you can reduce unconscious behavior. Being unconscious appears in many different ways. For example, if you believe a person doesn't like you, and that offends you, then you may be unconsciously defensive around them. Or if you are insulted by the lack of attention from a person, you may unconsciously ignore them in advance. Let's say you don't feel confident or joyful and, whether accurate or not, when you go to work your insecurities arise about your ability to perform. While at work you are listening to what is said and done around you from a point of view that "I'm not good enough and soon I will get dismissed." Therefore, regardless of what your colleagues do or don't do, you don't feel comfortable at your job because you don't feel comfortable in your own skin. You might be projecting by saying to yourself, "They don't like me" and unconsciously pushing them away from the beginning. If your spouse criticizes you, then you might start believing that (s)he doesn't love you when it could be constructive feedback. Granted, some people belittle to maintain control of a relationship, but conscious communication empowers you to ask questions eliminating ambiguity. Asking the simple question, "What does that mean to you?" reduces jumping to the wrong conclusion. If you know you have insecurities (and we all do in some form) then you may project your fears onto your partner, or others, without even knowing it. Consequently, this behavior unconsciously limits your connection to others. Don't expect others to anticipate your needs. Playing the victim with internal comments like, "They don't like me" keeps you preoccupied with a pessimistic point of view. If you want to be included in office luncheons, then invite them to lunch, or at least one of them. Don't expect them to invite you each time. If someone hurts your feelings, get clarity on what they really mean. Most people are not bullies. They just miscommunicate and others will not take the time or make the effort to understand the true message. Many people you meet over the course of your life will only remain for a short while ~ a month, a year or five. If you miscommunicate with someone early on, (s)he probably will not clarify it; (s)he may just stop calling you. Conscious communication skills give you access to a richness in relationships that is unlimited.

When we first married, my husband wouldn't say anything when I talked too much. He just stopped listening without telling me. This is very common for men. I had no idea that he was entertaining another mental task. With my head in the kitchen fixing a meal, I would ask a question and then realize he disappeared mentally while I jibber-jabbered. Oops! I realized I had a lot of words, and I stopped talking to focus on the meal at hand. I would relax into the silence and enjoy my task. When he reconnected, the focus would be on him, and he would talk about his day for awhile. Limit your sharing to about 10-minutes each of your daily highlights when you first reconnect with your partner at the end of the day. Don't force someone to listen to every detail about your day. It's inconsiderate.

We adopted a phrase from the Charlie Brown animation. Charlie Brown and fellow students couldn't hear their teacher. She stood at the front of the classroom and droned on and on "Wa Wa Wa." That became our sweet way of saying, "I can't hear you anymore." It might be due to inability to focus at that moment, or it might be due to location (physically out of range). If we can't hear each other we sweetly say, "Wa Wa Wa." We both laugh, and it works for us because we know that we will make time to listen later. Or maybe we don't even need to say those words.

Find a harmonious phrase that validates your unique style. Don't criticize the other for talking too much. Identify that you have a lot to share and choose the most important topics, not everything. Your spouse wants to talk too. We all *jaw-jack* at one time or another (or constantly for those who are really unaware), and finding a neutral word to bring you back together in silence maintains rapport. Keep it simple like, "Oops! I have a lot of words right now" or "I need some stillness right now, Sweetheart" or "Can we talk later?" or "I'm sorry. I'm having a hard time listening right now."

Sometimes you can reconvene later, sometimes you can't, but it's good to ask. Begin setting healthy boundaries at any stage of any relationship so that you're not rolling your eyes at each other or behind each other's back, especially if you've been the "listener" for years. Identify what you want and don't assume that because you've been together for ten or fifteen years that the other automatically knows what you're thinking. We go through phases in life, and it's empowering to continuously create new and healthy ways to stay connected. Don't expect others to anticipate your needs since those are always changing.

A few signs indicate you won't be friends or happily married in five years (maybe even divorced). Rolling your eyes at each other is one of them. Harboring resentments or dread in discussing certain topics or activities are indications of relationship trouble. Sexual anxiety is another, and conscious communication lifts a level of discord that you both want removed. (Sex is discussed in a future chapter.)

If you find that you're a little nervous when making love, talk about it. Ask if your concerns are a problem for the other. They might not be. Many wives feel uncomfortable sexually and don't indicate what feels good while the husband tries feverishly to please. Your vulnerability in communicating consciously is a mature way to stay connected and possibly even save your marriage. Attempting to communicate openly is honorable, even if the other doesn't respond to you in a tender loving manner. Many books are written in depth on this delicate subject.

World renowned psychologist Dr. John Gray authored a voluminous series entitled, *Men Are From Mars, Women Are From Venus*. It's a fun read explaining the natural differences of the opposite sex. We communicate in distinct ways, and Dr. Gray validates our unique styles. We experience the world differently but still value community equally. If you've been butting heads or avoiding your significant other, I strongly recommend reading the first book. Generally speaking, men relax and recharge when they watch sporting events or action films. Men recharge by spending time alone in their cave for 10-30 minutes each day. Women, on the other hand, regain their sense of self and their importance in the family or community through communication. Although there are exceptions, women need to verbally process at least some of their day. The significance of a best girlfriend should not be underestimated. Talking for 10-30 minutes truly relaxes women. There are many natural differences and knowing them can transform your relationships. Learning to accept our differences can be immensely helpful.

Be vulnerable and be honest in your relationships. If you're unwilling to risk and speak your truth, then you can't be upset when you don't get what you want. If you don't tell your boss why you think you're the perfect person for the promotion, then you can't be upset when you don't receive it. Surrender to the wisdom of uncertainty when asking for what you want. You're not expected to speak perfectly, just honestly. It takes courage to be authentic but the pay-offs are big. If you can't get what you want from your boss or partner (or whomever), then it's 100% your responsibility to find another resource to get your needs met. Communicating directly with integrity, kindness and authenticity attracts quality healthy relationships and maintains rapport.

Learning new conscious communication skills can transform your life. When you identify the facts of a situation just think about the "who, what, when, where" and postpone on the "why" until later. The brain is a meaning-making-machine, and it quickly decides the "why" of situations without all the facts. Journaling about a heated exchange or troublesome situation can be very helpful to identify this information analytically. Your outlook and your attitude are your choice.

 ZENERGY BOOST FOR BETTER RELATIONSHIPS
Monitor the time of your next personal phone call. Notice how much you talk and how much you listen. Become a better friend by balancing talking with listening.

BRAIN-DRAINS

Brain-drains are people who suck the energy out of you. You might not have labeled them before but consider the type. They are usually the nay-sayers or complainers in the group. They frequently are the ones voicing their negative points complaining about illness, disease or even spewing hate. *Brain-drains* are people who manipulate, dominate or intimidate. They appear as friends initially but with a little investigation you may find their real agenda. I'm referring to those who appear to be healthy and alert, even affable. They are active in the community or at work. They want to have lunch with you and get to know you better, but after being with them you feel depleted. Initially, you may not even realize what is happening because when forming friendships you want to share energy and connect, but after interactions with them you may need to recharge.

Some people are ill or weak and need compassion and extra energy. You visit them with the intent to share and provide support. You intend to help them out of an unfortunate situation. Possibly you're visiting the hospital to offer kindness and consideration so that they can get well quicker. In those situations you know in advance that you will be giving energy to them and truly expecting little in return. I'm not talking about them. *Brain-drains* lure you into their friendship, and then steal your energy with their cynicism or manipulation.

Cynics and skeptics have a difficult time seeing the good in people, situations and events. They look for the worst in life and often get it. Negativity can begin from a common cold, fatigue, trauma, hunger, or sleep deprivation. Even allergies can make you doubt the good in the world. For many, being a Debbie Downer is a temporary state of being, but for cynics it's a constant state of consciousness. Noticing the awful things in life on a daily basis drains energy and consequently pessimists are looking to restore their energy in some way–maybe from you. Sometimes reframing a situation offers a fresh look at a dismal circumstance but rarely does this help. A *brain-drain* will counter your positive approach, quickly sucking the life force from you with each excuse. You may find yourself jumping through hoops in an attempt to lift their spirit only to be disappointed by the end of your time together. And, not just disappointed, but exhausted. Dealing with a *brain-drain* depletes your vitality.

Psychological manipulation can influence others' perception through dishonest and deceiving methods. Forwarding the interests of the manipulator at your expense can be misleading, underhanded and drain your energy. Manipulative individuals often start a discussion inviting you to share your thoughts, beliefs and attitudes. They then can assess your perspective to detect your weak spots. This cues them to your weak points without being vulnerable themselves. Frequently a manipulator is evaluating your standards and principles in order to hit you where it hurts the most. An exploiter's ideal position of strength is to sway a decision in their favor or simply demoralize you to polish their own image by comparison. They may do it publicly or privately. In fact, a lot of toxic spouses (or family members) only abuse their partners in private where there are no witnesses. Your loss of self-esteem and uncertainty can derail you so that you won't have the strength to question them. Misrepresenting the truth by not disclosing all the information, embellishing or intentionally minimizing important facts can lead you to wrong conclusions. This behavior ultimately creates an unhealthy dependent connection that the *brain-drain* needs in order to siphon off your vital energy.

Brain-drains may not even consider themselves as such. Many don't even notice how negative or manipulative they are being. For instance, when you decline an invitation to a party, they will press you to join them anyway. They typically don't like being alone, and they don't like healthy relationship boundaries. Their need to control situations, whether by dropping a wet blanket on a joyous occasion or starting an argument to dominate, is due to a feeling of powerlessness at a deep level. *Brain-drains* don't encourage authentic self-expression since spontaneous behavior cannot be managed. They want you to be like them and validate their way of being. Initially, they may not seem like vampires, but after a day with one you are going to feel bled and drained.

Brain-drains cause mental fog and suck the joy out of you. Next time you notice you're with a *brain-drain* consider the following suggestions:

1. Ask if they want a solution to their problems. Typically *brain-drains* just want to gripe and that can go on for hours, days, years and decades.
2. Redirect and deflect sarcastic or cynical statements. Don't agree just because.
3. Do they have a victim mentality? Indicating what is good in life can slow down a cynic. Eventually, you will notice that you two are **not** on the same page. The more optimistic you are, you both may find that you're not only not on the same page, you're not in the same book or even in the same library.
4. Do you need a nap after you spend time with them? That's a sure sign you got drained.
5. Do they let you talk or do they dominate the conversation?
6. Do they use your empathic abilities to get you ingrained into their project?
7. Do you feel confused or imbalanced during or after spending time with that person? Manipulation feels like this in the aftermath.
8. Do you feel unsure of yourself or even insecure while with them or afterwards?
9. Did you pick up a bad habit by spending time with them?
10. Can you delegate and refer them to others? Manipulators will not like this approach and may try to guilt you into helping them more.
11. Can you delay in returning the call? Many problems work themselves out in a day or two.
12. Don't offer to assist. Monitor how much time you give, limit to 20-minutes when possible, and politely excuse yourself for your important projects.

If you've made some poor decisions because a *brain-drain* caught hold of you, begin to correct your behavior as soon as you can. You can't blame your unfortunate choices on anyone else, but you can modify and choose differently in the future. Recharge yourself appropriately, and be your healthy authentic self. Avoid that *brain-drain* in the future.

SLICERS

Spiteful toxic statements are called many things~backhanded compliments, back-stabbing, malicious or just plain mean. Catty is a sexist statement against women. Men equally deliver their stealthy cruel remarks. However, society says it's just "natural or territorial" for men to defend their turf. Regardless, sarcastic remarks with the intent to hurt are common for both genders, and *slicing* slams fall just as easily from a man's mouth as a woman's. A *slicing* remark is offered with an iron-claw handshake or a guarded grin. Probably the most familiar is, "beauty before age" as the men take the hand of a young lady entering the ballroom before older women.

When someone insults you, cuts you down or discounts your contribution, how do you handle it? Do you stomp your foot and talk louder to get your point across? Do you gossip about it to others without handling the situation? Do you shriek and slink off into the corner? There are many ways to handle competitive situations and finding the best one for you will change with each circumstance as you mature (age is irrelevant to maturity).

Society encourages being your best, getting the A, the promotion or the spouse. Once you have the prize, jealous acquaintances resist your new stature. If it's a rival you may expect a spiteful spin in their words, but when an acquaintance offers a *stealthy slice*, it can really throw you off-guard. Have you ever laid awake in bed and contemplated what you *should'a said…"should'a, would'a, could'a"*… reviewing an encounter where someone insulted you or tripped you right as you were walking on the stage? In the future, think about how important this situation will be in a month or a year. This can really put it in perspective. Consider praying for the assailant in order to remove the sting of what they've done to you. It might not change their behavior, but it will help you see the situation from a higher perspective.

It may be humorous on the screen, but reality TV stars use this type of sarcasm to stay edgy. Reality TV is not real. Those personalities are cued with precise *slicing* statements, and mimicking their behavior harms our society causing unnecessary competition and isolation. Generally, these *slicers* are self-conscious, perfectionists who may be familiar with duking it out. Many feel there is only one mountaintop to aspire to and only one spot to acquire when you reach it. This is clearly shortsighted, but you can't educate a foe. They don't recognize their own value.

If you're vibrant and healthy, someone may envy your vitality. They offer friendly cordialities initially and then wham you with their snide comment (and no telling what they say behind your back). They only knock you down so they feel better about themselves. She/he may make a *slicing* compliment like, "you look amazing. Don't gain an ounce." Meaning if you gained even one ounce you would look awful. Let the original statement ring in your ears; don't focus on the sting. If possible, try to add some levity to the situation since clearly they wish to dazzle like you. Avoiding a conflict, you could reply with, "what a great party." You've addressed them and changed the subject.

A spontaneous-sounding response can really throw a rival off course without making it worse. It's unlikely you will win if you stoop to their level. *Slicing* is unattractive, selfish behavior. Yet, it's easier and safer than slugging it out in a back alley like the guys. Next time you could respond with a raised or a furrowed eyebrow, or give 'em a look which says, "inappropriate." This indirect approach can allow you to save face and move on to another, more enjoyable, area of the room. You might be able to smooth the exchange with a nod and a quick departure instead of a snide retort. Think about something you could say that would diffuse the catty remark, something comical. It doesn't have to ignite a full round of uproarious laughter, just a smile. Another option is to ignore it or make a statement about what a nice color shirt they are wearing. You're not complimenting them, you're commenting on the color of the shirt or the jewelry they are wearing. In that way, you change the subject, and leave on a high note. You don't forget the exchange, but you can remove yourself from their presence. Both of you can be at the party and not talk. You can smile and move to the buffet table or the other side of the room in a positive and powerful strut.

Next time you see that person, you might even cringe mentally hearing the *slicing* comments replay as you see their face. Let your smile carry your words and feet away from those types of petty people. They aren't your friends; they may not be friends with anyone. A few good one-liners might make you feel better but only worsens your association, and it may even land you in the Human Resource department for counseling. Avoiding conflict and workplace drama is a great skill to possess. You can't really help *slicers* see their own value, but you also don't have to *slice* them down further. Usually you'll end up looking and feeling worse after one of those hollow contests. Eventually, everyone determines who is the assailant and excludes them. Acting calm and respectful disarms some adversaries.

Slicing contributes to feelings of anxiety and depression and can stoke the fire of negative *under-thoughts*. *Slicers* are typically unhealthy and they too have a whole host of unresolved feelings and unconscious behavior. People who make cutting comments are good at dirty debates. Remember they are jealous, prepared and determined to bring you down a notch. Shun these snake pits by refusing to slink down to their level with an equally bitter response. They want you to grovel in the pits with them so they can bite you again. Clearly, they are young souls who don't see how this type of spiteful malicious communication is destroying them and our society.

It's easy to get ticked-off and lament about it. At some point, you'll need to turn the whole situation upside down so that you can laugh about it and go on. You don't want to dwell on crap like that. Those types of people are a dime a dozen. If you were upset about all the snide comments made to you, you would feel miserable. Instead, laugh about how great you looked that day or how awesome you were during your performance (which is why the *slicing* remark was made anyway). The main reason those comments were stated was because you ARE so amazing. They feel that they can't measure up to you. If you sting back, then you're on their level. That's what they want. So, take the high road when you can. Sometimes just pretending you don't hear them is enough.

Consider some of these responses next time you get sliced:
• Sounds like it's been a tough week for you.
• I wish I hadn't heard that one.
• Laugh at what they said.
• I'm headed out the door now (only if you are).
• Say nothing, just look at that person. Let their nasty words linger in the air and stare neutrally at them.
• "This communication is so paltry (trivial)." By using an unfamiliar word you'll have everyone checking google and remembering your large vocabulary instead of the *slice*.

ADULT ADOLESCENTS

Do you know an adult who acts like a child? Don't be fooled by some wrinkles. Just because you grow older doesn't mean you mature. Some people still act like they are in high school even though they are 50-years old. Some people don't get wiser with age; they just get clever at avoiding responsibilities. You may find some of these adult adolescents in the dating scene, at work, driving on the roads or even within your own family. Don't assume that someone is an adult just because they look like one. You can save yourself all types of headaches and reduce your stress by quickly assessing your audience.

Now, this may be a bit Psychology 101 but it is helpful. Consider the following about your audience next time you're in a discussion at work, church, school or on a date.
Do they pass the buck?
Are they looking to blame someone else?
Have they been dependable over the last few weeks or years?
How punctual are they? If late, do they give long drawn-out excuses?
Are they argumentative or easily angered?
Do they complete assignments or keep agreements?
Do they miss deadlines very often?
How responsible are they with money?
Do they pay their monthly expenses timely?
If you loaned them $1000, would they repay it?

There are many questions to ask as you're evaluating the person before you. Of course, we all make mistakes or are late for an appointment once in a while. I'm talking about the habitual people. When you ask the above questions is there a litany of excuses from that person? Then yep, you got a child masquerading as an adult. Beware of these people because they really can do you harm. They don't know that they are still a child. So when interacting with them, remember that you are carrying the torch for both of you. Albeit, they may be able to contribute in a big way, but generally speaking, adult adolescents are better off on a team with strong leadership.

It's common for staff to transfer unhealed childhood emotions onto their managers and supervisors. Be mindful when a staff member is avoiding their responsibilities. They may be confusing you with someone who left a negative imprint in their past. Notice who blames and who resolves. We all need emotional healing, but managers are not Life Coaches. Managers are the motivators to get the job finished correctly and timely. Unfortunately, there can be an undeserving amount of stress at work because you're expecting someone to keep his/her word and participate like an adult; however, if you know you're dealing with a child camouflaged as an adult it makes it easier to cope. You don't get to decide with whom you work, but you can determine how you communicate with them. If you're considering raising your voice, think twice. These adult adolescents are skilled at out-maneuvering, pointing-the-finger and avoiding personal responsibility. They likely know exactly how to get your goat and pass the buck. Meanwhile they whine, cry, gossip, deflect, deny or out right lie to avoid direct communication. Notice their temperament, and consider that you may have to do some damage control after a disagreement with one of them.

When dating, figure out your potential mate's Emotional Quotient (EQ) early. Are they emotionally available or emotionally dependent? What are their abilities to manage the cards that were dealt them? How do they handle Plan B? Spend time with them in public places where you can see how they respond to your friends and strangers. If they are rude to the waiter or fly off the handle at the movie theater, then you know to expect the same behavior toward you eventually. Although no one is perfect, its beneficial to learn these traits about a potential suitor sooner than later. Knowing someone's background can be very helpful. Where did he/she grow up and how? What were some of the good, bad and ugly he/she had to deal with as a young adult? Listen to how the circumstances are replayed. Is there a lot of blame in their story or have they mastered some of those challenges? Few got the childhood they hoped for, but as we mature we come to realize that we received different opportunities that made us who we are.

PUNCTUALITY MATTERS

Workplace punctuality shows a strong work ethic, dedication to the company mission and competency in handling deadlines. It indicates that you are responsible, committed and capable of honoring your word. Is being late a disorder? Well, not exactly, but habitual tardiness is a non-verbal statement not just about inadequate time-management skills, but also about how much

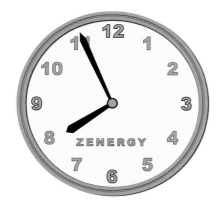

you value the job. You're definitely punctual for an airplane or a train. Why? Because there is a big penalty when you're late. Consider your motives when you're habitually late for work or social events. Being late 10 minutes daily over the course of one year costs more than the equivalent of one week's paid vacation (43 hours).

If arriving at work by 8:00a is a chore, renegotiate a flexible schedule with your employer (8-6 is the same amount of time as 8:15-6:15). Possibly you would enjoy working second shift, nights or weekends. Some people really enjoy working late and sleeping till noon. You might consider a night job in show business, radio or stocking shelves. Police officers, fire fighters, taxi drivers and fitness club managers provide good professions for those who enjoy working nights. A little bit of self-examination can offer the insight that may be necessary to find the right job at the right time for you.

Being late can be a way to non-verbally manipulate. You're forcing your friends and family to wait for you, like you're a king or queen, and everyone should wait for royalty to arrive. Smart people will assess and adjust. For instance, they may invite you to arrive an hour or half-hour early so that you're not late. Others will resent you and ultimately just stop inviting you entirely. Tardiness is an indication of being disorganized and incapable of completing simple tasks, and it can be a sign of passive aggressive behavior. Clearly, you don't value the person or the event very much or you would be timely.

When your friends or spouse are chronically challenged with punctuality, spend some time discussing it with them over dinner one night. Keep it upbeat and jovial. Make sure you don't have a tone of frustration or irritation. Be an investigative reporter to learn more about them. Ask questions about their schedule, and why they feel it's important to cram so many things into a 10-minute window. What's wrong with postponing certain activities, like stopping at the dry cleaners when you're already rushed? Why can't they delegate more? What does it mean to be calm and have clarity through the day instead of riding an adrenaline rush into home base each night? Measurements of productivity and achievement are very important to many people and forcing one more thing into the day may mean ultimate success to them. Learn more about their measuring system for achievement and how you both can benefit daily from their accomplishments.

Occasional lateness is understood because we have different watches and spontaneous events can arise to delay you five minutes, but repeat offenders generate animosity and resentments.

Setting your clock ahead 10 minutes or a reminder on your cell phone can be beneficial for those infrequent blunders that may arise. Track how long certain activities require. For instance, it takes me about 3 minutes to empty the dishwasher, but checking emails is uncertain. Never check email right before you're about to leave. Soon you'll enjoy the intrinsic value of walking through the door on time for an appointment. It feels so good every time.

ZENERGY BOOST FOR PUNCTUALITY
1. Monitor how long it takes to empty the dishwasher, vacuum or garden.
2. Track how long it takes to grocery shop (door to door).
3. Set an alarm when you only have one hour to complete a task.
4. Set your clock 15 minutes fast.
5. Take responsibility if you're late and acknowledge it ~ don't just shrug it off.

WIN/WIN NEGOTIATIONS

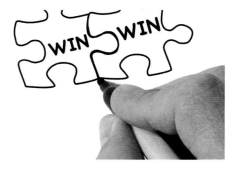

Have you ever walked away from a situation where you got the short end of the stick? It's unfair, unwarranted or just flat wrong. You don't like being taken advantage of and neither does anyone else. Learning to create win/win situations is a healthy skill and reduces tension among family, friends and colleagues. You can't generate integrity in others, but your evenhandedness can set the tone for your immediate environment.

It's important to maintain collaborative efforts in negotiations. Whether with a spouse, associate or employer, clearly you both want to participate together or you wouldn't even consider another discussion. State your obvious goals but keep them short and precise. Write this out in advance so you stay focused during the conversation and consider the expected outcome. Precedents set a standard that is generally enforced in a corporate setting but have more flexibility for a family. However, the past does not direct the future, otherwise we would never evolve. Be willing to ask for what you want even if you think you won't get it. Have a few rebuttals rehearsed prior to the meeting.

When you're asking for a raise don't refer to what others are earning. Focus on your skill set and continuing education to benefit the company. Comment on your attendance, punctuality and community efforts for holidays and birthdays. Introduce a new and exciting marketing idea to generate more profit for the company. Indicate how you could contribute to the fruition of that idea, but don't pile on more work for yourself without a raise or promotion. Sometimes a promotion means more work, more responsibility and the same income (which is a downgrade for you). Be mindful of what the outcome will mean for you both. If you need additional time to contemplate the new agreement, ask to reconvene tomorrow. Sleep on it for the night and decide in the morning. Oprah always asks God to assist her with business decisions and rarely decides in the moment. Give yourself a day or two to pray on the subject seeking advice from your Highest Council.

Identifying who has what power in the relationship and who controls which resources is imperative. Spouses share many different roles and lean on each other in unseen ways; it's the same with employers and employees. Know what power and resources you bring to the table that they enjoy. You need each other and agreements are a common part of everyday life, but in negotiations it's important to know who stands to win and lose more. This allows you to understand their point of view.

When you present choices, substitutes or even unconventional possibilities, you open the door for candid communication. Consider your relationship, shared history and the new path you are forging. Indicate your accommodating and cooperative nature to lower defensiveness. Consider all the choices each of you have and be willing to let go of something in order to find a compromise.

Keep in mind that change is uncomfortable initially and pushback can come from lack of clarity of the new arrangement. Change offers a mixed-bag of emotions. Be mindful of any unknown or hidden issues that may influence the negotiation. If your compromise presents potential frustration or additional workload for your associate, you may need to walk them through the new routine to acquire the final agreement. If you don't find a resolution, there will be a loss for you both, and that loss can cause a heated debate and hurt feelings.

For instance, when a wife needs a larger budget for the household operating expenses it's important for her to itemize all that she does each week. Identify the chores, beyond the 40-hour work-week, like grocery shopping, cooking, vacuuming, cleaning the house, discarding the trash, preparing the kids for bed, purchasing and mending their clothes, planning the budget, clipping coupons as well as exercising to stay toned and grooming. Although applying makeup and getting a manicure doesn't seem like something to negotiate, husbands benefit from having an attractive wife. Don't discount grooming as it takes at least one-hour each day for women to look lovely. Husbands can forget the effort a wife takes to maintain the home and her beauty. Even though some of this may sound antiquated, many women just don't realize how valuable they are to the family and making a list like this can really boost self-esteem. Be open to renegotiating the household budget every two or three years.

Negotiating with your parents can be precarious but setting realistic boundaries can restore the loving bond between you. If attending the weekly family dinner just isn't convenient anymore, and you sometimes even resent going, then consider compromising to only once or twice a month. If you used to take your parents to the doctor, but now you have your own children, then negotiating a new schedule can be empowering to maintain a healthy family dynamic. Don't short-change yourself. Your idea of a healthy harmonious family is just as valuable as what your parents think.

Setting healthy boundaries with a roommate is important. Have a list of expectations like rent due dates (usually the first of the month), shared chores, quiet time from 10p–10a and overnight guest privileges. Don't underestimate the stress associated with a messy kitchen or untrained pets. Be clear on what you will and will not tolerate in advance and put it in writing. Have all parties sign it. This type of clarity can save all kinds of potential hassles, and if you later need to discuss your living arrangements you can present that document as a baseline for the conversation. Maintain rapport with your roommates. You want your house to feel like a home.

Negotiating can be exhilarating and exhausting. It takes patience, creativity, inventiveness and resourcefulness. Go in rested and ready. Be prepared for something unexpected so that you don't feel ambushed if a new idea is presented. Also, you don't want the other to feel ambushed if they weren't expecting a renegotiation. Remember you can always reconvene the following day but don't bail too quickly. Sometimes a soft pinch on the arm (that no one can see) will ease nervousness in the moment and keep you present. Nervousness is scatter chatter and *under-thoughts*. Stay alert and aware of what is happening in the moment and not what your unconscious mind is interpreting. Take a few deep breaths and stay intuitive about all possibilities. Remember you want a Win/Win!

 ZENERGY BOOST FOR NEGOTIATING
Silence can be an effective negotiation strategy. If you need to entice someone to share more, remaining silent can open the door for more disclosure. Next time you're in a conversation or negotiation, after your partner finishes their statement, choose to remain quiet and attentive. See what bonus information you might allure them into revealing through your silence.

FORGIVENESS RELAXES YOUR GUARD

When you are angry with another, your mind is filled with repetitive thoughts of discord. Even if you know you should "let that go and think about other things," sometimes the mind hangs onto an injustice causing you to feel defensive. The subconscious mind's prime directive is to guard you. The ego can dwell in negative thoughts ad nauseum in order to protect you from future offenses, and your neurology generates biochemicals and hormones and stimulates, or impedes, your immune system making you physically stronger or weaker (depending on the thought). Forgiveness is like watering the seeds of love. Prayer, mindfulness, joy, laughter and kindness all create loving feelings that are measurable. Equally measurable are hostility, hatred, seething and resentments.

> *Anger is an acid that can do more harm to the vessel in which it is stored*
> *than to anything on which it is poured.*
> **Mark Twain**

Avoiding explosive anger can be a useful life skill but suppressing your authentic self can lead to all kinds of physical ailments like weight gain, acid reflux, ulcers or heart disease, to name a few. Frequently avoiding confrontation saves time, money and energy. You know when you confront someone, the communication gets heated and how uncomfortable it can be. Immediately, quarrelsome words like "you did this and that" come from both parties. Someone is going to win and someone is going to lose, and neither of you want to be the loser. Instead, you both end up experiencing a loss of friendship or at least loss of inner peace. You're both losers. Afterwards, maybe an hour, maybe a decade, you communicate with that person again. It's awkward and uncomfortable initially, but your intent is to find common ground. Why don't you just start with that? You can follow the status quo, be like the herd, and engage in competitive communication, or you can take the high road. Taking the high road is a skill you can learn.

Next time you're feeling angry toward someone or a situation, write down a paragraph or two (maybe one or two pages) to your opponent. Get into it. I'm not recommending that you ever send the letter, just write it all down. Periodically (after one paragraph or one page) measure your breath and heartbeat. You may notice that by journaling your anger you get stressed out, the heart beats faster and the breath gets shorter. It's safer to release your aggression in pen and paper than to unleash it on your spouse or other family members. Express either in writing or in an audio recording what's really on your mind. Again, do not send this communication to anyone. Being angry is a sign of feeling guarded. This exercise allows your internal guard to express concern and release anger in a controlled setting. Just pulling back from a situation and evaluating it from another's point of view can let your guard stand at ease. If you repeatedly tell yourself that someone or a situation offended you, then that will continue to be your outlook in the future. If you're focused on another distressing event or expecting one, then you might make a mountain out of a molehill, resulting in a loss of friendship or future friendships.

Initially, we forgive and remember and continue fighting. "Bury the hatchet and leave the handle sticking out," as Garth Brooks sings. You can set healthy boundaries and ask for what you need in the relationship, but people aren't going to change for you. They change for themselves because they see the value in it. What is the benefit for them in changing their behavior? You might think, "it will make me happier." Generally speaking, people don't really care if you're happy. It's not that they necessarily want you to live in discord, but they are more motivated by their own wellbeing, not yours. If you're angry or offended by something, then it's your responsibility to review your perspective and restore your inner harmony. It's not their responsibility. For example, if your boss annoys you, then walking into her office with an attitude won't really solve the problem. You need to alter your viewpoint so that you can perform the task properly. The last thing you should do is blog publicly about it. Be mindful when asking someone to give you virtually anything: a ride to a doctor's appointment or the airport, requesting your spouse to be quiet in the morning or a neighbor to maintain his or her home. Maybe the people in your life who upset you don't have the capacity to give you what you want. If you've asked three or four times then stop asking, and begin to realize that this person doesn't have the ability or desire to give you what you want. That may mean asking another, maybe God, for a new solution. (More ideas on this topic in the Spirit Section.)

Resentments can pile up leading to cynicism and bitterness. Forgiveness means, "to give as you gave before." You might not be able to do that today, but you can begin by moving to a neutral space. You could start with the repetitive affirmation, "I forgive you, I forgive you, I forgive you," even though you don't mean it initially. It's a start. This technique is easier to initiate with reckless drivers with whom you have little interaction with on the road. For instance, when you notice someone driving erratically you might say or do something defensively, and mostly you just get away from that car and continue your route. You're not expecting all drivers to operate their vehicles dangerously. Most people respectfully follow the road rules and are not trying to harm you or have a wreck. They're just preoccupied, distracted or late for an event. You can circumvent all kinds of tension by realizing that it's not about you. Their poor behavior, or dangerous driving, has nothing to do with you. When you quickly forgive or stop the repetitive expletives, you alleviate your stress quickly. You benefit from dropping the subject, stating a positive affirmation like, "I forgive you," and returning your attention to the street where most drivers are following the road rules. Most of us automatically practice this simple method of forgiveness. You're already good at it. We just want to transfer that skill to other, more significant, grievances.

Purge negative offenses from the previous day that deplete vitality and resilience, and soon you will notice a new sense of optimism. Recapitulation can be an empowering process to help you become aware of long-standing patterns and make conscious choices in the future. According to Dr. Deepak Chopra, recapitulation is a gentle rewind of the past 24 hours. When you lie down to rest at night, take 1-2 minutes to skim through the events of the day. Allow the images, sounds and memories to scroll through your mind quickly. Don't analyze or judge it; just review your recollections like eating breakfast, driving to work, completing tasks at your desk, enjoying lunch, etc. Review the day's events as a silent observer without any emotional commentary on the events. Then, you can safely store those memories away. This can free your mind of petty intrusions from the day so you don't get stuck on any one occurrence. Small offenses are easy to store away after recapitulation and to ultimately forgive, but significant emotional events may take extra time to resolve.

Dream of your brother's kindness instead of dwelling in your dreams of his mistakes.
A Course in Miracles

Practicing the forgiveness process with small offenses can open the door to forgiving more substantial wrongdoings. Over time, some negative feelings can be forgotten so that when you see that person again, you really will have forgiven them. There may come a time when you don't even remember what they did that upset you. However, some people are just plain selfish and inconsiderate, and you may need to remain cautious around them. Remember, when you process your inner world and resolve bitterness, you will feel better, but they may not have processed the experience. Don't expect them to have changed just because you experienced forgiveness. Setting healthy boundaries means asking for what you want, like restoring common ground, and if they can't give it to you, then don't spend a lot of time with those people. To forgive and forget is an advanced level of spiritual awareness that increases your happiness and inner peace exponentially. Plus, you don't have to take someone to lunch just because you forgave him or her.

You are in charge of your mind. You're not in charge of your spouse's mind, or your children's mind or your in-laws' minds. When you notice that things aren't going your way, try to stop and recognize what IS going your way. For instance, you have clothes, transportation, and you can read (that's a huge perk in life). Begin an attitude of gratitude. Then, if things go awry, you won't become resentful because you're in control of your mind, and you're focused on what IS working in your life.

Victor Frankl (1905-1997), a German Psychiatrist imprisoned for five years in a Nazi concentration camp during WW II, wrote the book *Man's Search For Meaning* in 1946. He states, "Everything you have in life can be taken from you except one thing, your freedom to choose HOW you will respond to any situation. This is what determines the quality of the life we've lived - not whether we've been rich or poor, famous or unknown, healthy or suffering. What determines our quality of life is how we relate to these realities, what kind of meaning we assign to them, what kind of attitude we cling to about them, and what state of mind we allow them to trigger."

Forgiveness can be liberating and help you release unresolved feelings. Resiliency is about maintaining a positive outlook regarding the past and a curiosity toward future events to come.

Reflect on your life at any age, review your past circumstances, revisit previous situations and, if appropriate, consider changing your relationship to the past. As you do, new neural pathways will begin to form releasing you from those heavy burdens, redefining the bondage to negative behaviors that no longer serve you, and allowing you to magnetize an unprecedented reality.

 ZENERGY BOOST FOR FORGIVENESS

1. Reflect on what you appreciate about your life, and reinstate positive feelings about the past to maintain optimism toward the future.
2. Practice recapitulation for one or two minutes each night.
3. Journal 1-3 pages about a past occurrence.
4. Pause. Take a moment and pause before interpreting a current painful situation to reduce judgments and knee-jerk reactions in the moment.
5. Replay in your mind what was factually said or done to whom, not your interpretation and side story.
6. Ask for clarity. "What did you mean by that?" Don't jump to conclusions.
7. Take a Time Out. Excuse yourself to the bathroom or another private location PRIOR to responding, if possible.

Making Amends

We will all make mistakes from the cradle to the grave. It's common to make errors in judgment. Knee-jerk reactions and negative blog bursts are now a common communication blunder and, sadly, many of those posts will remain online for decades.

Making amends with someone is different from an apology. Frequently, an apology can sound more like a band-aid than a real attempt to resolve something. Making amends for an error you've made is typically associated with the 12-step program (*www.12step.org*), but you don't have to be an anonymous member to apply the wisdom. When you've harmed someone, you could irreparably damage your relationship. If you feel ashamed, guilty or humiliated by your behavior, then personal coaching or therapy may be in order prior to resolving the situation.

When making amends there must be a commitment for your behavior to be genuinely different in the future. Acknowledging your mistake, allowing the other person to share their feelings and finding common ground could take time, or you may even need a mediator to assist. Don't be afraid to clean up the past and start fresh. The sooner you do, the quicker inner peace and joy will be restored.

Steps to Making Amends from WikiHow:
1. Take an objective view of what happened.
2. Face your mixed feelings.
3. Stand in the other person's shoes.
4. Write down the reasons why you need to make amends.
5. Make amends with a clear heart.
6. Decide what it will take to resolve the damage that was done.
7. Fearlessly create a new future for yourself and your relationship.

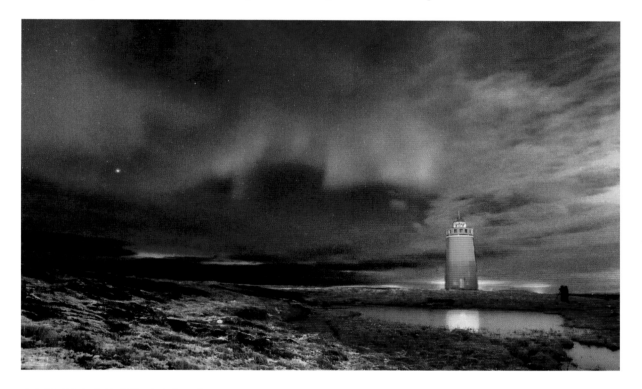

A TIME FOR REFLECTION

Take a day or two to reflect on the topics you've read thus far. This how-to book provides practical transformational methods to empower you. If you rush through this book you'll miss the application. Knowing isn't enough, you must apply what you know. Review the Zenergy Boosts in the previous chapters and practice some of those exercises now. Spend the rest of today journaling and reflecting on the recommendations. Transformation can occur in the blink of an eye but you must contemplate what you really want. Knowing what you don't want is a step on the path to knowing what you do want. What is your ideal mental outlook? Build it in your mind's eye now.

PEACE PROVOKING APTITUDE

STRESS MANAGEMENT SKILLS

Stress is a leading factor for all illness and disease. If you have any type of injury, illness or disease your doctor will ask, "What is your stress level?" Questions like the following are common...

Recently...
Have you moved?
Have you married or divorced?
Did you change jobs or relocate?
Did a loved one pass away?
Do you have teenagers living with you?
Do you have parents living with you?
Do you have a newborn child?
How much do you work each week?
Do you enjoy your job?
Do you have a hobby?
Do you have a social life?
Do you take an annual vacation or stay-cation?

Stress whittles its way into our lives. We create a comfort zone within the stressful perspective and circumstances until something collapses. Then, we don't know how to change. We just know we need improvement, and we need it today. According to Carol Ritberger, Ph.D., three types of stress are: physical, psychological, and psychosocial.

1. **Physical Stress** involves external stressors such as environmental pesticides and pollution, noise and extreme temperatures. It also includes injuries, allergies, surgery, prolonged exercise, and an inadequate supply of oxygen.
2. **Psychological Stress** is associated with the way we feel, the emotions we experience, the attitudes we have, and the way we react to anything that threatens us, whether the threat is real or perceived.

3. **Psychosocial Stress** occurs as a result of our interactions with other people such as conflicts with family members, neighbors, bosses, co-workers, friends, or other people around us. It can also occur when there's isolation due to inadequate social interaction and social phobias.

Identify your main source of stress. Is it physical, psychological or psychosocial? Reducing stress could be something simple, like purchasing a different type of chair for the office, or it could require more professional assistance with a marital counselor. Saying, "I'm stressed out" is vague and unnerving. Identifying that your low back hurts because you sit 6-8 hours daily is much easier to alleviate than trying to mitigate everything. Adrenaline (a stress hormone) motivates us to move faster, and it also taxes the adrenals, kidneys and low back. Inability to reduce stressful activities can occur because of an overwhelming need to perform, produce and achieve, and at times it can be difficult to shift gears or delegate. You can get addicted to the stress hormones just as much as the activity that causes the stress, and behavior modification can feel awkward initially. Craving the stress hormones can invite familiar behavior to return. Pretending that tomorrow will be better, or at least different, and then doing the same thing as yesterday is a sign not only of denial but also insanity. The definition of insanity is doing the same thing over and over and expecting a different result. In hopes of not being insane, one day this week try something different.

Reduce compulsive behavior by introducing some R&R into your schedule. Consider a 20-minute chair massage or a mani/pedi. Notice how a little bit of pampering can make a big difference in your outlook. Consider it an opportunity to tune into your body for a few minutes, and let someone nurture you for a change. Unplug from the hectic world, and revamp your outlook. Remember, during a sporting event a professional athlete sits on the bench briefly and recharges before rocketing back into action on the playing field. Conserving energy can restore your vitality and vibrant outlook quickly. Consider some of the following tips to reduce stress and build the muscle for inner peace.

1. **Breathe**–Become aware of the quality of your breath as often as possible. Place post-it notes in your car, at your desk or on your makeup mirror to remind you to breathe consciously. The reminder could be a paper clip. Only you know the suggested meaning behind the paper clip at the side of your monitor. Everyone else may see it as a paper clip, but for you it means breathe deeply and relax.
2. Play soft classical **music** or ambient groove in your home and at your office. Find a station (preferably without advertisements) that compliments your environment. Distracting music with lyrics or commercials can increase stress levels.
3. Add a **water fountain** or water sounds, like a waterfall or a soft rain, at your office and home. They are lovely to look at and delightful to hear. Underneath the noise of the office and your mind, you will hear the tranquil sounds of the water that lulls you back to your center.
4. **Stretch** once or twice a day. Standing at your workstation to stretch your legs and low back can reduce aches and pains. Simple stretches can improve overall vitality if you've been sitting at your

desk or in your car for prolonged periods. Yoga and Qigong are great ways to awaken the body and relax the mind. Attending a chair yoga class once or twice a week can be very therapeutic, but beyond a class, you can practice on your own some of the postures included in this book.

5. Eat more **vegetables and fruits**. The Father of Aerobics Dr. Kenneth Cooper of the Cooper Aerobics Center proclaims, "5 is fine, but 9 is divine!" Eat five to nine servings of vegetables and fruits daily and transform your mind-body-spirit.

6. Dr. Cooper also promotes, "walk your dog, even if you don't have a dog." **Walk** around the block, the office building or the park each day. You could even walk in place (or march in your chair) for five minutes. Walking is free and increases circulation throughout your entire cellular system offering more communication between the brain and body. Most everyone should walk at least one mile daily (2,000 steps). It can be intermittent throughout the day and you can travel at your own pace. Just walk daily.

7. Drink more **water**. Many people are dehydrated which exacerbates chronic diseases, like Diabetes. Think about beef jerky. It's dehydrated muscle. Your muscles get tough from lack of water. Add one large glass of water (10-12 ounces) to your intake by placing it next to your bed at night. Drink it immediately upon awakening in the morning. Instead of showering, bathe once a week in plain water, no bubbles. The skin is the largest organ in the body and is soluble. What goes on the skin goes in the skin. It will absorb some of the water while bathing.

8. **Aromatherapy** works. I performed fitness evaluations on 100s of people. Initially, I measured their pulse and then asked them to sniff lavender oil. After one or two whiffs I measured their pulse again and frequently it dropped by 8-10 beats per minute. One or two whiffs, now that is impressive. If you have high blood pressure, keep quality oils with you all the time (especially at work and in your car). At night, you can mist your pillows with lavender, sandalwood or rose oil and smell it all night long. Initially, the olfactory system recognizes a new aroma, but subsides rather quickly after acknowledging consistent odors. Just know you're still receiving the benefits even after you stop noticing it.

9. **Journal**. If something or someone is on your mind, journal about it. If journaling about it on the computer, password protect the document so you feel comfortable expressing authentically. Journal to release the jibber jabber in your head, and you'll focus better on your tasks afterwards. Journaling has proven results with processing grief and reducing symptoms of anxiety. Consider it an intimate conversation with yourself.

10. **Hug someone**. Have you hugged someone lately? Go ahead, open your arms and ask, "Do you want a hug?" Many people will take you up on the offer. We just don't receive enough healthy non-sexual physical contact.

Generally speaking, "when women are stressed they are not interested in sex, unlike men," states Dr. John Gray, author of the voluminous series *Men Are From Mars, Women Are From Venus*. Although both sexes want to be safe, successful and fulfilled, we look for peace in different ways. This is possibly due to the hormonal differences between us, but also because of our psychosocial upbringing. Women and men find relief from stress sometimes in opposite ways. Women often process their stress by talking to friends or their husband. She can increase her personal power by cooking a meal, lighting candles, receiving a mani/pedi or planning a fun family event. These activities help women relax. Conversely, men reduce stress by relaxing on the couch, watching a sporting event or action flick with explosions, and basically not talking. Men build their self-esteem and confidence by being alone in their man-cave or workshop area. Understanding and appreciating our differences can reduce all kinds of stress in any relationship with the opposite sex.

Decide who or what generates the most stress in your life, sometimes called *brain drains*, and begin to eliminate the easy ones first. Relocating the whole family to the sunbelt because you're tired of shoveling snow might not be realistic, but you can easily change the radio station to more uplifting music on your drive through the snow tomorrow. Evaluate your life over the next week; take note when you're frustrated, sad or fearful. Indicate the date, time and location when it occurred. Dictate voice notes, text yourself a memo, or try some of the Zenergy enhancing exercises in this book. Keep track and notice what stresses you the most, then you can begin to make some appropriate adjustments. Noticing is the first step.

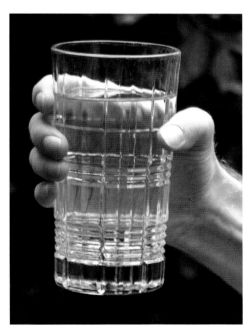

How Heavy is a Glass of Water?

A psychologist walked around a room while teaching stress management to an audience. As she raised a glass of water, everyone expected they'd be asked the "half empty or half full" question. Instead, with a smile on her face, she inquired, "How heavy is this glass of water?" Answers called out ranged from 8 oz. to 20 oz. She replied, "The absolute weight doesn't matter. It depends on how long I hold it. If I hold it for a minute, it's not a problem. If I hold it for an hour, I'll have an ache in my arm. If I hold it for a day, my arm will feel numb and paralyzed. In each case, the weight of the glass doesn't change, but the longer I hold it, the heavier it becomes." She continued, "The stresses and worries in life are like that glass of water. Think about them for a moment and nothing happens. Think about them for an hour and they begin to hurt." If you think about your problems all day long, you may feel overwhelmed, frustrated or even incapable of doing anything. Find balance between solving problems and enjoying the fruits of your effort. It's important to let go of your stresses as quickly as you can, and put your burdens down momentarily. Remember to set the glass down! (Author unknown. Reprinted on the internet many times.)

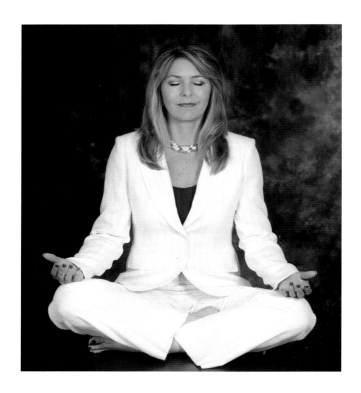

MEDITATION 101

Meditation offers a systematic approach to mind-body-spirit wellness. Meditation is a mental practice with tremendous emotional and physiological benefits and even a path to inner peace. Meditation is a fourth state of consciousness, distinct from waking, dreaming or sleeping. While sitting or reclining motionless and settling down the mental activity, the mind moves into restful awareness. Not thinking or sleeping but resting allows the body to rejuvenate at a deep level. A growing body of scientific research supports the health benefits of meditation. Stress and inflammation are specifically linked with every type of disease. Practicing a few relaxation techniques daily could be quite useful not just in decreasing your heart rate, blood pressure and stress hormones, but also improving your brain health and mental cognition. Meditation slows down the internal dialogue so that you can disseminate the data, discard the fear and regain clarity of insight.

Studies found in the *American Heart Association Journal* indicate that a regular meditation practice reduces risk of heart attacks and strokes (vol 6, no. 10, 2017). According to Transcendental Meditation Leader Dr. John Hagelin, "regular meditation lowers risk for cancer by two-thirds and provides a 93% reduction in mental nervous disorders. Daily meditation normalizes blood pressure without the negative side effects and dependency on hypertensive drugs by providing the body much needed rest to eliminate the stress that is the cause of a majority of diseases. Metabolic Syndrome (a combination of high blood pressure, obesity and diabetes) has overtaken millions of Americans, and meditation has a proven positive effect on this epidemic by lowering the levels in all three diseases" (YouTube, 2012). Stress-driven behaviors like smoking, vaping or over-eating also decrease due to regular mindful practices. When more attuned to your body, you will naturally want to take better care of yourself. Meditation can even reverse aging. For example, hearing and vision decline with age and improve with meditation. Those who regularly meditate for five years or more show to be 10-12 years younger than their chronological age through physiological tests from their doctors (tests on cholesterol, blood pressure, vision, hearing, etc.). Additionally, reaction time, learning capacity, recall, memory and aptitude decline with age and improve with meditation. Educator Dr. Hagelin further proclaims, "it has been proven that you can, in fact, increase your IQ at any age through the use of regular meditation."

Even rank beginners experience the benefits of pain management after only a few days of practicing. A study published by the *Journal of Neuroscience* showed that after four days of meditation training, meditators reported reduced unpleasantness of pain by 57% and decreased intensity of pain by 40% (April, 2011). It's so simple and it's free! Imagine reducing years of pain and discomfort in just four days. You don't need an education or religious understanding; you don't need insurance, an attorney or a stockbroker to make your life easier and more manageable. All you need to do is sit back, relax and watch your body breathe. Regular meditators Richard Gere, Jennifer Aniston, Bill Gates, Ellen DeGeneres, Jerry Seinfield, Paul McCartney, Katy Perry, Andrew Chert, Arianna Huffington, Will Smith and Oprah Winfrey, to name a few, endorse the profound benefits of meditation.

The Mayo Clinic suggests that meditation may help such conditions as allergies, anxiety disorders, asthma, binge eating, cancer, depression, fatigue, heart disease, high blood pressure, pain management, sleep problems, and substance abuse. The heart rate slows, the hormones balance and the endocrine system naturally improves increasing the body's autonomic immune system. Be sure to talk to your health care provider prior to initiating a meditation practice. For some, meditation can worsen symptoms like feelings of isolation associated with certain mental health conditions or even a sense of dizziness linked with low blood pressure or vertigo. Meditation isn't a replacement for traditional medical or psychological treatment, but it is complimentary. Meditation benefits the mind, body and spirit. Taking just 15-20 minutes a day can radically improve your physiology over the course of a few months and certainly over a few years.

World-renowned pioneer in integrative medicine and personal transformation Dr. Deepak Chopra states, "Meditation takes us beyond the mental prison of doubt, anxiety, and judgment to the silent field of expanded awareness in which we remember our essential nature as peaceful, centered and creative. Just a few minutes a day allows us to experience wholeness in our lives, which supports balance, healing and transformation." Dr. Chopra likened meditation techniques to a taxi. The intention is to carry you to a different location. Once you're there, you don't need the taxi, or the technique, anymore. Meditation techniques are a pathway to inner peace, and the feelings associated with meditation are likened to the soft floaty feeling you have first thing in the morning when returning to your body after a good night's rest.

Meditation is also an umbrella term for mindfulness. There are many ways to become consciously aware and finding the right method for you is fundamental. Attempt each of the following disciplines at least two or three times before you decide you don't like it. Guided meditation, mantra meditation, mindful breathing, Qigong (CHEE-gung), Tai chi (TIE-chee), yoga, fitness, running, dance, expressive movement, cooking and even playing an instrument (as in playing with abandon) can take you deeply into the present moment. I frequently hear those who are highly analytical (left brainers) say they can't quiet their mind and stop trying. This group may find mindfulness activities or moving meditations more appropriate at the beginning. After a month or two you may be ready for sitting still. Moving meditations do not replace sitting still; they are the precursor. You can escape the prison of your mind through a regular meditation practice.

Spiritually, meditation takes us to higher realms as we learn to become dispassionate toward the outside world. Even your thoughts are of the outside world. Meditation connects you with your Higher Self and God, and you begin to feel the mental-emotional side more and less physicality. You feel the energy moving within. This pure conscious awareness can guide you in countless opportunities allowing synchronicity to occur in unimaginable ways. According to Edgar Cayce, "Meditation is the emptying of ourselves of all that hinders the Creative Force from rising along the natural channels of our physical bodies to be disseminated through the sensitive spiritual centers in our physical bodies. When mediation is properly entered into, we are made stronger mentally and physically (Reading 281-13). The *Bible* states, "The Kingdom of God is within," (KJV, Luke 17:21) and meditation opens the door within you. Regardless of your religion, you can sit in a chair and call upon your personal prophet to guide you daily on your personal path. Meditation provides spiritual inclusiveness. Christians, Muslims, Jews, Hindus and Atheists can meditate in the same room while still maintaining their religious (or non-religious) identity. Taking time for relaxation transforms your life spiritually, and a regular meditation practice can take you to the holy of holies within yourself.

One of my clients with a Type A personality, Lisa, attended my meditation class. Everyone could tell she was a demanding businesswoman who got results in the corporate world; unfortunately, she was quite unhappy even with her extraordinary financial results. After attending my class for three weeks and meditating most days during that time one of her colleagues commented on her improved attitude. The associate sheepishly said, "Well, you're not as edgy as usual." My client admitted she was meditating. It was clear to everyone in the class (as well as her coworkers) that she had gained a new inner silence that she didn't have just three weeks prior. Over time you will naturally become calm, confident and centered from meditating regularly.

Understand in advance that various thoughts, feelings, and sensations will arise from time-to-time while meditating, and you may lose concentration on the breath. Remember, the mind will think like the heart will beat. If you notice your brain drifting, don't criticize yourself because you're thinking, that's only natural. Gently come back to your breath and feel your lungs rise and fall again. Thinking is like the sea. Your thoughts are floating around the ocean of the mind. Individual thoughts are similar to a droplet. Like Wi-Fi with a mass of information floating around, you search the Internet for one topic and that one becomes your focus, like a droplet. As you concentrate on one thought a droplet is formed. The thought-droplet receives your attention for awhile as you formulate that thought completely. For instance, the mind thinks about driving, and driving is the droplet while in the car. Then, you arrive at the grocery store. Grocery shopping becomes the droplet. You're not thinking about driving anymore, you're thinking about produce, soup and paper products. When you get home your thought-droplet is cooking a meal. You're not thinking about grocery shopping or driving. You're thinking about preparing the recipe. Clearly, thought-droplets arise about a wide variety of things. You are sitting in the sea of thinking while attempting to meditate, and you're trying not to create droplets. When a droplet is formed, your mind begins to focus on one thing. The rambling begins distracting you from the meditation technique. All you need to do is return to the meditation method (discussed next). Let the technique be the droplet for those 20 minutes. Insist that your attention stay on the technique. Discipline your mind to pay attention to one thing for 20 minutes and not 20 things for one minute each. The mind will wander, that's ok, just return to the technique as quickly as you notice that you're not doing it. As soon as you notice that you're creating thought-droplets, drop them and return to the meditation method. It's a practice. You won't ever be perfect at it, but trying will make you perfect at other things–like being relaxed, centered, calm, collected and focused.

Create A Meditation Space
Initially, it can be challenging to recognize where to meditate, but you really only need to sit with the spine upright. You might choose your dining room chair or even the floor, if your hips and knees don't ache while in that position. You don't want to be distracted by your body during meditation. If you lie down to meditate, you will most likely fall asleep (especially in the beginning). So choose a comfortable chair, not a recliner, and position it in a quiet space. If you have an unsupportive

spouse or active children, you might consider purchasing noise reduction earplugs or earmuffs. You could sit in your car at the park; just lock your doors prior to closing your eyes. Choose a safe space that is inviting for silence.

Place a few sacred objects nearby where you can see them just as you close your eyes and upon first opening them, like a photo of your favorite ancestor, a locket, crystal or bouquet of flowers. You might locate a rare painting of your prophet, a cross, deity statute or icon that connects you to the Creative Forces. Having your grandmother's hand-knitted afghan or prayer scarf on the chair is an open invitation to sit and be comforted. Find revered items that you admire and keep them on or near the location of your meditation chair. Create a special space for rest and rejuvenation.

Making Meditation A Daily Practice

Sit at the same time every day. Most people like meditating first thing in the morning because there is less mental activity at that time. 4:00-6:00am is considered the Guru Hour as that is the customary time to meditate. However, some caregivers might find 10am or noon to work just as well once everyone is fed and kids off to school. If you meditate in the middle of the day (1-2pm) you may end up napping, which has many medicinal benefits; however, meditation is not sleeping. You want to remain in restful awareness, creating the neurological network for inner peace. If you have insomnia, meditate right before bedtime. Position the chair near the bed and draw the sheets down so you're not stirring much before going to sleep. In this situation, you could use the meditation techniques while lying down in bed since the intention is to sleep, but first meditate in a chair. Meditating 30 minutes has similar benefits to sleeping for 8 hours so if you just can't sleep one night practice meditating then.

Locate a cell phone with a stopwatch and notepad on it. Sit down and write your to-do list. Whatever you think you might forget while meditating, write that down before you begin~ groceries, chores, favorite stocks to purchase. Purge your mind and set your cell phone to ring in 5 or 15-minutes. Choose a soft ring tone to bring you back. You don't want a blaring alarm to awaken you from the peaceful feelings you just created.

Chair exercises prepare the mind for relaxation. Meditating is typically easier after any type of exercise because the body fidgets less when fatigued. Once seated, practice a few shoulder rotations in each direction to increase circulation. Then move to neck spirals in each direction. Loosen the jaw, relax the shoulders away from the ears and begin small neck rotations at the beginning increasing the circumference with each circle. Lower your ear to each shoulder stretching opposite sides of the neck. Sit up straight and lower chin to chest elongating the back of the neck. Then close your eyes and focus on your breath.

The techniques listed here guide your brain to quiet down so the inner wisdom of your Soul can be heard. Prayer is talking to God; meditation is listening. Be gentle with yourself throughout the process. Anytime your thoughts distract you, acknowledge that you are postponing thinking at the moment and return to your breath. Acharya Pema Chödrön, an Ordained American Tibetan Buddhist Nun and leading exponent of teachings on meditation, recommends when you notice you are thinking, quickly label it "thinking" and return the breath. Don't spend any time with the distracting thoughts once you notice you're lost in scatter chatter. Label it and focus on the breath again. Remember, meditation is not the technique; it's the feeling behind the technique. It is likened to the soft floaty feeling experienced upon awakening in the morning when you're coming back into your body but haven't moved yet. There is a subtle sensation upon awakening. You will notice it tomorrow morning. Deep meditation feels like that. Embrace the practice; don't demand perfection.

MEDITATION PRACTICES

Mindful Breathing/*Vippassana* ~
Sit in a chair with the crown of your head over the tailbone. Close your eyes and softly focus on the point between the eyebrows. Hold a steady gaze at the third eye. Keep the ocular muscle relaxed and the gaze intentional. Follow the rise and fall of your lungs. Feel the lungs expanding gently. Relax from your temples to your toes. In your mind's eye gently scan your body for tension and release it on the exhale. Do not attempt to control or manage the breath by inhaling deeper; your silent observation will slowly begin to balance your breathing naturally which, in turn, will calm your mind. Marvel at the miracle of the breath-of-life flowing in and out of your body. Notice the rate at which your heart beats. Slow down your mind and literally feel the heart beating. Intend that your heart beat slow and steady. Feel your skin and relax your skin, the largest organ in the body. Release the need to understand or to be understood for just a few minutes.

Yoga Nidra/Relaxation from Temples to Toes ~
Simply put, yoga nidra means to soothe your entire body. Set your intention for how calm or focused you would like to be and proceed in systemically relaxing each part. Lie down and settle the body from your temples to your toes. If that didn't calm you enough, proceed back up from the toes to the temples. This is particularly useful for those with disease, illness or injuries as it allows you to gently focus on the entire body and not just the injured part.

Counting ~
Count your breaths. Begin at a number, say 10, 54 or 99, and count down. If you lose your place, just begin again. This simple technique diverts your brain from those rambling thoughts temporarily.

Understand in advance that thoughts, feelings and sensations will arise, and you will lose count periodically. Just begin again. Counting numbers is a technique; clearly it's not the goal. You won't realize the goal until you master the technique. Practice mindful breathing and counting down for 1-3 minutes daily. Do this for as many days or weeks as necessary until you can be conscious of each number with very little effort. This is also a useful technique for insomnia.

Busy Your Brain with a Task ~
Slowly moving one finger is the least amount of activity you can do. With the palms up and your arms gently resting on your lap, softly move the index finger on the right hand by bending at the knuckle on the inhale and straightening the finger on the exhale. Maintain a small subtle movement throughout your meditation. You can add a mantra to the movement for additional benefit. When you zone out, your body will naturally stop moving. That's when you're in the gap. Being in the gap is ineffable, meaning there are no words for it. When you start describing what you're feeling you're not in the gap anymore. When you catch yourself periodically coming out of the gap then just begin any of these techniques again until you complete your allotted time.

Mantras, A Silent Song ~
Silently affirming one to three words can be very sensible in quieting the scatter chatter. If you're muttering words in your mind, then mantras can disrupt that pattern. A simple phrase like "I am peaceful" can guide the brain and redirect your attention. When you first sit down and the mind is active recite "I am peaceful...peaceful...I am peaceful." As you settle down and become relaxed, silently affirm "peace" on the inhale, and on the exhale silently affirm "full." Silently sing with a gentle tone, "I am peaceful." You might choose practical words like "tran-quil," "lov-ing," "bal-ance," "heal-ing," or "let go." A spiritual phrase like "I AM" or the Sanskrit equivalent "So Hum" or "Om" generates an uplifting feeling. Silently singing a spiritual word like "Jesus, Buddha or Krshna" can inspire you to surrender anxiety while strengthening your faith. Simple mantras help resolve resentments and build self-esteem quicker than you think. Silently saying, "I forgive you" or "I accept this [situation]" can offer a bit of solace if you're stewing. Allow the main word to carry you as you affirm, "forgive, accept or dissolve." Create a tag line for the day. "I am feeling calm, confident and centered!" "I am smart and prepared!" "I create the solution now!" "I am focused." Again, allow the main word to carry you by affirming, "confident, smart, create, focus." Simple and short are the best type of mantras.

If you are meditating to eliminate insomnia, choose two different mantras~one while sitting upright in your chair and a different one while lying down to sleep. Your chair mantra could be "peaceful" and your bed mantra could be "sleep now" because the intent of the bed mantra is to help you fall asleep. You don't want to nap when you meditate. You want to be awake in restful awareness during meditation; at nighttime you want to fall asleep.

Begin meditating just 5-10 minutes per day. Keep the goal small and achievable. Increase your meditation time by a few minutes each week until you reach 20-30 minutes once or twice daily. Consider meditating once for your work life and once for your family life each day. Decide how long you are going to meditate in advance. When you decide to meditate for 10 minutes don't sit for 11 minutes. Sometimes, the ego can be a bit rebellious when we force it to do certain things or renegotiate midstream. When you make an agreement with yourself to sit for 10 minutes and then you change your mind in the middle, next time it may be harder. The rebellious spirit might say, "well, last time you said 10 minutes and you made me sit 15 minutes so I don't want to do it again." If you want to meditate longer, then do so later in the day or the following day. When you are ready to meditate longer, ask yourself in advance if you can increase the time and wait for an answer. This interaction will strengthen your intuition. Listening to the small wise voice within is a skill, and meditation can aid you in becoming more intuitive.

Be gentle with yourself throughout the process. Don't get stuck with the notion that there are rules. Meditation is basically about quieting down the alert and active beta brain. Eventually, you will desire that private silence with the Divine Mind creating feelings of faith, confidence and courage. Conscious awareness builds over time making life more peaceful and productive. Buddha was asked what he had gained from meditation. He replied, *"Nothing! However, what I lost was anger, anxiety, depression, insecurity, fear of old age and fear of death."*

BREATHING TECHNIQUES FOR RELAXATION ~ *PRANAYAMA*

Pranayama is the formal practice of controlling the breath,
which is the source of our prana, or vital life.
Yoga Journal

"The ancient Indian system of yoga identified prana as the universal life force or energy which distinguishes the living from the dead, and flows through thousands of subtle energy channels they called 'nadis' and energy centers called 'chakras.' These original yogic seers observed the power of the breath to increase one's vitality and developed special breathing techniques to increase life energy, maintain health and create a calm, clear state of mind that is conducive for meditation" (*The Art of Living.org*).

When you learn to manage, massage and direct your breath, you gain more clarity and wisdom for your mind, body and spirit. Your breathing naturally changes throughout the day. When the scatter chatter is heightened, the breath is short and choppy. When the mind is relaxed, your breath is slow and steady, like while sleeping. The mind chatter redirects the breath just like the breath can refocus the mind. For instance, when you have anxiety, you can take a deep breath, retain the breath for two seconds and exhale. Altering your breath instantly influences how you feel and what you think. When you notice your breath is short and shallow, like when fearful, begin long deep breaths and lift out of that lower state of panic. First and foremost, you have to WANT to be different (relaxed, peaceful, centered, calm, wise), and then you can try some of the breathing techniques listed below. I only mention four methods here, but there are many that you can research online.

Edgar Cayce suggests in *A Search For God Book 1* (1942, 2018) varied breathing techniques. The simplest method is:
• Inhale through the right nostril and exhale through the mouth three times.
• Inhale through the left nostril and exhale through the right nostril three times.
  Practice this simple technique at the start of meditation. Then rest hands on lap for remainder of meditation while beginning "incantations [or mantras] which carries the self deeper into a sense of oneness with the Creative Forces of Love, and enter into the Holy of Holies."

Alternate Nostril Breathing ~ *Nadi Shodhana*
Approximately every 90 minutes to 2½ hours, the body naturally transfers which nostril dominates the breath, silently and rhythmically moving back and forth behind the scenes. The length of the cycle indicates natural rhythms and the mental and physical state of the individual. The body works harmoniously underneath daily living. Frequently, we force ourselves to do a few activities that move against our natural tendency (i.e. glued to a chair staring at a computer monitor or TV for hours each day). This behavior lends itself toward further imbalance. Flowing with our fundamental rhythms naturally provides more vitality.

When the left nostril is dominate (which is connected to the right side of the brain) the intuitive, spiritual, creative, artistic, emotional side is activated. You're likely to be more receptive or introverted during that time. Activities like using your imagination,painting, drawing, creating a work of art,addressing your feelings, or even sleeping are preferred. The right nostril is connected to the left side of the brain. A good time for home improvements, solving crossword puzzles, handling the budget, exercising or giving a presentation is when the right nostril dominates. The breath usually flows evenly through both nostrils while meditating when we experience calm inner peace. Approximately every two hours consider doing a different task like standing at your desk to work instead of sitting. A quick visit to the water cooler or bathroom every two hours or so supports the natural changes of your physiology. If you're drinking enough water you should go to the bathroom every hour or two depending on the size of your bladder, and movement accommodates your natural rhythms. It's not healthy to sit at your desk for several hours with very little movement. Improve creativity and concentration with one-to-three minutes of alternate nostril breathing periodically throughout the day. If you're having a sinus infection then you only breathe through one nostril or your mouth. Obviously, you cannot do pranayama practice until you clear that infection but you can do the cooling breath and humming bee breath.

Breathing through the left nostril:
- Feminine receptive energy or creativity
- Cleansing, eliminating and digesting
- Improving sleep, tranquility & sensitivity
- Reduces anxiety and calms you down
- Curbs appetite

Breathing through the right nostril:
- Masculine active energy or taking action
- Revitalizing and energetic
- Focuses attention
- Encourages logical thinking
- Will power (or won't power)

When you are nervous or depressed or even trying to fall asleep use this simple alternate nostril breathing technique. It provides a direct connection for balancing the sympathetic (fight-or-flight) and parasympathetic (rest-and-relax) branches of the central nervous system that can reduce blood pressure, improve immunity, increase respiratory function and enhance attention. It's a simple technique to reduce mind chatter prior to an exam, first date, board meeting or anytime you want mental clarity.

Alternate Nostril Breathing Technique ~ *Nadi Shodhana*
This method involves alternating the breath through each nostril. Use your right hand with the right thumb on the right nostril and the right ring finger (next to the pinkie) on the left nostril. The breath is always relaxed, smooth and steady.
1. Touch the third eye at the point between the eyebrows with the index finger and middle finger. Gently gaze, with the lids closed, at the point between the eyebrows where you are touching.
2. Thumb to right nostril, breath **in** through the **left** nostril for about 4 seconds
3. Ring finger on left nostril, breath **out** through the **right** nostril for about 4 seconds
4. Ring finger on left nostril still, breath **in** through **right** nostril for 4 seconds
5. Thumb returns to right nostril, breath **out** through **left** nostril for 4 seconds
   Simply Stated: In left, out right, in right, out left for 3-30 minutes.

During this practice, you force the shifting back and forth between the yin and the yang, the internal and external, the female and the male, the creative and analytic aspects of the mind-body connection. This creates more connections through the corpus callosum (midline in the brain connecting the right and left hemispheres). After only 2-3 minutes typically you will notice a slight feeling of euphoria (slight feeling, nothing like a martini). You can miss it if you're not expecting it. You can calm down, get centered and create a new outlook in just a few minutes through alternate nostril breathing.

One day I was on my way out the door when I noticed I didn't have my cell phone. I rushed through the house spinning papers, clothes and dishes to find the device. I didn't want to be late for my appointment, and I needed my phone. I ran up and down the stairs as fast as I could. Then, thinking about this tip that I usually only do during my yoga practice, I decided to put it into action. I noticed my breathing was short and choppy and the anxiety building. I began doing this simple alternate nostril breathing technique while rushing through the house. It slowed down my mental activity but not my bodily movements. I still moved rapidly around the house, but the anxiety disappeared. I found my device, hit the road and arrived on time. Incorporating these techniques into your every day life can transform your outlook quickly. While rushing through the house doing this technique, I just used my thumb and first finger (the pinchers), and I typically use the pincher method when trying to return to sleep in the middle of the night. However, at the beginning of your regular seated meditation, I recommend using the classical method with the thumb and ring finger of the right hand (as directed above).

Alternate Nostril Breathing Technique ~ Expanded Version
This slow forced and retained breath helps reduce symptoms of panic attacks or similar stressful situations. Preferred practice in seated position; however, the benefits are the same whether sitting, walking or lying down. You can calm down quickly using this method.
1. Touch the Third Eye at the point between the eyebrows with the index finger and middle finger. Gently gaze, with the lids closed, at the point between the eyebrows where you are touching.
2. Thumb to right nostril, breath **in** through **left** nostril for 4 seconds,
3. Keep both nostrils closed for 4 seconds (softly pinch your nose closed)
4. Finger on left nostril, breath **out** through the **right** nostril for 4 seconds
5. Retain the breath out for 4 seconds, (softly pinch nose closed)
6. Breath **in** through **right** nostril for 4 seconds
7. Keep both nostrils closed for 4 seconds (softly pinch your nose closed)
8. Breath **out** through **left** nostril for only 4 seconds
   One Round Simply ~
   In left for 4, retain for 4,
   out right for 4, retain out for 4,
   in right for 4, retain for 4,
   out left for 4.

Cooling Breath ~ *Sheetali/Sitkari Pranayama*
Have you ever gotten so mad you almost couldn't breathe, fussing and fretting and ready to blow a gasket? Try this method next time you get upset (big or small). *Sheetali* means cooling, which explains the effect it can have on your mind and body. When you're aggravated or irritated, you're hot and ruffled under the collar. This simple technique can shift your outlook quickly. It's simple and you can do it just about anywhere. Curl your tongue like a straw and inhale. If you are unable to

curl your tongue, practice a variation known as *sitkari*. Relax your lips and jaw and inhale through the teeth, with the tongue softly touching the gum line just behind the front teeth. You'll feel the breath flowing around the tongue. Notice the breath instantly cools the mouth and ultimately the rest of your body. It's especially helpful while in hot climates, while driving in rush-hour traffic or if you're having a hot flash, Ladies.

Humming Bee Sound ~ *Bhramari*
During the *bhramari* breathing technique create a buzzing sound like a honeybee to obscure the continuous scatter chatter that energizes emotional suffering. It's a powerful centering tool, especially for those busy bees that just don't have time to meditate. You can do it right now while reading this text. On your next exhale start making a honeybee sound. Do that for six breaths. The sound waves gently vibrate your tongue, teeth, and sinuses and even your entire brain. Now, try it again but silently. Imagine making the sound for six more breaths. Continue noticing your internal experience. Can you sense the vibration in your face and sinuses? Return to your normal breathing pattern. The silent buzz is great for when you just don't want to be obvious about how stressed you really are.

Humming, silently or verbally, "Om" or "Ah" (like in God) diverts the attention away from random unbridled thoughts to focused intention. The sound "ah" is found in many religious or inspirational words like Buddha, Jehovah, Mohammad, Kabala, Krshna, Amen. Sound frequency connects you with your divine nature.

Breathing is one of the most natural things we do. It is a potent gift and awareness of it creates more grace and poise. Focusing on the breath allows you to break from common stress, physical exhaustion and toxic emotions that promote human suffering. When you return to a neutral state you reboot, feel invigorated and boost your enthusiasm. These are just a few wonderful reasons to initiate a pranayama practice into your daily activities.

Benefits of Meditation
• Reduces irritating thoughts that lead to arguments
• Rebalances the brain from flight or fight to acceptance
• Produces feelings of confidence and inner peace
• Automatic reduction in stress levels
• Generates greater efficiency
• Improves concentration and focus
• Improves digestion
• Boosts immune system
• Gives a natural facelift
• Harmonizes relationships
• Increases contentment

MEDITATION FRUSTRATION

You're noticing that you want to be quiet but the brain is not behaving. Discipline your brain like you discipline your body. Meditation frustration is an indication that you're ready for change. Resistance to a new behavior is common in the beginning.

1. **Can't Shut Up?** Instead of pushing away the thoughts or suppressing them, examine what you're actually saying to yourself. Sit like a cat at a mousehole and ask, "I wonder what my next thought will be." Then watch each thought that passes through your mind on the stream of consciousness. Frequently, the mind doesn't want to "get caught" and, ironically, more space between the thoughts, or silence, occurs.

2. **Looking for Quiet?** The world will never be quiet for you to meditate, but you can choose to be peaceful at any time. Get some earbuds or noise reduction earmuffs. Learn to see certain noises, like the neighbors mowing their lawn, as an advantage for you. Think instead, "property values are going up since the neighbors take care of their land." Recognize and label whatever the noise is and then return to your breath. Name it, "AC turning on and off," and return your awareness to your breath; "a car door shutting," and return to your breath; "dog barking," and return to your breath.

3. **Keep Falling Asleep?** Clearly, you're tired. Napping is good for you, but that's not meditating. If you fall asleep, upon awakening sit and breathe consciously for another 5-minutes. You want to create a neurological network for inner peace. Sleeping is autopilot.

4. **Bodily Discomfort?** Initially, make sure your location is comfortable and safe, and that you're clothes are loose. Meditation is a great tool for overcoming distress, aches or pains. Go deeply into the pain don't avoid it. Narrow down the discomfort to the size of a quarter or dime. For instance, if you have a headache, it's not your whole head. Identify the precise location, possibly behind the left temple. Ask pertinent questions about the body or mind tension. What message is the body conveying to you through the ache? How can you better manage the strain? Also, be sure not to eat prior to meditation, as the digestion process can be distracting. Equally important, don't go hungry.

5. **Haven't Experienced Enlightenment Yet?** Me either. Keep trying. Lower your expectations to the mastery of the technique before expecting to attain the ultimate achievement.

 ZENERGY BOOST FOR MEDITATION
Set your alarm to ring with soft chimes in 5-10 minutes. Sit in a chair with eyes closed and let your mind wander where it will. In the beginning, discipline your body not to fidget and sit motionless until you hear the chimes.

RESOLVING SCATTER CHATTER

When I recommend meditation I often hear my client say, "I can't quiet down and relax. I'm too busy and agitated. It's loud inside my brain." In fact, many people will not meditate past the first few attempts because they have too much scatter chatter. The mind's relentless commentary on daily activities generates tension, fatigue and overwhelming feelings. All meditation beginners start there. Me too.

April 1, 2000, I attended a 10-day silent retreat (*Vippassana*) at Suan Mokh Monastery in the jungles of Thailand. We spent 45-minutes in seated meditation and 45-minutes in walking meditation all day for 10-days. We practiced yoga at sunrise, completed basic community chores and received two vegetarian meals before noon. No eating after lunch. I slept under a mosquito net on a cement bed with a woodblock pillow. While meditating in the shala (outside assembly hall) I noticed how loud it was inside me and at times I was certain I was quietly muttering. Sheepishly, I opened my right eye to see if anyone could hear me. I quickly peered around the room to see everyone silently meditating and was relieved to know they were not listening. I returned to my feeble attempt at silence. I'm pretty sure when I closed my right eye someone opened their left eye to see if I could hear them. It was agonizing to try to be silent, when in fact I was not at all. There were approximately 150 people attending the retreat and only half of them finished.

Scatter chatter keeps you stuck in the past or lost in worry about the future. The perpetual swirl of repetitive thoughts (looped thinking) occupies the mind and distracts from the precious present moment. Worrisome thoughts about health, finances, career, parenting and personal interactions are common. When you decide to be quiet is when you will notice just how loud you are, but what are you really thinking anyway? Is there a valuable message or is it jibber-jabber? Observe your stream of consciousness to gain clarity into how turbulent the waters of your mind actually are. Your brain is never going to "turn off" until the successful completion of your life (death), but you can postpone entertaining the thoughts. Thoughts can be distracting and the moments of silence so small that you rarely notice them; however, there is a small pause between each word and between each breath. Tell the brain that you will think those thoughts at the end of the meditation. I assure you they will wait.

The mind will think like the heart will beat.

Some of my clients are runners and they frequently say with relief, "My brain turns off while I'm running. My body catches up to my mind when my feet hit the pavement." Eventually the body is going to collapse if you force it to keep up with a frantic mind. I'm not just talking about runners either. Those who chose a demanding schedule, working 12 hours daily, could easily buckle from mental anguish.

The Heart-Math Institute (HMI) completed extensive research over the last 40 years investigating the correlation between the brain and heart. An electroencephalogram (EEG) measures the electrical activity of brain wave patterns. Small metal discs with electrodes placed on the scalp send signals to a computer to record the results. The brain moves into EEG coherence during the meditation process. Meaning, the left and right hemispheres profoundly connect, the frontal lobe and occipital lobes correlate, and the temporal and parietal lobes all fire together, causing unity throughout the entire brain. HMI found that just by thinking of someone you love, a treasured pet or favorite hobby, you uplift your spirit and improve overall physiological health. Studies prove that the brain is receiving just as much, if not more, information from the heart as vice versa, and emotional stress, such as anger, frustration, and anxiety, gives rise to irregular and erratic brainwave and heart wave patterns.

"Positive emotions send a very different signal throughout our body. When we experience uplifting emotions such as appreciation, joy, care, and love, our heart rhythm pattern becomes highly ordered, looking like a smooth, harmonious wave. This is called a coherent heart rhythm pattern. When we are generating a coherent heart rhythm, the activity in the two branches of the autonomic nervous system is synchronized, and the body's systems operate with increased efficiency and harmony. It's no wonder that positive emotions feel so good. They actually help the body synchronize and work better" (*HeartMath.com*).

Research shows that meditation increases emotional stability, mental clarity and physiological balance. We perform more efficiently in the moment and later in the day just by relaxing and thinking good thoughts. Initially, if your mind is too busy to focus on the meditation method then consciously think about someone you love, your treasured pet or favorite hobby. This may be the needed pathway for beginning meditators to release the relentless commentary of scatter chatter.

 ZENERGY BOOST FOR BALANCING HEAD AND HEART
Set your alarm clock to bring you back with soft chimes in 5-minutes. Close your eyes, feel the body breathing and think about someone you love for a few minutes.

CHARTING YOUR FUTURE

MAGNETIZE YOUR HEARTSONG

What will it take for you to get impassioned about your life? Do you know what makes your heart sing? Do you know how to attract it? Is something missing, but you don't know what? Even if you have fabulous things like health, wealth, family and belonging, career and contribution, you may still feel unfulfilled. Don't be so arrogant to assume you don't need to do this exercise. If you're not singing upon awakening each morning then you don't really know what you want. Designing your life and getting the most out of it is a skill that you can learn. You may not know your ultimate life purpose beyond your main responsibilities, but if you're looking for more meaning in life, below are a few steps to harmonize with your heartsong.

Write down the skills, education and jobs you've held in the past (include the short, temporary and volunteer assignments). Use only one sentence each and go fast; it's not a resume. For this exercise it's better to write down what comes to your mind first and not analyze too much. Continue your compilation with your favorite hobbies and interests (even if you've never put any physical time into the idea). If you've been thinking about it for more than a year, include that on your list.

Create a list of professional contacts, friends or neighbors with whom you've worked or those who could confirm your abilities. Add to the list the top ten people you admire (there may be some overlap from the previous list or you could include celebrities). Add three words that describe each person. Prioritize from the one you admire the most to the least (even though you admire them all). Here's a few words to get you started: honest, kind, respectful, driven, creative, carefree, rich, alluring, trusting, pensive, eloquent, elegant, fashionista.

Dedicate 20 minutes a day for one or two weeks on this research. It doesn't have to be all at one sitting. Spending five minutes four times daily works just as well. Review the list periodically and add a word or a phrase. Remember, you are looking for clues to your life passion and what makes you sing with joy. After a week or two, analyze your list. It might appear that there is one major thing or a complete hodge-podge of activities. Both are great. Notice what you enjoy the most and whom you admire most. Look for repetitions on the list. What person or qualities attract you? Qualify your list from the most important behavior traits to the least important. Do you express those qualities? Rank yourself on a scale from 1-10. Add to the list of qualities the ones you express the most and those qualities that you express the least. Notice what is natural for you already. You most likely have many positive qualities in your favorite areas, and this exercise will help you identify what is already working in your favor.

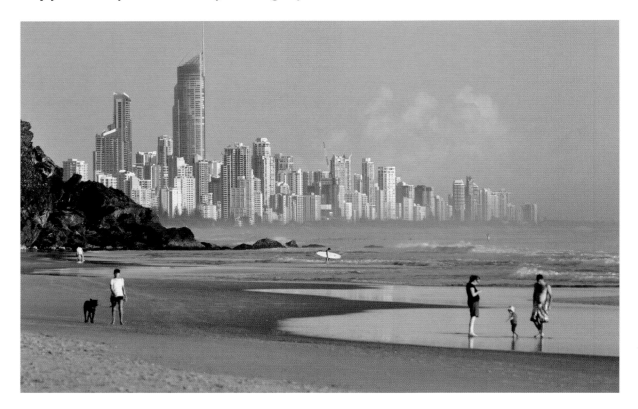

What do you really want? Is it a different job or a better paying job doing the same thing? Is it a new partner, vehicle or home? Don't concern yourself with how you will acquire it. Just ask the basic questions to determine what you really, really, really want in life. (It's the answer to the third "really" that we're looking for.) This can be a difficult exercise for some, because many people don't know what they want. Once you know what you don't want then you can deduce what you do want. If you know you don't want to sit behind a desk most of the day, then you can add "kinetic, moving, athletic, variety or traveling [representative or salesperson]" to your list. Some people want to live in an exotic environment, but don't know how to handle all the details with relocating. In this exercise, I invite you to think about what you want and not how to obtain it. That's jumping the gun. Think about your favorite things to do and your fantasy location to do them. Where would you choose if you could live anywhere?

Let's say you love the water. Ask the following questions~beach, lake, river, pond, fish tank? Get specific with your ideal environment. If you want to be near the water yet you live in the desert then consider a fish tank. Daily viewing of a fish tank or even posters or paintings of the ocean can be very nourishing. If you have good social skills or a knack for computers, then you might find many opportunities at marinas or hotels around the world. You could find a quality hotel chain that can provide stability with plenty of locations to explore. Generally speaking, they're usually located in touristy areas near the water. Knowing that your heart sings while building sand castles isn't going to produce additional income, but identifying your connection to the beach can transform your outlook. You will feel harmonious and joyous once you're in that environment or viewing pictures of that environment. Identify your favorite activities and your dream location. If the mountains inspire you, and you have a business skill set in marketing, then consider working at ski resorts. Once you're in your ideal location where you can practice your favorite activities, melodious inner contentment is soon to follow. Focus not necessarily on the best but the next avenue to express your interests, skills and abilities. They may not have the exact job for you but, once your foot is in the door, you have a chance to prove yourself. Don't be complacent, pick up the tempo, and call that resort today.

Finding your life purpose doesn't mean you need to relocate, but you can contemplate it. You may not want or need to move, but an annual vacation to that type of location could harmonize the rest of the year. Just imagining a new environment can help you access more opportunities that are already within reach.

Imagination is more important than knowledge. Knowledge is limited.
Imagination encircles the world.
Albert Einstein

How do you identify success? Many people link money with success. "The person with the most toys wins!" Wins what? What is your favorite toy? When you have that toy will you really "win?" What does "winning" mean to you? Gain clarity on what you're really thinking. If you want a lot of money, then purchasing a lot of toys is not winning, that's spending. Our current method of trade is to exchange a skill and time for currency; however, for thousands of years we exchanged services, skills, food, beads, land, gold and greenbacks. Today we commonly exchange "currency" through debit charges. Basically money is now just a digital number on your computer while banking online or using a credit card. If you add another zero to your bank balance will you then feel successful? Is it all about another zero? The external criterion for exchange of services keeps morphing. If success is just plain greenbacks then there will never be enough. Craving more and more money, however you identify, will never satisfy. Discover what financial security means to you and how it feels.

Magnetizing your heartsong is part physical (identifying your goal and moving toward it) and part emotional. If you don't feel that you deserve what you want then you cannot attract it. Under-thoughts and scatter chatter steal successful feelings away through self-sabotaging behavior. You must feel worthy and deserving of your heartsong to draw it to you. Contemplate manifesting your goal. When you close your eyes and state silently what you really, really, really want, then you can notice the feelings you have around that goal. For instance, if you want a million dollars but secretly you think money makes people greedy or spiritual people shouldn't need money, then you're going to resist what you desire. Many times we don't even know we're resisting something we're requesting. You don't need your eyes to hack into this other realm. Sit down, close your eyes and state silently what you truly want and notice your feelings and inner dialogue surfacing. Maybe you're saying you want a significant relationship when really you want a baby. Possibly you're thinking you want a better job but really you like your job you just want more money. When you close your eyes and notice your feelings deep inside you will acquire clues as to what is resonating within. We are constantly surrounded by the iCloud, WiFi, Bluetooth, radio waves, cable, etc. Your thoughts, emotions and feelings also encircle you like a personal iCloud. Tap into it. Imagine receiving that new job, home or marital proposal. Do you feel expansion, shrinking or shrieking? It is during the silence that you access your feelings more and then you'll know what you believe you deserve. If you don't currently possess it, then you know you're blocking it in some way. Silent contemplation is a way to hack into the makings of your own mind. Notice your current vibration (calm, uncertain, scared) and tune your antenna to the right frequency to attract what you truly want.

You may be successful at earning income, but can you save some too? Squandering your salary on things you don't need due to enticing advertisements can lead to major dissatisfaction in life. Consuming dissipates your wealth. Consume, consume, consume… unnecessary trinkets, festive decorations, cars, boats, electronics, clothes, eating in restaurants…. all lead to a loss of not just money but also valuable life force. Enslavement to your credit card company paying for things long after the thrill is gone can be exhausting and overwhelming. It depletes your vitality. We need money. Money is energy. Money gives choices. Are you wasting your energy at a job where you feel like a slave, in a city you dislike and therefore purchasing things you don't need to regain some sort of fulfillment? One good question to ask is, "Will this be in the landfill next year?" If yes, then don't buy it. Success, wealth and abundance don't necessarily revolve around a bank account. You can be a successful team player, have a wealth of friendship and an abundance of good health.

Identify what you want to feel and experience versus just buying something to sit on the shelf. Learning to resist purchasing things you don't need is a valuable skill to possess.

What would you do with your money if you were financially independent? Many people want to be rich so they can travel and yet they never leave their own hometown to visit a nearby city. If you want to travel more, there are many economical ways to experience the zest of an adventure in a new city without it costing a small fortune. Consider an outing to the nearest suburb or a daytrip to a nearby town. Even pretending to be a tourist in your own town can be an economical and exciting occasion. Visit your local park, museum or library. These activities are usually free and many times provide enjoyable entertainment. Trying new things can spark your motivation and evoke a new line of thinking. Observing what you currently have while also imagining what is possible can induce a new level of appreciation. If you stay on autopilot you will surely continue getting what you've always gotten. Do the same things, get the same things. Exploring new locations, cultures and events opens your mind to original ideas of making your heart sing.

Consider your best pace and time of the day to contribute your talents. Many people can't stand the grind of corporate combat in a large city with hectic traffic. They just don't have the interest in offering their time and energy to that type of discord day after day. Others find the corporate world and big city living provide an ideal place to cultivate teamwork and challenge the mind in rhythmical ways. They feel the synchronicity with the diversity of people and cultures, kinetic energy, variety of aromas and a symphony of sounds. Studies show that more patents are developed in large cities. Maybe you could design the next revolutionary patent, like the weather machine (US Patent 20030085296), cloaking device (US Patent US20150365642A1) or the black hole contraption (US Patent 20060073976A1). Thinking audaciously moves you beyond your own mental programming and into a dynamic way of experiencing life whether in a fast-paced city or in the relaxed country environment. (See the glossary to learn more about these patents.)

Maybe your heartsong is a melodic steady waltz. You may be more interested in a slow and easy pace at this stage in your life. Or, you might be interested in performing on the stage. Many entertainers, their managers and their critics work nights. That's a whole different opus. Knowing your energy level (slow, medium or allegro) and when it is vibrant (morning, noon or night) can help you choose an appropriate career and suitable hobby.

Once you accept what you truly love doing, reach out to others who share your passion. Find like-minded people or groups who share your interests. Create community and build rapport with your social base online and in your neighborhood. Offer your skill, trade, barter or sell your services to the quality people in your network and on your lists. Facebook, Linked In, Instagram,

Pinterest, Meet Up, Next Door and numerous other online resources can connect you to a nearby group immediately. Hosting a neighborhood wine tasting party or volunteering at the dog park is a great way to network and build organizational skills. Locating lead positions outside your full-time job cultivates new strategies for embracing your heartsong.

If you applied for a management role but were denied, consider finding a mentor in your chosen field. Tap into the resources that are at your fingertips. A leadership role at your church, homeowners association or professional organization builds communication skills and can increase business prospects. Developing competency and efficiency prepares you for promotions in upcoming years. Additionally, look the part you want to play. Be congruent in your appearance. Your attire is seen well before you speak. For instance, bankers wear suits, chefs wear black-and-white houndstooth patterned pants, and plumbers wear jeans. Don't apply for a banking position in blue jeans. If you are a laborer choose clean dark blue jeans. Even pressed jeans and clean shoes indicate you've put some effort into your appearance. You would be surprised how a smart outfit and a full face of makeup impart a good first impression. This, in turn, can attract new people and new opportunities preparing you for your next promotion.

When you magnetize a metal material you rub the object with the magnet in the same direction, not opposite directions. Stroking in the same direction, or moving in the same direction, keeps your eye on the prize. Magnetize your heartsong by staying the course regardless of uncertainty or criticisms. Don't stop midpoint and focus in a different direction because you lack confidence or conviction. That's self-sabotage. Focus on what you want even when you feel tentative, fearful or vulnerable. You become stronger or more magnetic when you are clear about what you want. Once you know, then find one, two or ten like-minded people with whom you can share your talent and strategize for achievement. Zest and vigor weaken when sitting on the sidelines or hiding on the fringe. Brainstorming and collaborating with a small group can strengthen your conviction and enthusiasm; however, if you shared a secret goal with someone who doesn't understand, (s)he may say the wrong thing and that interpretation can throw you off course. Privately you can still walk toward your goal in silence even if you don't have the confidence for fulfillment. Being vulnerable is actually an act of courage, and sometimes friends just don't know what to say. Don't take your eye off the prize of achievement because of something one person said. Find others who affirm your goals with you and don't share (again) with someone who is not on the team with you. The act of being vulnerable and sharing your goal shows confidence even if you don't feel it deep down. Momentum is soon to follow as you keep your eye on the prize!

Imagine what your ideal day looks like. Where will you work and in what city? What does your house look like? Who are the key players dancing through life with you? Just reading these words is not enough, you must intimately ask yourself these questions and review your answers several times. You have something wonderful to contribute to this fantastic existence and there will be a harmonious exchange with others in your ideal life.

Being healthy, wealthy and wise is the key. Many millionaires would give their money if you could restore their health or sense of belonging. Frequently, it's the chase for money that takes its toll on our heart and soul, and that lifestyle can steal health, quality family time and inner peace. There is nothing holy about sitting on a mound of gold alone and lonely, just like there is nothing holy in poverty. Continue seeking your inner calling. Remember, the average human lives less than 80 years, but tomorrow could be your last day. Magnetize your heartsong now!

 ZENERGY BOOST TO MAGNETIZE YOUR HEARTSONG
Sit down in a quiet environment and envision a mystical key opening the door to your vibrant, joyful and passionate life. Feel the key in your hand. See the door before you. Notice any outside markings on the door. Is there a shingle or sign indicating what type of business it is? Do you hear any sounds or voices from the other side of the door? What do you hear? As you turn the key you feel the anticipation of something wonderful about to happen. You know that the experience on the other side of the door is just perfect for you. Allow all your senses to come alive toward your new life and fantasize fully now. Unlock the door and walk over the threshold. Use your unlimited imagination now! Feel successful now as if you are already living in that new life. Allow that vision to come alive and know the excitement of your dreams coming true. Offer gratitude for what you're seeing and sensing. Discovering what you love creates a deep meaningful life with lasting happiness. What's on the other side of the door? Close your eyes now; See it, Feel it, Hear it, Know It Now!

MAGNETIZING YOUR HEARTSONG WORKSHEET

This form is for your eyes only. Invest about 20 minutes a day for one to two weeks completing the steps. You could take 5 minute increments, but dedicate about 20 minutes each day contemplating your passion(s). Return to the list periodically to add a word or a phrase. You may need additional paper to complete this exercise. Keep these worksheets private at least until you completely finish.

STEP 1
List all your skills, like waiting tables, plumbing or typing. Include a list of all software programs you know.

_____
_____
_____
_____
_____
_____
_____
_____
_____
_____
_____
_____
_____

STEP 2
List the jobs you've held in the past (include short, temporary and volunteer assignments). Keep it brief; this is not a resume.

_____
_____
_____
_____
_____
_____
_____
_____
_____
_____
_____
_____

STEP 3

List your education. Include any personal development classes, continuing education courses or weekend marital retreats (as these teach you how to relate and communicate with the opposite sex).

_____
_____
_____
_____
_____
_____
_____
_____
_____
_____
_____
_____
_____
_____
_____

STEP 4

What do you like to do in your spare time? List your favorite activities, hobbies and interests, even if you've never put any physical time in the idea. If you've been thinking about it for more than one-year, include that on this list.

_____
_____
_____
_____
_____
_____
_____
_____
_____
_____
_____
_____
_____

STEP 5

Make a list of your top 10 locations/environments to live. Your answer could be the beach or Fort Lauderdale, mountains or Montana. The more specific you are the better but don't get lost in the details. Get some ideas on paper first.

_____
_____
_____
_____
_____
_____
_____
_____
_____
_____
_____
_____
_____
_____
_____
_____
_____

STEP 6

What's your pace?   _____

Slow and easy, little traffic, country living   _____

Moderate with relaxing weekends   _____

Big city, fast living, comfortable with traffic   _____

Other   _____

STEP 7

What's your favorite time of day?   _____

Morning   _____

Afternoon   _____

Evenings   _____

Wee Hours   _____

STEP 8

On vacation, do you spend your time inside or outside? Do you prefer museums or hiking?

_____

_____

_____

_____

_____

_____

_____

_____

_____

_____

_____

_____

_____

_____

STEP 9

What talent do you not have, that you admire in others? Could you take a small step in finding that within yourself? If you like to paint, purchase a canvas and make the first brush stroke. Surprisingly, a second and third are sure to follow.

_____

_____

_____

_____

_____

_____

_____

_____

_____

_____

_____

_____

STEP 10

Create a list of professional and personal contacts and 1-3 words of their admirable traits.

Name	Contact Information	Admirable Traits
Ex: Former Supervisor	JaneSample@gmail.com	helpful, kind, motivator
Next Door Neighbor	Neighbor@gmail.com	friendly, gardener, trendy

_____   _____   _____

_____   _____   _____

_____   _____   _____

_____   _____   _____

_____   _____   _____

_____   _____   _____

_____   _____   _____

_____   _____   _____

_____   _____   _____

Here's a few words to get you started...

Kind	Driven	Spiritual	Reliable
Respectful	Out-spoken	Optimistic	Elegant
Generous	Free-spirited	Playful	Pensive
Financially-Secure	Frugal	Wise	Alluring
Artistic	Jovial	Dependable	Dedicated
Loving	Compassionate	Genuine	Relaxed
Committed	Worldly	Trusting	Rich
Honest	Responsible	Joyful	Wistful
Transparent	Healer	Sexy	Wise

Spend about 20-minutes a day for one or two weeks on this research. It doesn't have to be all at once. Take 1-5 minute increments to complete this assignment.

STEP 11

Create a list of the Top Ten people you admire.

There may be some overlap from the previous step or they could be celebrities or professors. Add 1-3 words that describe each person on both lists. Even though you admire them all, rank them from 1-10 (#10 being the most admired). See list of qualities previously presented to get started.

Rank	Name	Admirable Traits
Ex: 10	Barbra Streisand	singer, creative, driven, audacious
9	Dr. Wayne Dyer	orator, motivational, innovative author
8	Jillian Michaels	fitness expert, focused, service-oriented

STEP 12

After reviewing and answering the above questions for at least one to two weeks move forward to unlocking your passion with the remaining questions.

Now, narrow down the qualities that are most important to you from Step 11. What qualities do you naturally express? Include other qualities not listed above. Of course, this changes over time but we're looking at what you're doing today. Rank your choice from most admired quality to least, even though you appreciate all the attributes. Do you have these character traits? Rank yourself on a scale of 1-10 (#10 being the highest) as to your ability and frequency in articulating that quality.

Rank Quality	Name the Quality	Self-Ranking
Ex: 1	creative	4
2	social	7
_____	_____	_____
_____	_____	_____
_____	_____	_____
_____	_____	_____
_____	_____	_____
_____	_____	_____
_____	_____	_____
_____	_____	_____
_____	_____	_____
_____	_____	_____
_____	_____	_____
_____	_____	_____
_____	_____	_____
_____	_____	_____
_____	_____	_____
_____	_____	_____
_____	_____	_____

STEP 13

What is your favorite activity and why?

_____
_____
_____
_____
_____
_____
_____
_____
_____
_____
_____
_____

STEP 14

What is your favorite season? Where is your favorite location? It could be spring in the mountains or a specific city and state.

SEASON _____

LOCATION _____

STEP 15

What was the last city you visited? Where is your favorite location to visit? Have you visited a nearby city recently? When can you do that?

_____
_____
_____
_____
_____
_____
_____
_____
_____

STEP 16

With whom and what skills can you barter?

Find like-minded people or groups who share your interests on Instagram, Facebook, Linked In, Pinterest, Meet Up, Next Door and numerous other online communities. Get connected to a nearby group immediately.

Who will Trade Ex: Neighbor	What Skills Roof repair for car repair	Location/Connection Next Door Online
_____	_____	_____
_____	_____	_____
_____	_____	_____
_____	_____	_____
_____	_____	_____
_____	_____	_____
_____	_____	_____
_____	_____	_____
_____	_____	_____
_____	_____	_____

STEP 17

What do you really, really, really want in life? (It's the answer to the third "really" that we're looking for.) Is it a different job or a better-paying job, a new partner, vehicle or home? What makes your heart sing?

_____

_____

_____

_____

_____

_____

_____

_____

_____

_____

_____

STEP 18

Tomorrow, if you won the lottery or received an unexpected inheritance, what would you do? What would your life look like next year? Even if you said, "quit my job," you still need to fill up 24 hours each day. What else would you do with your time if you didn't have to work at the same old job? Identify what your ideal day looks like. Where will you spend your time and in what city? What does your house look like? Who are the key players enjoying life with you? Review your lists from above knowing you have something wonderful to contribute to this fantastic existence.

_____

_____

_____

_____

_____

_____

_____

_____

STEP 19

Look at the patterns in your life for the past 5, 10, 15 years. What is a recurring theme? For instance, you may be an accountant, but everyone stops by your office for counseling. Counselor might be another career option for you. Review the major occurrences in your life and note what events or activities periodically return.

_____

_____

_____

_____

_____

_____

_____

_____

_____

All these questions lead you to know yourself better and get on track for your Divine Life Purpose. We each have a specific purpose in life and when you're moving toward your purpose you will feel joy and enthusiasm everyday. Ask these questions throughout the days and weeks to come. Find out what really makes your heart sing. Return to this process several times until you find what you love to do. Feel your success now as if you've already achieved it. Allow that vision to come alive and know the excitement of your dreams coming true. Offer gratitude for what you're seeing and sensing. See it, Feel it, Hear it, Know It Now!

TAKING ACTION

You've found your passion. You know what you want to do with the rest of your life (or at least the next direction), but how do you get inspired to make the necessary changes? Many people slink down into a rut because they don't know how to change and already feel overwhelmed. It's a challenge to uproot inertia. Thoughts of changing a job or relocating to another city can appear daunting initially. Starting a new company or having a baby will completely change your life forever. So, before you head to the nearest U-Haul outlet, apply some of these techniques while you're still in your comfort zone. Taking action can look and feel awkward in the beginning. Start with easy things that you can't really mess up or at least the things you can correct without spending a fortune.

There is an order to everyone's morning ritual (e.g. shower, coffee, makeup, breakfast, drive to work). Tomorrow, notice the sequence of events in your morning ritual. Start switching it up. If you awake and have coffee first, tomorrow shower first. When applying makeup or shaving, start on the other side of your face first. If you normally feed yourself last after everyone else in the family, then eat first for a change. Shifting a ritual can be liberating and a bit comical. Drive a different route. For each activity, take a different street than your usual path. There are countless ways to get from point A to B. You might find a secondary artery in the city is less congested than the highway, and arrive at work in the same amount of time with less stress. Driving the opposite way on a familiar road presents a different experience too. That counts!

Consider altering your appearance. Thinking that you have to look a certain way, like the way you looked for the last decade, may be the only thing that needs enhancing. When you style your hair differently, even parting your hair on the other side, a few people will notice. When you change the color, everyone will notice (most importantly you). I'm not just talking to the ladies either, Guys. You, too, are due for an appearance and fashion intervention. Revamping your hairstyle or clothes can have an immediate impact on how you are perceived in your community and that influences how you feel in your own skin. Everyone notices your eyes and then your smile. Whitening your teeth or getting dental work can update your appearance for an emerging new you. Remember, you can always return to the old you if you don't like the new look. The point of these small gestures is for you to get out of your comfort zone before doing something really serious.

Pare down. Look at each item in your home and start selling things that aren't important to you. Each picture on the wall, each piece of furniture, old electronics, clothing, shoes, unnecessary kitchen gadgets, and clutter in your garage is worth something to someone. It might just be a few bucks but downsizing can be very liberating. Save the money in a special account (or piggy bank) so that you can monetarily identify how much you gained by what you lost. You might find there is a bigger gift than money behind this exercise.

Rearrange your furniture, move the artwork or reposition a lamp. Change it up so that when you walk into your home, it feels and looks differently. The living room will have the most impact but you may need to alter a less important room first. Notice how you feel with the new layout for at least one month. Give it time to wear on you or you'll miss the point. The point being– you're looking for inspiration, action and invention in your life. These are the easy ways to build confidence for change and inspiration to take risky action in the future. If you are uncomfortable with some of these suggestions, then other changes, like relocating to a new city, finding a new job, or getting married, might stay out of reach for a long time. Remember, change is not for everyone. You might just need to settle into what you've already got and hang on until the end arrives. The End? Yes, just wait for the end of your life until you start something new. How ridiculous you might think. I concur. Don't wait until you're nearly dead to try something new.

Finding your heartsong is rewarding. If you love your job, you'll never work another day in your life. When you're impassioned by a goal, you keep moving upward and onward. You don't hear objection or rejection; you automatically notice a different door of opportunity. You continue climbing to greater heights frequently even requiring less sleep than usual. These periods in our life can carry us to unforeseen mountaintops.

When your compass needle alters direction due to catalysts like job changes, loss of a loved one, divorce, trauma, illness, floods, fires or forced relocations, don't continue driving forward while looking in your rearview mirror. Create a new GPS location with an accurate trajectory toward your next aspiration. Dream a New Dream!

When you are inspired by some great purpose,
Some extraordinary project,
All your thoughts break their bonds
Your mind transcends limitations,
Your consciousness expands in every direction,
And you find yourself in a new, great and wonderful world.
Dormant forces, faculties and talents become alive,
and you discover yourself to be a greater person by far
than you ever dreamed yourself to be.

Pantanjali, Author of the *Yoga Sutras*

WRAPPING UP THE MIND SECTION

When you take time to contemplate your life, manage stress, and develop a wellness program, your inner world becomes balanced. Acknowledging and accepting your emotional state, and being willing to transform unnecessary habits is a mature outlook to life. Setting appropriate boundaries and communicating consciously prepares you for quality long-term loving relationships. Learning how to ask for what you want and creating win/win situations lifts needless layers of stress off your mind and off your plate, giving you time for what you truly love. Avoid people and activities that drain your vital energy, and strengthen that place of peace and wisdom inside through simple meditation techniques. During meditation you can unlock your true calling, giving your life new meaning and restoring enthusiasm. Reflect on some of the questions on the Heartsong Worksheets to solidify your next successful steps. Your output depends on your outlook and spending quality time with yourself rebuilds happiness.

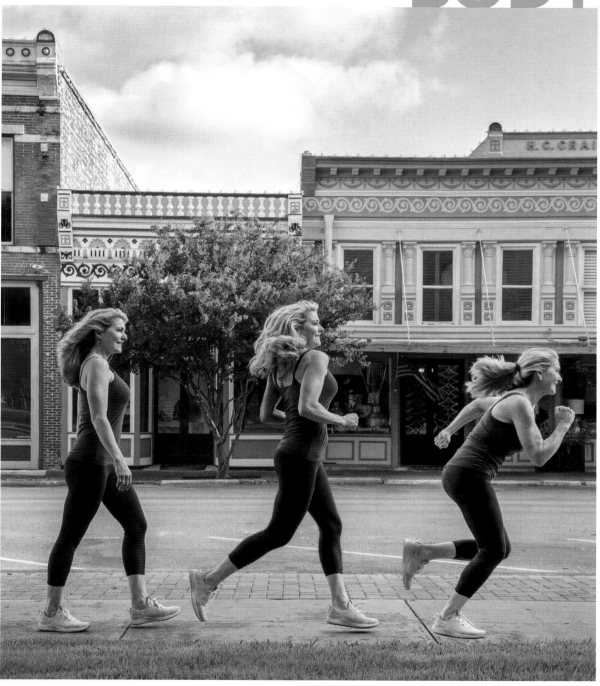

BODY

NUTRITIONALLY STARVED AND PHYSICALLY FAT

Most people will admit they aren't as healthy as they would like to be. Many say they could lose at least 10 pounds, maybe 30, yet they do absolutely nothing different to achieve that goal. Some eat and never give a second thought to what is happening to the food they just ingested, focusing on the taste buds and not on the nutritional needs of the body. Consuming poor quality food is directly linked to a higher risk of weight gain, obesity, Type 2 diabetes, emotional imbalances, depression, common colds, acid reflux, abdomen discomfort, digestive issues, hardening of the arteries, heart disease, stroke, cancer and even early death. Junk food is unusually high in added sugars, salt and saturated fats that can lead to addiction and even Type 2 Diabetes. Doing nothing about being overweight or obese can lead to many of the above-mentioned diseases plus kidney, liver and colon cancer not to mention sleep apnea, gout and bladder control problems. Illnesses and diseases compound by doing nothing. Dr. Mark Hyman, Director of Cleveland Clinic Center for Functional Medicine states, "What you eat is the single most important thing you do each day to effect the health of your body and mind. Eating the right food is the key to having more energy, a clear mind and maintaining healthy weight." The more processed foods you eat, the less likely you are to receive essential nutrients that your body relies on for vitality and vigor. So if you feel sluggish, lethargic or even emotionally charged, consider your intake. Your body needs high-energy, nutrient-rich foods to maintain good health. Your human body is like a cave. Yeast from breads can turn into Candida in the intestines, which is likened to mold. Parasites from cheap meat are the creepy crawlers found in digestive disorders. Creaky knees are the stalagmites. If you do nothing to your organic cave it's going to get messy in there.

When you value your body more than your automobile you will offer better care to it. Like a vehicle, the human body needs fueling, lubricating, cleaning and long-term maintenance. Do you ever sense that your "check engine" light is on in your body but you're just ignoring it? Simple signals like aches and pains, inflammation, migraines, foggy brain, insomnia, weight management issues, sugar cravings, emotional imbalances and acne, are all signals from your body asking you to pay attention to it. Imagine if you just went under the hood of your car, disconnected the "check engine" wire and continued driving. How far do you think you would get? What type of damage to your car would occur over the next few days, weeks and months?

You may not notice being a little sluggish or lethargic until it's too difficult to get out of bed. You might write-off having emotional outbursts or road rage as other's faults. Consistently poor nutritional choices, excessive use of tobacco, alcohol or coffee can drive you off the cliff. Are you at risk for a stroke? Do you have high blood pressure, diabetes, high cholesterol or poor cardiovascular conditioning? Possibly being a little curvy, soft or overweight doesn't bother you until you are pre-diabetic, pre-hypertensive or pre-high cholesterol. These are disturbing diagnoses but pre-anything just means "eat less junk." "Pre" doesn't mean ingest pharmaceuticals and stay the course; it means wake-up and be mindful of what you're eating and how much. Keep a food journal to remember your daily intake. Don't drive your vehicle into a cave. Bring it out and polish it. Make it shine!

For most people just consuming less would be a step in the right direction.

Think about your body being a chemistry vial. You choose foods your taste buds enjoy but after you swallow, what happens? The body has to sort through all the food particles that arrived and decide how to distribute those nutrients to nourish the tissues. The stomach produces HCl (hydrochloric acid) to digest food. Adding something like ice water or ice tea or ice sodas completely changes the contents of the vial. Warming the food for digestion is one of the jobs the stomach does so that nutrients transfer into the small intestines. If you saturate your stomach with water (and ice water or cold sodas are even worse), you slow the assimilation and absorption process. Once the food particles become molecules for distribution, the intestines decide which tissues shall receive the proper nutrients and, keeping it simple, the large intestines purge the waste. Healthy bodies naturally eliminate daily.

Disease isn't inevitable. Frequently, what you're eating is causing your disease. We did an experiment with "healthy" bread and confirmed that after two months no mold formed. There are many well-documented and circulated photos and videos online of years-old McDonald's hamburgers that never aged. You can do this experiment with almost any type of processed food. Some genetically modified brands of tomatoes, zucchini and other vegetables rarely mold. If you leave a bucket of margarine outside, no insects will touch it. Folks, that's not real food. Real bread, real vegetables and real food molds and rots. Food manufacturers are not required to indicate all the ingredients (i.e. "spices" and "natural flavoring") or when the product was made. They tell you when it expires but many foods today never perish regardless of the expiration date.

GENETICALLY MODIFIED ORGANISMS/FOODS (GMOs)

"GMOs are living organisms whose genetic material has been artificially manipulated in a laboratory through genetic engineering. This relatively new science from the 80s creates unstable combinations of plant, animal, bacteria and viral genes that do not occur in nature or through traditional crossbreeding methods," according to the Non-GMO Project (*NonGMOproject.org*). Genetic modification, biotechnology, biotech seeds, genetic engineering and GMO are all terms that indicate a change was made to the DNA of a product or organism. Soy is the most common GMO and you can find it in livestock, poultry and fish feed, pet food, vegetable oil, lecithin, soymilk, soy sauce and almost any product in a box or jar.

Unbeknownst to you, you might have gobbled a GMO ear of corn, tossed back a few GMO cherry tomatoes or lathered some GMO mayonnaise on GMO Wonder Bread (wonder what's in it). Possibly you've enjoyed a power bar, candy bar or protein shake once or twice. GMOs are common and the general populace is becoming more aware of the damage that genetically modified foods wreak upon our human DNA. We have more allergens, epidemic illnesses, autoimmune diseases, and more childhood obesity today than ever before. Children are especially susceptible. According to the Institute for Responsible Technology, "Several animal studies indicate serious health risks associated with genetically modified (GM) food, including infertility, immune problems, accelerated aging, faulty insulin regulation, and changes in major organs and the gastrointestinal system." The American Academy of Environmental Medicine (AAEM) called on "Physicians to educate their patients, the medical community, and the public to avoid GM foods when possible and provide educational materials concerning GM foods and health risks." According to the Environmental Working Group there are more than 85,000 man-made chemicals approved for use in the United States alone. No wonder you're fatigued. You are constantly being exposed to toxic chemicals through the air you breathe, the water you drink and the foods that you eat.

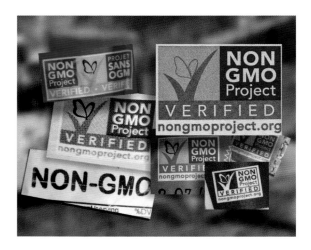

Many developed nations around the globe do not consider GMOs to be safe, and there are considerable restrictions or outright bans on their cultivation, import and sale. The   United States government approved GMOs based on studies conducted by the same corporations that created the GMO and profit from their sale. It is estimated that GMOs are in at least 75% of the processed food in America, like soybean, corn, sugar beets and canola. You may not be able to afford organic food, but know that most fast food is GMO. Unfortunately, even though polls consistently show that a significant majority of Americans and Westerners want to know if the food they're purchasing contains GMOs, the powerful biotech lobbyists succeeded in out-ranking the general consumer. Although new US legislation beginning in 2020 requires food manufacturers to identify the accurate contents of the product, there is some speculation about the verbiage on the labels. Instead of using the commonly recognized term "GMO" the labels will state "bioengineered" and, unfortunately, soy, sugar and sugar beets can be excluded.

Taking matters into their own hands, many are choosing to opt out of being the proverbial guinea pig for the GMO experiment by purchasing organic produce or growing their own. 70-80 years ago many families had their own vegetable garden. If you have a severe illness, rare or unusual disease, and/or desire to lose a significant amount of weight, I strongly encourage you to eat only whole foods, lots of vegetables (preferably organic) or packaged items that have less than 10 ingredients on the label. Consider it a vote with your pocketbook. Nowadays, that seems to be what's actually heard.

ZENERGY BOOST FOR GROWING A VEGETABLE GARDEN
Purchase a large bag of soil (about a yard), poke a few holes in it and add a few tomato or vegetable seeds. Watch them grow straight from the bag! You don't need a lot of space to have your own vegetable garden.

According to Neil Levin, "Biotechnology, by turning living crops into 'intellectual property,' increases corporate control over food resources and production. Rather than alleviate world hunger, biotechnology is likely to exacerbate it by increasing everybody's dependence on the corporate sector (large patent-holding multinational biotech corporations angling for their next quarterly profit) for seeds and pesticides" (Who's Afraid of GMOs? Me! Neil E. Levin, CCN, DANLA, June, 2005). Is the world hungry because of a lack of patented genetically modified crops? That's like saying you're aspirin-deficient and therefore you have a headache.

Many of my clients struggle with weight loss. Prior to our sessions, they tried a variety of different methods, but none reduced their size. Disease generally follows excessive and/or long-term weight gain. In the past, diseases like diabetes, hypertension and cancer were a problem but never like today. "Fat children are an investment in future sales," said Tim Lobstein of the World Obesity Federation. He argues, "the food industry has a special interest in targeting children, since repeated exposure to processed foods and sweetened drinks in infancy builds taste preferences, brand loyalty and high profits." (Pat Thomas, *BeyondGM.org*, February 2015) Think about your favorite comfort food from childhood. Even if it's unhealthy it still brings a sense of emotional grounding because you relate that taste with a more innocent time in your youth.

STRAINS, GRAINS & BRAIN FOG

Starchy foods like bread are highly processed, simple carbohydrates with little or no vitamins, minerals, fiber or phytochemicals. That's what the body needs to thrive. Because bread is high in carbohydrates (which can turn to sugar) and low in micronutrients, soon after ingesting it the blood sugar spikes, straining the metabolic process. Most people could lose an inch or two just by reducing or eliminating bread from their diet. Fresh bread has significantly fewer chemicals and subsequently less weight gain, but I recommend reducing intake to only one piece every other day (only 3-4 pieces per week).

According to the Celiac Disease Foundation, "Gluten is a general name for the proteins found in wheat, flour, rye and barley. Gluten helps foods maintain their shape, acting as a glue that holds food together." Typically, we find it in pizza, pasta, noodles, cereal and bread. It's also hiding in frozen vegetables, like frozen corn, zucchini and yellow summer squash. Processed meats, like hams, hot dogs and sausages, and snack foods, like donuts, cookies and ice cream, contain some form of gluten.

Approximately 3 million Americans have Celiac Disease, and they frequently experience doubled-over gastric distress. More than 80% are undiagnosed or misdiagnosed. Those with gastric distress should avoid gluten and wheat products at all cost. That may mean only eating at home because you cannot control the cross contamination found in most restaurants. Millions have been gluten-free for the past decade. The numbers continue to grow. According to Global Market Insights, "gluten free food market size exceeded USD $7.4 billion globally in 2018 and is estimated to grow at over 9.4% compound annual growth rate between 2019 and 2026." The consumer shift is not so much because of an increase in Celiac Disease but more for the weight loss factor. If you stop eating gluten for two weeks, you will notice a decrease in your measurements. And hey, after age 30 that just doesn't happen so easily.

If you're gluten sensitive you may notice some of the following symptoms that frequently go undiagnosed or misdiagnosed. Many arthritic aches are gluten aches.
• Headaches
• Nausea
• Trouble sleeping
• Bloat
• Gastric pain
• Joint & knuckle aches

Dr. David Perlmutter wrote the International Bestseller, *Grain Brain* (2013). Since then, his book has been translated into 34 languages for more than 1.5 million readers. His studies show how "grains and carbohydrates are destroying your body and brain," and he guides on basic changes to alleviate or even reverse brain disease. You can learn how to eliminate brain fog symptoms, improve memory and energy levels. Diseases like depression, dementia, ADHD, autism and more are soaring due to the consumption of grains, sugars and processed foods. His nutritional program (which to keep it simple, basically excludes bread) boosts brain functioning, demonstrates the advantages of using quality fats as a main fuel source, and offers the most compelling evidence to date that a non-GMO, gluten-free, and low-carb diet is vital for cognitive functioning and long-term health.

The following grains and other starch-containing foods are naturally gluten-free (it's recommended to only eat these twice a week):
• Buckwheat
• Rice (brown, white, wild)
• Millet
• Quinoa
• Corn
• Amaranth

Consider these cost-effective, healthy and naturally gluten-free food groups:
• Fruits
• Vegetables
• Meat and poultry
• Fish and seafood
• Dairy (only eat twice per week)
• Beans, legumes, and nuts
• Tapioca

SUGAR SHOCKER

Do you enjoy orange juice with breakfast? Did you know that 8 ounces of quality orange juice has 23 grams of sugar and 26 grams of carbohydrates, which turn into sugar, and then spike your insulin levels? Your body uses insulin to move blood sugar from digested food into cells, where it is stored until your body needs it. If you don't exercise very much then it can be stored for a very long time. Diabetes can begin when you ingest too much sugar and don't exercise properly.

Americans eat over 100 pounds of sugar annually (*TheDiabetesCouncil.com*). The last quarter of the year we consume most of it. Don't fool yourself into thinking that you're actually drinking an orange. Orange juice is basically sugar water and it is tasty, but it's not healthy. If you want orange juice, eat an orange. If your kids have ADD or ADHA, on behalf of your children and their teachers, please don't give your kids sugar water (orange juice) prior to school. Sugar exacerbates attention deficit. Interestingly, drinking coffee can balance attention deficit.

You might not be able to control all the candy and junk food your children eat, but at least you can curtail it at home. Find a couple of healthy treats and keep those in the house. Being prepared is the key to staying healthy. Don't wait until you're famished to eat, and don't go grocery shopping when you're hungry; that's typically when poor choices are made. Read the nutrition labels while shopping at the grocery store and become aware of what's hiding in your cupboards. (See Reading Food Labels in next chapter.)

Sugary Foods to Avoid or Minimize
There are products that list sugar as the very first ingredient—which of course means that by weight, there's more sweetener than any other ingredient. Read the labels.
• BBQ sauce
• Fat free salad dressing
• Pretty much "fat free anything"
• Hot cocoa
• Milk chocolate covered nuts (reach for dark chocolate instead)
• Lemon flavored ice tea
• Ensure
• Chocolate hazelnut spread
• Kid's cereal (should be criminal)

KICKING THE CAN

In the 1960s Americans were encouraged to drink diet sodas to lose weight. This brought about a billion-dollar explosion of artificial sweeteners in the 80s. We devour copious quantities of these substances, mostly in the form of aspartame (NutraSweet), sucralose and saccharin, which are used to enhance the taste of everything from diet sodas to crackers to vitamins. "Artificial sweeteners may favor the growth of bacteria that make more calories available. Calories that can then find their way to our hips, thighs and midriffs," says Scientist Peter Turnbaugh of the University of California, San Francisco, and an expert on the interplay of bacteria and metabolism. According to Harvard School of Public Health, "one study of 3,682 individuals examined the long-term relationship between consuming artificially sweetened drinks and weight. The participants were followed for 7-8 years and their weights were monitored. After adjusting for common factors that contribute to weight gain such as dieting, exercising or diabetes status, the study showed that those who drank artificially sweetened drinks had a 47% higher increase in BMI than those who did not."

Research also availed that drinking diet sodas taxes your kidneys and liver and lowers bone density potentially leading to osteoporosis. The product dehydrates the body and can cause skin and muscles to whither which can also lead to bone density issues. The active ingredient in sodas is phosphoric acid with a pH of 2.8. It will dissolve a nail in about four days and a steak in two. Not surprisingly, irritable moods, even depression and pregnancy issues have been linked to diet sodas. Sometimes just having a glass of water can lift your spirit and improve your outlook. The study further found increased risk for diabetes, high blood pressure and heart disease from drinking sodas (*TheDailyMeal.com*, February 2019). You might find it disturbing to know that when the trucks carry soda syrup (the concentrate) the commercial truck must display a warning that they are carrying "highly corrosive materials." So, if you have a six-pack in your refrigerator and are unsure what to do with it, then clean your car battery. All sodas are great for removing corrosive battery discharge.

Benefits of Kicking the Can
• Fewer headaches
• Reduced insulin levels (and potential elimination of diabetes)
• Calmer sympathetic nervous system
• Decreased blood pressure & heart rate
• Decreased LDL cholesterol & triglycerides
• Reduced inflammation
• Less acne

FAST FOOD FRENZIE

Fast food companies, specifically McDonalds, were called out in the famous 2003 documentary Super Size Me where Morgan Spurlock, an American independent filmmaker, went from super healthy to nearing cardiac arrest. As a result, the then 32-year-old Spurlock gained 24 pounds, a 13% body mass increase in one month, increased his cholesterol to 230 mg/dL, and experienced mood swings, sexual dysfunction, and fat accumulation in his liver. Spurlock lost the one-month weight gained from his experiment in 14-months using a vegan diet. The doctors repeatedly stated they knew that type of liver toxicity was possible with alcohol but not from junk food. Spurlock proved that saturated fat, loads of salt and tons of sugar, as found in most fast foods, could cause the same damage to the human body as a tequila binge.

If you find that you're addicted to junk food (including food you didn't know was junk) wean yourself off of those disease-producing foods over the course of a few months or even one year. Eating fried foods can lead to weight gain but losing weight is the easy part compared to combating a disease when you've taxed your system too much. It's more challenging to restore health after the onset of an illness. It's much easier to eat less now than taking all the medicine needed to control a disease not to mention the side effect concerns.

You might find that your plate begins to look a little odd. A typical meal is chocked full of toxins and processed foods. Eating eggs over medium with sautéed garlic spinach for breakfast might be unusual, but you'll feel much better at 10 and 11am when it's time for another quality meal. When you reduce carbohydrates in order to lose weight, increase quality fats and proteins, like salmon and avocados, to avoid sugar cravings. If you continue eating what you've been eating, you will continue feeling the way you've felt in the past. If you've tried many food & fitness fads and are still having trouble shedding those pounds, consider watching documentaries like *Fed Up* (2014), *Fat, Sick and Nearly Dead* (2011), *Knives Over Forks* (2011) and *Food, Inc.* (2008) available on Netflix and Amazon. Many trailers are available on YouTube. In these documentaries you will learn that the Food Lobbyists appeal to Congressional Members, Senators and the Food and Drug Administration to change the laws to serve their corporate greed. These films identify how the food industry continues their marketing campaigns to keep us addicted to food that has minimal nutritional value.

With all the information available why do we keep ingesting junk food? Due to marketing, many people think that eating at home is more expensive than eating in a fast food joint but not anymore. Conventional fruits and vegetables may not be as healthy as organic, but they are better for you than fast food. Depending on the items, they can cost about the same for a family of 4. Even if you live alone, you can cook for four and freeze the leftovers. Remember, most restaurants serve GMO food, microwave it and charge you extra for it.

There is so much to say on this topic, but the documentaries listed above will stimulate your outlook in a whole new way. If nothing else let me add, should you be having a problem kicking the junk food diet, don't guilt yourself to death. Just note that the type of food you're eating is causing many problems. Many people live on a high caloric diet while remaining nutritionally starved, and processed foods are chock full of sugar. Sugar lights up the brain just like cocaine does. So, if you're addicted to junk food and sugar, you should feel normal, not guilty; however, only you can control what you put in your mouth. This book is designed to get you thinking and acting differently, and if you still choose to eat junk food, please counter it with some additional wellness steps included in this book. Knowing the right path isn't enough; you must walk it too.

Move away from the notion that certain foods are good or bad and reframe food choices as economical or expensive. Vegetables, fruits and legumes are easy to digest for most people. Let's call those items economical. Fried foods, heavy cream sauces, pasta, candy and cake require more organ output to digest. Instead of identifying say, lasagna, as bad, label it as expensive to digest. Meat and meat products are expensive for vegetarians to digest, but many people can burn through those nutrients easily. You decide what is economical for you based on how you feel after you ingest it. Rethink your relationship to food and consider having a nutritional budget. When you know you're going to splurge on a special event, then budget appropriately earlier in the week or the following day. Don't make yourself wrong or bad because you ate pizza or biscuits and gravy. And, certainly don't require your organs to output that much daily. Live inside your dietary budget and choose economical foods.

 ZENERGY BOOST FOR BETTER FOOD CHOICES
Create a list of your favorite foods. Instead of identifying products as "good or bad," label them as "expensive to digest" or "economical to digest." Resolve to eat the "expensive items" less often.

HOW TO READ NUTRITION LABELS

GROCERY SHOPPING

Reading nutritional labels can prevent avoidable digestive discomfort. Educate yourself on your favorite items and learn what's hiding in your cupboards. Select quality products in the future and choose fresh organic produce whenever possible. Prepare to spend 30 minutes extra reading labels at the grocery store next time you shop. Confirm you are purchasing food that is appropriate for you and your family. Once you find the right brands you won't spend as much time grocery shopping in the future. Visiting your local health food store or natural grocer can be quite a shopping experience. Some health food stores are more expensive than regular grocery stores, but they offer reduced rates on organic produce, as it's moving toward its expiration date. Additionally, they provide bulk items that are more economical than popular name brands. I really appreciate that the sales associates are more educated around organics, supplements and natural care products, and can answer questions on the fly. Consider perusing the outside edges of the grocery store where the produce, fresh meats and dairy are located. Processed foods are stored in the middle of the supermarket; you will feel better when you eat less manufactured foods.

Looks for items that indicate the following:
- Low calorie items have 40 calories or less per serving. How many servings per container? Lower calories can help you reduce weight but may mean that you stay hungry and that can lead to cravings.
- Find items that have low cholesterol, less than 20 milligrams per serving and stay under 200mg for the day.
- Low-fat items have 2 grams or less of saturated fat per serving.
- Reduced calories mean that the product has at least 25% less of the specified nutrient or calories than the usual product. Look to see what they are comparing the item to. Margarine has reduced calories compared to butter but it's fake food. Philadelphia soft cheese has fewer calories than butter but you typically use three times as much. Whipped butter or coconut oil might be a better choice.
- Words like good source of indicates approximately 10 to 19% of the Daily Value of a particular vitamin or nutrient per serving.
- Low sodium products contain 140 milligrams or less per serving.
- An item high in a nutrient means 20% or more of the Daily Value per serving.

Ask these questions while shopping:

- If the product is sugar-free or fat-free (less than ½ gram of sugar or fat per serving) then which artificial sweetener is used in its place? Are you allergic to that one? You can add honey to many unsweetened products for a flavorful burst.
- Calorie free typically means less than five calories per serving, but is it loaded with trans fats or other chemicals? Read the entire label with this type of provocative marketing scheme.

If you have food sensitivities or digestive disorders, look for items with the least number of ingredients and make sure you can annunciate all of them. If a product has ingredients that you cannot pronounce, then it's probably a chemical. Ingredients are listed in descending order by weight. Those in the largest amounts are listed first. Many people are allergic to soy, and it's in almost every processed product now. Unfortunately, items like monosodium glutamate (MSG) and artificial sweeteners, like aspartame or NutraSweet, hide under numerous names. If possible, avoid products with words like "natural flavoring" and "spices." American food manufacturers are not required to list all the ingredients and can mask toxic items under these general terms. Thanks FDA.

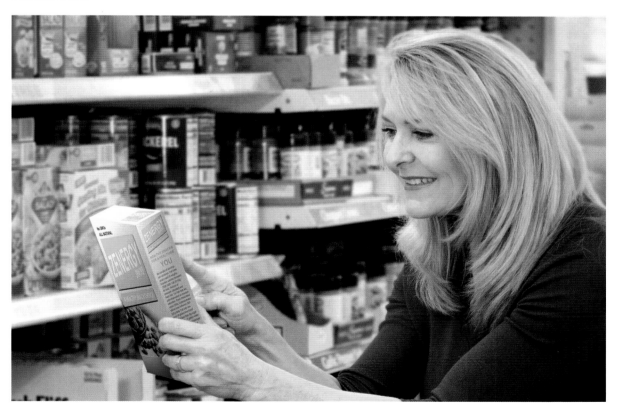

READING LABELS

Serving Size: Identify how large one serving is.

Serving Per Container: Be mindful of the number of servings per container. Frequently 1 large drink is two servings. If you eat the whole package, increase the calories and nutrients appropriately.

Saturated Fats: "I sat and got fat." Limit saturated fats.

Trans Fats: Eliminate Fake Fats created to increase shelf-life of packaged foods.

Polyunsaturated Fats: Good fat found in salmon, nuts and seeds.

Monounsaturated Fats: Unsaturated fats are good for you-Poly or Mono. Reduces cholesterol and risk for heart desease. A quality product may have 6g of fat but 5g are unsaturated fats. Eat this type of food more often.

Cholesterol: A waxy fat-like substance your body makes naturally. Important for proper brain functioning and cellular repair. Maintain total cholesterol under 200mg. Eat under 200g daily to maintain proper numbers. Limit animal fats to reduce LDL (bad cholesterol), and eat fatty fish, nuts, beans, 1 Tbsp extra virgin olive oil daily for HDL (good cholesterol).

Sodium: AHA recommends 1500-2300mg (about 4g or ½ tsp or less) daily. Reduce sodium if you have high blood pressure; increase sodium if you have low blood pressure.

Potassium: Mayo Clinic recommends 1600-2000mg daily. Too much sodium or potassium strains kidneys.

Carbohydrates: Important source of energy every day. 45% to 65% of daily caloric intake. For a 2000-calorie diet, aim for 225g to 325g daily. Simple carbs (white bread, pastries) turn into sugar and spike glucose/blood sugar levels. Eat more complex carbohydrates like vegetables, fruits, beans, brown rice, quinoa or oatmeal. Limit only one piece of gluten-free bread daily or preferably every other day. Diabetics should eat about 45% of daily caloric intake.

Dietary Fiber: 25-30g daily. Subtract grams of fiber from total number of carbs.

Soluble Fiber: Vegetables, green leafy veggies, avocados. Important for elimination.

Insoluble Fiber: Mostly breads, pasta and crackers that remain unchanged during digestion. Limit insoluble fiber to maintain good health.

Sugar: WHO recommends 10% of daily calories or 6 tsp or less could be sugar.

Protien: Multiply your weight times .36g to lose weight or multiply your weight times .82g to gain weight. 150 pounds X .36 = 54g daily to lose weight. 150 pounds X .82 = 123g protein daily to gain weight. Eat approximately the size of your palm (minus the fingers) in animal protein daily. Aging population should increase protein, possibly through protein shakes.

*Specific nutritional requirements vary for each person. Above are suggestions by the FDA (Food and Drug Administration), American Heart Association (AHA) and World Health Organization (WHO) for Recommended Daily Allowances (RDA). The FDA has not evaluated these statements. This chart is not intended to diagnose, treat, cure or prevent disease. See your healthcare provider for your exact numbers.

Nutrition Facts

Serving Size 1/2 Cup (56g)
Servings Per Container about 7

Amount Per Serving

Calories 240
Calories from Fat 50

	% Daily Value*
Total Fat 6g	9%
Saturated Fat 1g	5%
Trans Fat 0g	
Polyunsaturated Fat 2g	
Monounsaturated Fat 3g	
Cholesterol 10mg	3%
Sodium 1830mg	76%
Potassium 180mg	5%
Total Carbohydrates 9mg	12%
Dietary Fiber 4g	16%
Sugars 13g	
Protein 5g	

Vitamins

Vitamin A	2%
Vitamin C	7%
Calcium	4%
Iron	8%

* Percent Daily Values are based on a 2,000 calorie diet. Your daily values may be higher or lower depending on your calorie needs.

LOSE WEIGHT

Be mindful of servings per container. Eat less and exercise more to lose weight. Maintain calories between 1200-1800. Eat under 25g fat daily. Reduce or eliminate saturated and trans fats. Eat fats that are polyunsaturated or monounsaturated. Keep cholesterol under 200g. Limit carbohydrates to 50-150g daily. Eat more vegetables. Limit or eliminate bread, pasta, white rice and white potatoes. Drink ½-1 gallon water daily. Limit daily sugar intake to under 6g. Appropriate amounts of hydrochloric acid (HCl) are essential to digest food properly. Acid reflux is a sign that you don't have enough HCl. See "Reading Labels" to calculate daily proteins properly.

GAIN WEIGHT

Be mindful of servings per container. Eat more protein and lift weights. Maintain calories between 2500-3000. Eat 35-50g fat daily. Reduce or eliminate saturated and trans fats. Eat fats that are polyunsaturated or monounsaturated. Keep cholesterol under 200g. Carbohydrates should stay between 300-325g daily. Eat only one piece of gluten-free bread daily. Eat less than 9g sugar daily. Drink ½-1 gallon water daily. Choose proteins/protein shakes that have essential amino acids. See "Reading Labels" to calculate protein consumption for best results.

The FDA has not evaluated these statements.

FOOD JOURNAL

When you log what you're eating you will naturally eat less or better, but even if you don't change your nutritional habits, you will become mindful of what you eat day-to-day. Consider photographing your meals, using a food journal app or the following food intake form. Keep it simple and write down everything that crosses your lips including a handful of nuts, 1 piece of candy, a bite of someone's food, water, other drinks…

Breakfast   Time: _____   All 6 Tastes? _____ Y/N

Mid Morning Snack   Time: _____

Lunch   Time: _____   All 6 Tastes? _____ Y/N

Mid Day Snack   Time: _____

Dinner   Time: _____   All 6 Tastes? _____ Y/N

Evening Snack   Time: _____

Quality of Sleep (Rate 1-10)   How Long: _____

Bowel Movement & Consistency   When: _____

Daily Mood?
Chipper/Upbeat, Anxious/Worried, Goal-Oriented/Focused, Grumpy/Impatient, Kind/Community-Minded, Tired/Lazy

Water Intake: How Many glasses/ounces?

Sweet, Sour, Salty, Bitter, Pungent and Astringent are the 6 Tastes.
Eating all 6 Tastes at each meal, or each day, can make a difference in your overall health.

Adding cardamom, garlic, ginger, rosemary or turmeric covers several Tastes with one spice.

INTRODUCTION TO AYURVEDA

INTRODUCTION TO AYURVEDA ANCIENT WISDOM

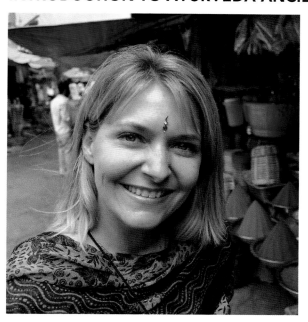

Ayurveda is Ancient Wisdom thousands of years old. Ayurveda is annunciated "Ah-u-ve-dá," and it means *the science of life*. The medical profession of India practiced Ayurveda by oral tradition well before recorded time but has been written for the last 5,000 years. It is a healing gift to us from the ancient enlightened Vedic culture. It is a health and healing system that treats not just the mind and body but also the senses and spirit to maintain vibrant health and balance. The tradition is rooted in the idea that each of us is born with an entirely personal blueprint for optimum health. Ayurveda is a sophisticated yet intuitive system in establishing balance through nutrition, exercise and mindful practices that lead to empowerment of your natural characteristics. It provides a system that recognizes the subtle energies making each of us unique, yet still indicates categories (called doshas) for better understanding of human nature. Thinking of food as medicine, knowing what to eat and which spices to use, improves your health in numerous ways. Simple methods are used for maintaining good health physiologically and psychologically to improve outlook and output throughout one's life. This system provides a path to balance the brain, central nervous system, and hormonal secretion from different glands that influence a person's mental makeup, and enhance your life through the natural Ayurvedic approach.

Today most Western doctors are allopathic who focus on the pathogen or disease (allo means to move away from; pathic indicates the pathogen/disease). Allopathic Western Doctors and the scientific community are disease-care physicians, and are only now recognizing integrative and complimentary approaches to health and healing. Incorporating simple things like the time of day that you take medication, the importance of meditation to balance blood pressure, and proper nutrition to reduce inflammation have been embraced by many doctors in modern medicine. There are numerous warning signs prior to the onset of a full-blown disease. Ayurvedic Doctors have known this and recommended natural healing techniques for centuries. West meets East.

Digestion is a key role to optimal health. Good digestion, called *agni*, indicates a strong digestive fire and maintaining it is imperative for disease-free, long term vitality. Digestive heat and energy are responsible for all transformative processes of the body. Three important components of correct digestion are strong digestive fire (*deepana)*, correct assimilation (*pachana*) and timely elimination (*anulomana)*. When these three function normally, the body is vibrant and healthy with an abundance of energy, called *ojas*. Your mind is clear and happiness prevails. A weak digestive fire creates toxicity called *ama*. *Ama* is a product of improper nutrition, sluggish digestion, slow metabolism and negative emotions. *Ama* builds up at the weakest point in the bodily tissues ultimately causing disease. Negative thoughts and emotions can lessen clarity of mind by reducing mental *agni* and subsequently physical *agni.* This means that our unprocessed (undigested) experiences become just as toxic to our body as indigestible foods. *Ama* has similar qualities to *kapha* heavy, sticky, cold, slimy, and dense, and can block any dosha. Ayurvedic Doctors see *ama* as the underlying cause of all medical conditions. Digestion has two parts. It starts in the mouth, and finishes with expelling wastes through the anus, and takes about 24 hours. The second part of digestion continues to the seven tissues where the cellular structure obtains the nutrients and expels the bioproducts from one tissue to another. The final product of this transformative process is immune fluid and the flow of the immune system. It takes approximately five days to complete the process. The seven tissues are plasma, blood, muscle, fat, bone, grey matter and reproductive tissues.

According to the Ancient Traditions of India, life is composed of a master plan for vitality including the five basic elements: space/ether, air, fire, water and earth. From these elements three mind-body metabolic types are formed, called doshas. They are a tangible functional intelligence that governs bodily tissues and its capacity. The *vata* dosha is a combination of air and space, and comprises the brain, the central nervous system, circulation, colon, pelvic region and thighs. The *pitta* dosha constitutes fire and water, and regulates the metabolism, heart, liver, spleen, gall bladder, small intestines, blood, skin, eyes, and lower part of the stomach. The *kapha* dosha is a blend of water and earth, and governs the structure, bones, tongue, larynx, pharynx, esophagus, sinuses, chest, lungs, bronchi, senses, joints, joint lubrication, spinal fluid, and the upper part of stomach. There is some overlap as to which dosha governs each organ and gland, and Ayurveda centers on restoring balance in all three doshas rather than focusing on symptoms of disease. For instance, achy joints indicate the joint is dry from too much *vata*. Rheumatoid arthritis points to inflammation from excessive *pitta*. And, loose joints denote too much *kapha*. Illness is a manifestation of disharmony and restoring balance impedes the root pathway of disease. While we each have a dominant dosha the other two also influence. Some people are equally bi-doshic or most balanced is tri-doshic, but that is rare. Our mental, emotional and physical characteristics generate our personality based on our dosha. Think about calming *vata*, cooling *pitta* and stimulating *kapha* to stay balanced.

Doshas are a mind-body principal indicating a basic quality of expression. We each hold qualities of the mind and body so we have two doshas, one for the mind and one for the body. You're not necessarily imbalanced when you have a different mind dosha from your body dosha; however, you may have a high propensity toward one characteristic and a healthy dose of another versus being two distinctive doshas. For instance, you may be a good communicator and leader (*pitta*) but find it difficult to manage proper height-weight balance (*kapha*). Possibly, you are tall and lean (*vata*) but are prone to fits of road rage (*pitta*). You may be very compassionate with friends and family (*kapha*) but completely disorganized at the office (*vata*). It's not fair to reduce a dosha down to a generalized example, but when your dosha becomes imbalanced the door opens for frustration, loss of direction or even disease.

Doshas, Your Body's Blueprint
Primary Characteristics of the Mind

Vata	*Pitta*	*Kapha*
Creative, Fluid	**Focused, Type A**	**Structured, Supportive**
Artistic, Enthusiastic	Leadership, Joyful	Grounded, Steadfast, Calm
Impulsive, Quick	Fast, Organized	Orderly, Stable, Serene
Spontaneous, Adventurous	Perfectionist, Orderly	Inability to Accept Change
Wind, Air, Space, Floaty	Fire, Water, Steam	Earth, Water, Mud
Mood Swings	Picky, Sharp Speech	Stuck, Sticky, Stagnant
Architects, Marketing Dir	CEO, CFO, Big Picture	Dir of Ops/Admin/Provost
Decorators, Remodelers	Direct, Pejorative	Loyal, Compassionate, Kind
Scattered, Worried	Driven, Focused	Hoarders, Like Possessions
Long Talkers, Social	Sweet Natured	Takes Direction Well
Imaginative	Generous	Mensch, Kind, Considerate

Primary Characteristics of the Body

Vata, Thin	*Pitta, Athletic*	*Kapha, Curvy*
Ectomorph	**Mesomorph**	**Endomorph**
Sleek, Lanky, Wiry	Medium Bone Structure	Larger Bones, Curvy, Soft
Small Bone Structure	Muscular, Svelte	Overweight, Obese, Diabetic
Forget to Eat Sometimes	Strong Digestion	Tolerates Pain Well
Constipation, Deer Pellets	Should Not Skip Meals	Good Stamina, Slow-Moving
Dry Skin, Chapped Lips	Heartburn, Heart Disease	Chronic Sinusitis, Mucus
Arthritic or Achy Joints	Acne, Bloodshot Eyes	Over-Sleeps, Slow-Starter

You might find yourself in all these categories but what is your basic nature? Look for your commonly expressed qualities. According to Dr. Deepak Chopra there are three reasons why knowing your body type is so important. "First, the seeds of disease are sown early. Second, body types make prevention more specific. And third, body types make treatment more accurate once a disease appears" (*Perfect Health*, 2000). Taking the simple dosha questionnaire below will help you identify yourself better for the conversation over the next few pages, and glean the tips for your master plan for vitality.

 ZENERGY BOOST FOR DOSHA QUIZ
Take the Dosha Quiz on the following page and read the Ayurvedic Section with self in mind. Practice two or three dosha-specific techniques to stay balanced. Answer the Expanded Dosha Quiz at *KiBrowning.com.*

DOSHA QUIZ

Find your dosha type by ranking the characteristic in each row with a number 5, 3, or 1 in the box. **5=Most like me 3=Somewhat like me 1=Least like me.**

Do not use the same number twice in the same row. When you have ranked each statement with a number, total the numbers at the bottom. You should have a final number for each *Vata*, *Pitta* and *Kapha* Dosha. When you add the totals across at the bottom they should equal 90.

CHARACTERISTIC	VATA		PITTA		KAPHA	
BODY TYPE	I am thin and lean with boney joints.		I have a medium build and am muscular.		I am curvy or overweight.	
WEIGHT	I do not gain weight easily		I can lose or gain weight easily.		I have a hard time losing weight.	
EYES	My eyes are small, dry and active.		My eyes are sharp with an intense gaze.		My eyes are big, soft and pleasant.	
SKIN	My skin has a tendency to be dry, thin and prone to cracking.		My skin is smooth, oily and is prone to redness.		My skin is thick and prone to be oily or moist.	
PHYSICAL MOVEMENT	I move fast.		I move at a moderate speed.		I move slowly and deliberately.	
SLEEP	I am a light sleeper and awaken easily.		I am a sound sleeper and fall asleep easily.		I sleep deeply and long. I awaken slowly.	
BODY TEMPERATURE	My hands and feet are often cold, and I like warm temperatures.		I am warm or hot, and I like cool temperatures.		I am adaptable, but I do not like cold and damp.	
SPEECH	My speech is quick and sometimes unclear.		My speech is sharp and direct.		My speech is quiet, and I mostly listen.	
PERSONALITY	I am active and enthusiastic. I tend to be anxious.		I am organized and purposeful. I tend to be impatient.		I am calm and easy going. I tend to be depressed.	
DIGESTION	I am often constipated, gassy and feel bloated.		I have acidity and heartburn.		My digestion is sluggish.	
TOTAL	VATA TOTAL _____		PITTA TOTAL _____		KAPHA TOTAL _____	

Once you know your dosha a new sense of self and wellbeing begins to form. For instance, one person may prefer routine (*pitta*) while another enjoys a variety of spontaneous events (*vata*). If you know that you work better as a team player with supervision (*kapha*) then you shouldn't bother with self-employment, as it can be quite isolating at times and that can be disempowering. On the other hand, if you enjoy being the leader of an organization and excel as the Lone Ranger (*pitta*) then entrepreneurialism might suit you just fine. Again, I'm generalizing the doshic qualities so you can get the gist.

Remember, we have two doshas, one for the mind (as mentioned above) and one for the physical form. The expanded dosha quiz provides more details about yourself. Regarding the body-dosha, if you have a curvy body (*kapha*) then you can accept that about yourself instead of trying to be model-thin like *vatas.* While not all *vatas* are skinny, they typically have small bones and a thin frame. On the other side of the coin, when you accept your bodily frame as slender and wiry (*vata*) then you're not criticizing it to get brawny and muscular (*pitta*). Generally speaking, *pittas* enjoy the middle ground with a natural ability to gain or lose weight. Typically, athletes are *pittas* who enjoy a strong constitution.

Signs of a Balanced Dosha & Healthy Metabolism, Ojas
1. Sleep well & feel rested upon awakening
2. Tongue is pink and clear
3. Body feels light, regardless of weight
4. Digestion is strong
5. Elimination is easy
6. Feel energized and enthusiastic
7. Mind is calm, clear & focused
8. Body has a pleasant smell
9. Rarely get sick

Signs of an Imbalanced Dosha or Toxicity, Ama
1. Bad breath or coated tongue
2. Dull appetite or delicate digestion
3. Sensitivities or allergies to foods
4. Sluggish or irritable elimination
5. Generalized aches and pains
6. Fatigue
7. Depression
8. Susceptibility to infections
9. Difficulty manifesting intentions

When you observe the transformation of your body from day to day you will become aware which foods or activities are good for you. Look at your eyes–are they clear or bloodshot? Look at your tongue–is it pink, coated or raw? How does your skin appear–dewy or dry? Physical stress and emotional trauma throw us out of balance. Your body is communicating with you daily about its ability to handle stress.

You may be surprised to know that in Ayurveda it is recommended not to eat raw foods, certainly not every day. For years I ate loads of raw salads and smoothies, and my digestion became more sensitive with each passing week. I thought I was doing the right thing for my body, and it just needed to "catch up." What I learned is that steamed or lightly sautéed vegetables improve overall digestion. Once I shifted my cooking style, the stomachaches disappeared and my elimination improved. I'm not saying this is the hard and fast truth for everyone but consider the importance of the digestive fire to burn food into nutrients for your cellular structure. Your stomach produces hydrochloric acid and the gall bladder delivers bile creating the chemical process of transforming food into energy. Now, think about placing a cold wet log on a fire. What happens? Certainly a lack of fire, possibly steam or even mold occur in that cold damp environment. Condensation or steam, not combustion, occurs from eating raw and/or cold food. This steam can lead to rot gut, food putrefying in your stomach or taking days to move through the intestines. If digestion is not right in the stomach then it's not right in the seven tissues (plasma, blood, muscle, fat, bone, grey matter and reproductive tissues), and that leads to dis-ease. And, as we know from our current statistics with the National Institute of Diabetes and Digestive and Kidney Disease, "60 to 70 million Americans are affected by digestive diseases annually." How many are drinking a cold smoothie daily? Smoothies and vegetable juice drinks at room temperature are far more effective than cold ones, but most people need to eat warm lightly cooked foods. If you don't have the vibrant health you desire then do something different today. *Physician Heal Thyself*!

A different example of seeking balance takes us to another client, Marsha, who had a very sharp *pitta* mind and slow *kapha* body. She was about 60 pounds overweight. Her slow metabolism (*kapha*) betrayed her focused mind and outgoing personality (*pitta*). Through the use of mindful practices she came to learn more about nutrition, exercise and stress management tools; however, she wasn't getting the results until she had an emotional breakthrough. Her parents depended on her as a mediator (*pitta*) in their failed marriage, and that had been the triangle with them for decades. Once she realized what she was doing and how deeply incongruous it was for her to be in the middle of their conflict, she set a loving healthy boundary with her parents. She returned the conflict resolution responsibility to her parents to handle their own dealings. She regained focus on her own affairs and stopped solving their problems. She learned that by intentionally being involved in their disagreements, she used the weight gain as a form of protection. It took some time, as new habits do, but over the course of six months, she weaned herself from their daily interactions, and they found new support. It was a win/win for everyone. She talks to her parents once a week now, and today she is naturally height-weight proportional. How much of your weight gain is directly related to an unhealthy relationship?

You can see from these two very different examples (my eating raw salads for years and Marsha's emotional breakthrough with her parents) that becoming aware of your mind-body connection can restore vibrant health. Frequently, we have to start in one area before getting balanced in another. You might find that you don't have road rage (*pitta*), but you can sit and sulk for hours (*kapha*). Possibly, you are a controlling parent (*vata*), but you do it with compassion (*kapha*). Maybe you're a good collaborator at work (*pitta*) because you introduce new creative strategies for efficiency (*vata*), but you don't have the structure to meld the ideas into a cohesive order (*kapha*). Identifying what is working and what needs improvement in your life puts you back in the driver's seat.

Ways to Get Unstuck
Likened to the butterfly, *vata* has a hard time getting grounded. If you awaken anxious for no reason or dread commitments (*vata*) then find a friend to help you set strong boundaries (*pitta*) with a few key people in your life. Sometimes fear can come from taking on other's emergencies like they are your own, leaving you little energy to handle your own responsibilities. Get a game plan and stick to it. *Pittas* are good at seeing the big picture. If you have constipation (*vata*) then eat warm soothing comfort foods (*kapha*). Most people, especially *Vatas*, should not drink cold smoothies. Try room temperature drinks in the future.

If your anger and impatience charred your colleagues at the water cooler (*pitta*) then contact a compassionate massage therapist (*kapha*) for some quick RnR. Stress can cause heartburn (*pitta*) just like spicy food can, so drink a little apple cider vinegar and meditate for 10 minutes. Ease up on the competitiveness (*pitta*) by sharing a personal story of your life that you rarely tell anyone with a trusted compassionate friend (*kapha*). This builds a level of intimacy and vulnerability inducing connection and reducing isolation. *Pittas* need to learn to delegate to someone who can provide the structure (*kapha*) for manifesting ideas. Switching your athletic outlet to vinyasa yoga or hot yoga can move a *pitta*'s physical prowess of competitiveness (even against yourself) to daily personal achievement. Learn to stop comparing and competing and just participate in athleticism.

If you get into the dumps, stuck and stagnant (*kapha*) then go dancing with an artsy fartsy type (*vata*). The enthusiasm and joy that a healthy *vata* emanates is contagious. *Kaphas* are frequently trying to lose weight but typically find more comfort on the couch. Washing your car or getting your nails done gets you out of the house and shifts inert energy. Find your Idea Man or Creativity Chick (*vata*) to reposition your furniture or artwork, or hit the park for a walkie-talkie with an athletic outdoorsy friend (*pitta*). Strolling works as well as a fast-pace, just get moving.

114

Steve Jobs, Co-Founder and Innovator, frequently walked with his staff while they collaborated on the next successful step in the Apple and Pixar Empires.

Imbalance in one area can lead to unhappiness in many areas of your life and take away from your natural personality. One-third or more of America could be described as a *pitta* (driven workforce) with a *kapha* imbalance (overweight or diabetic). Many of those people don't even think they're fat because they are so focused on achievement. *Pitta* imbalance increases emotional outbursts, frustration, sarcasm, manipulation or judgmental statements. *Kapha* imbalance leads to congestion, over-eating, over-sleeping, laziness, loss of enthusiasm to achieve and even depression. *VVata* imbalance reduces your ability to create, leaving you scattered, off-in-the-clouds, victimized or anxious. You move away from your natural personality when you are imbalanced. Eating properly and exercising at least every other day offers a heightened level of contentment. Be the person you were meant to be.

BALANCING TECHNIQUES FOR EACH MIND DOSHA

Signs of *Vata*/Anxious Mind Imbalance
Anxious, nervous, apprehensive
Flighty, head in the clouds
Inability to finish projects
Fear of commitment, commitment-phobe
Disorderly, disorganized desk, cluttered
Talkative, mind racing or jumping from one topic to another
Overly sensitive, sensitive to high pitch noises
Lack of punctuality, lack of coordination & skipping meals

Recommendations to Soothe the *Vata*/Anxious Mind
Vatas generally make great Marketing Executives, Artistic Directors, Teachers, Taxi Drivers because they embrace change. They do well with upheaval, spontaneity or even emergencies but need to maintain an organized lifestyle to reduce anxiety. Routine restores balance.

1. Make a short to-do list (3 items) to finish each day.
2. Plan a company picnic or family vacation.
3. Listen to soothing, grounding music (no lyrics).
4. Look at pleasant grounding images of the beach or garden.
5. Look at, decorate with, or wear pastel shades & earth tones.
6. Aromatherapy: floral, fruity, geranium, lemon or eucalyptus.
7. Don't over-commit; feel free to say NO occasionally.
8. Slow down the tendency for shallow breath; be aware of breathing.

Signs of *Pitta*/Angry Mind Imbalance

Cynical, sarcastic
Angry, hot-tempered
Irritable, frustrated
Road rage, impatient
Controlling, demanding
Pejorative, critical
Intense, sharp, judgmental
Quick to push people away

Recommendations to Pacify the *Pitta*/Angry Mind

Pittas can be enterprising, good leaders, and excellent communicators that know how to get results. Typically, CEOs, Entrepreneurs, Sales Executives and Professional Athletes fall into this dosha. When out of balance they unleash a verbal onslaught with costly repercussions. *Pittas* typically love seeing results from their efforts, but too much pressure from work deadlines challenge their balance. Try some of the following activities to maintain proper footing.

1. When you feel angry, practice *pranayama* (explained in meditation section).
2. Delegate and reduce micro-managing.
3. Stop cramming too much into one day & create better time management skills.
4. Listen to soothing, uplifting music with flutes & wind instruments.
5. Look at pleasant uplifting images of the stars or northern lights.
6. Look at, decorate with or wear cooling colors like blue, green & white.
7. Aromatherapy: cooling fragrances like sandalwood, rose or spearmint.
8. Wear cool fabrics, like linen or cotton, to cool down.
9. Keep a fan mister nearby to stay cool.
10. Avoid stimulating activities & pressures when you're out of harmony.

Signs of *Kapha*/Stagnant Imbalance

Clingy, dependent, whiney
Depression, sadness
Lazy, lethargic, slow or dull
Inability to set healthy boundaries
Unmotivated, loss of achievement
Hoarding things and food
Over-sleeping, over-eating
Stuck, stagnant
Dreamy, withdrawn

Recommendations to Appease the *Kapha*/Stagnant Mind

Kaphas are great at providing cohesiveness to a corporation, community or family. They best serve as Counselor, Chief Operating Officer, Human Resource Director, Non-Profit Office Manager or Daycare Worker. When out of balance, *kaphas* become clingy or inactive or even so fatigued they can't get out of bed timely. Try some of the following activities to restore balance.

1. Listen to upbeat motivating dance music & sing along.
2. Look at exciting images–people celebrating, fireworks or graduation images.
3. Look at, decorate with, or wear bright colors (red, orange or purple) with strong sharp shapes.
4. Aromatherapy: cinnamon, musk, juniper, nutmeg or clove.
5. Stop wearing your heart on your sleeve & managing everyone's problems; let them find other resources to resolve their issues.
6. Trying to fix others' problems can, at times, be depressing and unfulfilling~limit your free counseling services.
7. Setting healthy boundaries provides more mental-emotional protection than eating a donut.

ENJOYING ALL 6 TASTES PACIFIES THE BODY DOSHAS

For thousands of years Ancient Ayurvedic Doctors observed six tastes and their attributes. The knowledge is still relevant today. Sweet, sour, salty, bitter, pungent and astringent are the six tastes. Including foods with all six tastes at each meal in proper proportions allows the dosha to remain balanced. Reflect on your body-dosha type now. Which one are you ~ *vata*/thin, *pitta*/athletic or *kapha*/curvy?

Think of food as medicine and consider using spices as a form of natural healthcare. *Pittas* frequently have acid reflux and adding mint, dill or yogurt to the dish can reduce this imbalance. Spicy foods like jalapenos are great for diminishing congestion, which is typical *kapha* imbalance. Warm oily foods, comfort foods, can nourish those with dry skin, a common *vata* imbalance. Generally speaking, spicing up your coffee with a little cinnamon or your eggs with a little cayenne pepper increases your metabolism (provided you're not allergic to those spices).

As with any new diet or exercise program, begin slowly and monitor your progress. Use these suggestions as a natural map for proper nutrition. Document your nutritional choices and corresponding physiological changes in a food journal provided over the course of two-to-three months to monitor your improvements. If you're not improving, choose different foods within the appropriate category. A diet that works for your spouse may not work for you even if you have the same dosha. It's good to remember that everything can be beneficial or toxic. Do not stay the course and keep eating the wrong foods because you "think they are healthy for you." Your body will tell you that it likes those foods by feeling healthy and energized, or it doesn't like those foods by excessive belching, acid reflux, farting, constipation, etc.

Six Tastes

Sweet	Fruit, nuts, oils, flour, pasta, bread, dairy, meats
Sour	Citrus fruit, lemons, berries, tomatoes, yogurt, cheese, pickles, vinegar, alcohol
Salty	Sea salt, seafood, sauces, dressings
Bitter	Most veggies, broccoli, kale, chard, tea, coffee
Pungent	Spicy foods, cayenne, ginger, radish, thyme, basil
Astringent	Fiber, beans, mung lentils, dark green veggies, parsley, red cabbage

The body feels satisfied when you eat all six tastes at each meal or at least throughout the day. Most people crave sweet, sour and salty when they don't consume all six. (Example: fries with ketchup.) Cravings are a sign of being minerally depleted, and eating all six tastes at each meal reduces binging. Think of food as medicine and consider eating the right foods for essential balance. Eat the rainbow of colors of food at each meal and stop eating when you're full. Close your mouth while eating so that saliva can form properly around the food. Since digestion starts in the mouth, chew your food completely or chew five more times than usual per bite. Slow down while eating and set down your utensils periodically. Mush the food in your mouth before swallowing to improve overall digestion.

Quality Oils are essential to a balanced diet, and we cook with them everyday. Many people see oils as the culprit to weight gain, but oil is one of the building blocks to every cell in your body. Reduce or eliminate trans fats like margarine. Avoid using cheap cooking oils like canola or soy oil. Canola oil is derived from rapeseed and traditionally used to lubricate machine engines. It is claimed that the harsh-tasting toxin with high erucic acid was reduced to a safe level for human consumption, but with all the quality oils easily accessible today why would you risk ingesting something that was intended for a machine. And, almost all soy is GMO now. Exchange chemically processed canola oil for butter, and exchange butter for healthy oils like sesame, avocado, coconut, olive and ghee. Ghee is a clarified form of butter and suitable for all three doshas. Commonly used in Indian dishes, it increases digestive fire and enzymes in the body, but does not increase *pitta*. It is efficient for liver functioning as it doesn't clog like other oils and animal fats can. Ghee is ideal for those who have allergies or are lactose intolerant. Anti-inflammatory and heart-healthy, it is particularly healing for the subtle tissues in the body such as reproductive, bone marrow and nerves. Used in preparation with dosha-specific herbs, it provides a good carrier for absorption into the tissues. It can also be used on the skin to reduce dry skin and in the hair to reduce dandruff and increase growth.

Make Your Own Ghee ~ Melt butter slowly. The solids, casein and lactose, will sink to the bottom, and a foam will form on the top. The ghee floats in between the two. Strain the liquid into a jar or bottle, and let it cool to solidify. Leave the sediment in the bottom of the pan. It may not return to a full solid state unless you store in the refrigerator. Ghee is good for up to one year in the refrigerator.

Be mindful of the oil's smoke point. According to the Cleveland Clinic, overheating the oil not only degrades the nutrients but also releases free radicals. Free radicals are a toxic byproduct causing significant damage to the body. Cheap oils, saturated fats, processed meats and alcohol are examples of some products that release free radicals into the body. If you burn the oil, wipe it out and begin again. Choose sesame, almond, avocado, and olive over canola, palm or corn.

Low smoke point
Coconut Oil
Sesame can handle a higher heat than coconut oil but still has a low smoke point.
Virgin olive oil is a wonderful all-purpose cooking oil and can handle a higher heat than coconut and sesame.

Medium-high smoke point
Grapeseed, macadamia nut, pumpkin seed or hemp.

Highest smoke point
Highest in saturated fats, use these sparingly or eliminate.
Best for frying; typical oil found in most restaurants.
Canola, corn, soy or palm oil.
Ghee.

No heat oils like flaxseed, wheat germ and walnut are best for salad dressings, marinades and dips.

Albeit, you may not be able to eat dosha-specific oils at each meal because it's rare that the entire family will be the same dosha, but you can alternate which oils you use from day to day and even within each meal. Sesame oil and ghee are great for all three doshas. Choosing dosha-specific oils can strengthen your constitution and improve overall digestion.

Dosha–Specific Oils

Vata:	Sesame, almond or avocado. Bhringara oil has proven benefits as a support for the liver, skin related diseases and hair growth.
Pitta:	Sesame, olive, sunflower or coconut. Bhringara is helpful for *pitta*'s common skin irritations.
Kapha:	Sesame, almond, olive, grapeseed, sunflower, safflower or mustard.
All Three:	Ghee and sesame.

BALANCE YOUR BODY THROUGH SUITABLE NUTRITION

Vata/**Lean Body** ~ Those who are more lean and lanky are characterized by the air and space elements, and are highly affected by wind, cold and dryness. More prone to constipation, hard stools or deer pellet stools, *vatas* should consider choosing warm, oily, heavy, cooked foods. Eat more sweet tastes like grains, lean cuts of meat, sweet potatoes and dairy. Add avocado oils and proteins to the diet. Sour foods, which stimulate digestion, and salty foods, which promote appetite, aid in staying balanced. Since *vata* has a tendency to be dry, consider adding 1-2 teaspoons of quality oil over each meal, like avocado or sesame oils. Warm sesame oil self-massage on a daily basis nourishes the skin. Avoid caffeine, white sugar or stimulants. If you have fine or small-bones but are overweight, you are likely *vata* with a *kapha* imbalance. So exercise more and sit down while eating. Dashboard dining can lead toward constipation or other digestive disturbances. Imbalances in *vata* can create about 80 different body disturbances. Typical *vata* disorders include breathing conditions, asthma, fibromyalgia, nervousness, mental illness, and irregular heartbeat. For these reasons *vata* must be addressed first!

Signs of *Vata*/**Lean Body Imbalance**
Bloating, dry, hard stool, deer pellets
Constipation, gas
Undesired weight loss
Disrupted sleep, light sleeper
Troublesome female cycle
Dehydrated, dry skin or chapped lips

Recommendations to Balance *Vata*/**Lean Body**
Like increases like & opposites reduce.
Vata person eating *vata* food experiences more *vata*.
When aggravated, a *vata* person may experience dry achy joints or undesired weight loss and therefore eating *kapha* foods restores balance.

1. Eat all 6 tastes at each meal.
2. Favor foods that are sweet, sour and salty.
3. Eat warm cooked food in sesame or avocado oil with enough protein.
4. No cold raw food or cold smoothies or ice.
5. Stay warm.
6. Sit down to eat and don't talk too much.
7. Spices: basil, cumin, cinnamon, vanilla.
8. Receive a soothing Swedish massage with warm sesame oil.
9. Learn to focus your mind by participating in Tai Chi exercise.
10. Wear an eye mask and ear plugs to bed.

Pitta/**Athletic Body** ~ Those with a medium build, who can gain & lose weight easily, are highly affected by heat, warm air and spicy foods. Regulate your natural elements, fire and water, by choosing cooling foods, even room temperature vegetable juices, with sweet, bitter and astringent tastes, like watermelon, spinach, celery, ginger and apples. *Pittas* have a tendency toward heartburn, rashes or inflammation. Consider eating less spicy, salty and sour foods, and reduce red meat that causes excess heat in the body. Be sure not to skip meals as this can leave you hangry (hungry and angry). *Pittas* like a healthy competitive camaraderie, mentally and physically, but can overdo it trying to win at all costs. Imbalances in *pitta* can create about 40 different body disturbances including inflammation, heart disease, metabolic disorders, liver problems, hormonal imbalances and skin conditions.

Signs of *Pitta*/**Athletic Body Imbalance**
Inflammation, rashes or acne
Swelling in body or joints
Repetitive neck pain
Heartburn, acid reflux, ulcers, heat in body
Hot flashes, distressful menopause or painful periods
Dislike missing meals
Easily get hangry (hungry & angry)

Recommendations to Pacify *Pitta*/**Athletic Body**
Like increases like & opposites reduce.
Pitta person eating *pitta* food experiences more *pitta*.
When aggravated, a *pitta* person might experience heartburn and therefore needs to eat more *vata* or *kapha* foods to restore balance.
1. Eat all 6 Tastes at each meal.
2. Favor foods that are sweet, bitter & astringent.
3. Do not miss meals, especially lunch.
4. Drink cooling beverages like cucumber water or tepid peppermint tea.
5. Minimize pungent/spicy foods and add avocados or mangoes.
6. Avoid fish, alcohol and very sour foods.
7. Receive a nurturing muscular massage with coconut oil.
8. Rhythmical mechanical movement of weight lifting calms the mind.
9. Moderate intensity exercise increases agility and coordination.
10. Enjoy brisk walking, skiing, mountain climbing, biking & swimming.

***Kapha*/Curvy Body** ~ Does better with more pungent, bitter and astringent foods (which dries out accumulated fluids and congestion) like vegetables, greens, peppers, eggplant, garbanzo beans and spicy foods. Grains, like barley or quinoa, have a lower glycemic index, which is better for Diabetics than other types of starchy carbohydrates. Whole grains, fruits and berries are preferred. Eat less sour, salty and sweet tastes like cheese, roasted nuts and creamed sauces. Try lighter, dryer foods to reduce weight and decrease lethargy like spicy beans and rice with avocado slices. Imbalances in *kapha* can create about 20 different body disturbances. Typical *kapha* disorders include mucous condition, fluid imbalances, prostate conditions, rheumatism and obesity.

Signs of *Kapha*/Curvy Body Imbalance
Diabetes
Undesired weight gain, obesity
Increased cholesterol and triglycerides
Congestion, colds, sinus infections
Lethargy, laziness, slow or dull
Over-sleeping or slow to awaken in morning

Recommendations to Appease *Kapha*/Curvy Body
Like increases like & opposites reduce.
Kapha person eating *kapha* food experiences more *kapha*.
When aggravated, a *kapha* person may get congested or have sinus infections and therefore needs to eat more *vata* or *pitta* foods to restore balance.
1. Eat all 6 tastes at each meal.
2. Smell your food before eating. Smells are very important to *kaphas*.
3. Favor foods that are bitter, pungent and astringent.
4. Choose foods to increase metabolism like smashed cauliflower with cayenne.
5. Avoid bread, pasta and potatoes and increase caffeine to two cups daily.
6. Receive an active massage, Thai or Shiatsu with upbeat music.
7. Move your furniture or artwork once or twice a year to avoid stagnation.
8. Gardening is a slow movement inspired by nature and will suffice for those with limited mobility, but rigorous activity is recommended; a visit to the library gets you off the couch.
9. Vigorous vinyasa yoga to emphasize strength, endurance & concentration.
10. Basketball, biking, swimming, aerobics and weight training are preferred.

SIX TASTES SHOPPING LIST
Include all six tastes and a rainbow of colors at every meal

SWEET

Apples
Avocado and Asparagus
Carrots
Beets and Bell Peppers
Grains, Pasta and Rice
Bread
Mushrooms
Nuts and Seeds
Oils and Meats
Honey and Sugar
Mango and Melons
Papaya and Peaches
Sweet Potatoes

SOUR

Alcohol
Apricots and Berries
Cheese
Citrus Fruits
Lemon and Lime
Mango
Tomatoes
Papaya
Pickles
Soy Sauce
Vinegar
Yogurt

SALTY

Celery
Chips
Crackers
Salted Meats
Sauces
Sea Veggies
Seafood
Taste of the Ocean
Pickled Olives

SWEET SPICY

Basil
Cardamom
Fresh Fennel
Mint
Nutmeg
Vanilla

SOUR SPICES

Tamarind
Caraway Seeds
Oregano

SALTY SPICES

Bragg Liquid Aminos
Garlic
Soy
Tamari
Salt

PROTEINS, CARBS & FATS

Soothing Effects on Physiology
Builds Tissue
Diuretic, Anti-inflammatory
Increases Weight

Pacifies *Vata* & *Pitta*
Aggravates *Kapha*

ORGANIC ACIDS

Stimulates Stomach Acids
Promotes Appetite
Improves Digestion
Can Cause Heartburn

Pacifies Vata
Aggravates *Pitta* & *Kapha*

MINERAL SALTS

Stimulates Digestive Juices
Salt Water Can Be a Mild Laxative
Can Increase Blood Pressure
Combat Dullness and Depression
Guards Against Tumors

Pacifies Vata
Aggravates *Pitta* & *Kapha*

Some foods fall under two categories. Adding cardamom, garlic,
ginger, rosemary or turmeric covers several tastes with one spice.

SIX TASTES SHOPPING LIST

Include all six tastes and a rainbow of colors at every meal

BITTER

Almonds
Asparagus
Broccoli & Bok Choy
Kale
Chicory
Celery
Dark Chocolate/Cacoa
Lettuce & Spinach
Tea
Aloe Vera
Sprouts
Yellow Squash

PUNGENT/SPICY

Black Pepper
Garbanzo Beans
Coffee & Cocoa
Cooking Spices
Eggplant
Horseradish
Mustard
Onions
Peppers
Radishes
Salsa
Spinach

ASTRINGENT

Apples & Bananas
Beans & Legumes
Corn & Popcorn
Cabbage & Cauliflower
Tofu & Tempeh
Zuchini
Cucumber
Dark Greens
Mushrooms
Pomegranates
Red Wine
Seeds & Nuts

BITTER SPICES

Turmeric, Cumin, Pepper, Barley, Basil, Fenugreek, Dill

PUNGENT SPICES

Bay Leaf, Cayenne, Cloves, Cinnamon, Ginger, Asafetida (Hing), Nutmeg, Cumin, Fennel, Paprika, Rosemary, Thyme

ASTRINGENT SPICES

Turmeric, Dill, Basil, Parsley, Coriander, Cilantro, Oregano

ESSENTIAL OILS

Detoxifying
May Cause Gas
Increases Bile
Supports Liver
Promotes Weight Loss

Pacifies *Pitta* & *Kapha*
Aggravates *Vata*

ALKALOIDS/GLYCOCIDES

Improves Digestion
Promotes Sweating
Clears Sinus
Increases Metabolism
Promotes Weight Loss

Pacifies *Kapha*
Aggravates *Vata* & *Pitta*

FIBROUS FOODS

Helps with Elimination
Healing & Drying
Absorbs Water
Tightens Tissues

Pacifies *Pitta* & *Kapha*
Aggravates *Vata*

Some foods fall under two categories. Adding cardamom, garlic, ginger, rosemary or turmeric covers several tastes with one spice.

COMPONENTS OF AN AYURVEDIC DAILY ROUTINE

1. Awaken 5-6a (preferably without an alarm). Waking before 6am offers natural boost of energy.
2. Drink one large glass of water first thing (hot/ warm is better).
3. Meditate for 5-30 minutes while you're still in the sleep-time serenity.
4. Gentle stretches or yoga for 15-60 minutes.
5. Shower, clean teeth & use a tongue scraper.
6. Eat breakfast, if hungry.
7. Work.
8. Midday–eat a hearty lunch in silence, no technology, no liquids.
9. Sit for 5-minutes to digest.
10. Walk for 15-minutes.
11. Sip apple cider vinegar about 30-minutes after meal to assist with digestion.
12. Sip hot ginger/ lemon water throughout day.
13. Drink ½ gallon (2 qts) of water daily.
14. Meditate around 5-6pm for 5-30 minutes.
15. Eat a light dinner, if hungry–no technology at dinnertime.
16. Keep activities light and easy in the evening, watch less violence before bedtime.
17. Enjoy a warm Epsom salt bath and use dosha-specific oil on skin afterwards.
18. Get to bed around 9 or 10p.
19. Read inspirational material prior to sleeping.
20. No technology in bedroom, if possible.
21. Recapitulation of day's activities for 2 minutes as you close your eyes.
22. Leave a 10-12 oz glass of water by bed & drink first thing the following morning.
23. Lights out by 10:30p.
24. Say your prayers, count your blessings and begin your mantra while drifting off to sleep.
25. Listen to your breath as you silently repeat in a gentle voice "Sleep Now."
    Another good mantra for sleep is "I Am" or the Sanskrit equivalent "So Hum."
26. Keep room dark and quiet or use an eye mask and ear plugs.

If you're not an early riser, then consider exercising after work but before dinner. Room temperature vegetable juice drink or fruit smoothie may be enough as an evening meal once you're eating a hearty lunch; however, consider keeping dinner light and reduce or eliminate bread and dessert on a regular basis. The exact hour isn't as important to me as the spacing of intake and activities. If you awaken at 10am then keep the same schedule, just push the times down a few hours. You should awaken feeling refreshed and invigorated, or after your shower you should feel enlivened and eager for the day. If not, go to bed earlier.

HEALTHFUL HINTS

- Eat only when you feel hungry.
- Eat in a peaceful environment (not near computer or TV).
- Do not eat when you're disturbed or distressed.
- Slow down to eat and pay attention to how your food tastes.
- Set your silverware down three or four times within each meal and notice that you are filling up.
- Stop eating when full; don't overfill stomach. Satiated and satisfied not stuffed.
- Wait 3-4 hours between meals.
- Sitting down to eat offers more circulation in stomach.
- Avoid dashboard dining.
- Don't consume iced drinks with meals.
- Take a short walk after you eat when possible.
- Reduce processed foods, frozen or canned foods & TV dinners.
- Eat more organic food from the Farmer's Markets.
- Intermittent fasting is encouraged. If you finish eating dinner at 7pm, then don't eat breakfast until 7am or later. A 12-hour fast allows the organs to rest.
- Fasting one-day a week or one-day per month reduces toxins.

 ZENERGY BOOST AT THE GROCERY STORE
Use the 6-Tastes Shopping List next time you grocery shop. Consider different nutritional choices to obtain optimal health and emotional wellbeing.

THE GOODNESS OF FOOD

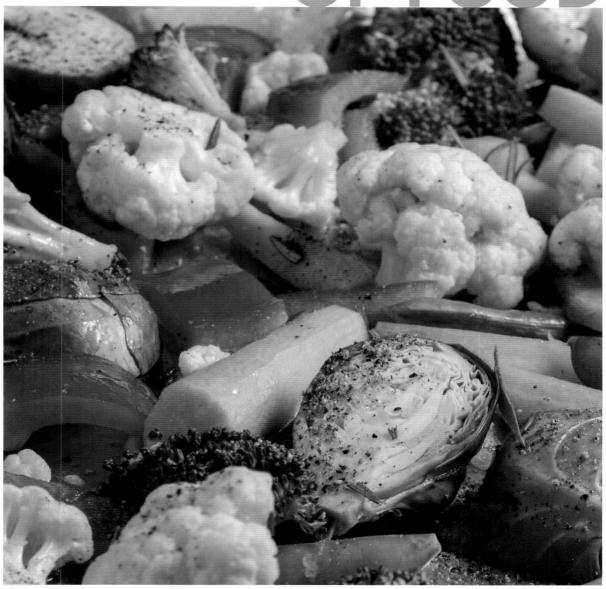

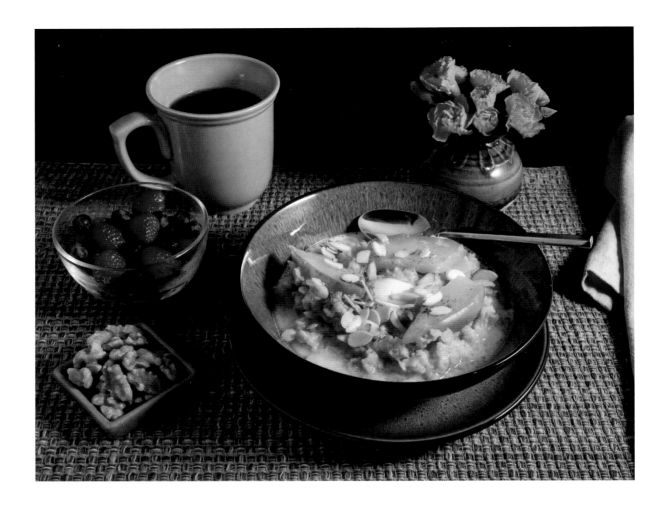

CINNAMON OATMEAL WITH APPLES

Oats are a warm hearty breakfast, ideal to get you grounded and start the day. Oats are nutritious, rich in fiber and B vitamins and lower cholesterol. Include oats in your nutritional plan only two or three times a week if trying to lose weight. Choose regular oats or steel cut oats. Instant oats have low nutritional value. Plain cooked and cooled oats can be used as a comforting treatment for those with itchy or inflamed skin (*pitta* imbalance).

CINNAMON OATMEAL WITH APPLES

Use all 6-Tastes to Maintain Healthy Balance ~

Sweet	Oats, Butter, Nuts, Honey
Sour	Blueberries, Raspberries
Salty	Salt
Bitter	Almonds
Pungent	Cinnamon
Astringent	Apples

RECIPE

½ c oatmeal
¼ c berries
1 T honey
dash of salt
¾ t cinnamon
½ medium sized apple
(You can eat the remaining portion of apple with nut-butter for mid morning snack.)

Dice or slice ½ medium-sized apple and cook with ½ cup oats into ¾ cup water. Add ¾ teaspoon cinnamon. Cook according to directions on oatmeal container and add 2 tablespoons extra water for apple.

Top with nuts, butter, honey and/or berries to taste. Butter has 100 calories per tablespoon so use it sparingly if you're trying to lose weight. Coconut oil is sweet and adds a nice texture to the oats. Berries are sour so consider a bit of local raw honey to sweeten the meal.

Abbreviations:
T=Tablespoon, t=teaspoon, c=cup

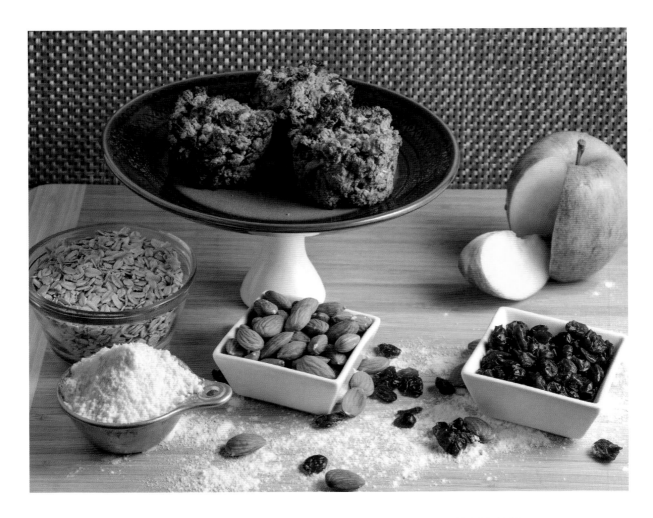

6-TASTES MAGIC MUFFINS

Oats numerous healing properties make this a healthy snack for the whole family anytime of day. Rich in fiber, low in fat, improves digestion, lowers cholesterol, loaded with nutrients and minerals, it's a heart-healthy food for just about everyone. Try gluten-free coconut flour for a delicious substitute. They crumble more but are still very tasty. Also, 1-to-1 Gluten Free Baking Flour is a good substitute. Apples supply antioxidants, fiber, vitamin C and K, potassium and encourage glowing skin. Apples promote weight loss and offer a pre-biotic effect supporting good gut health. Remember the adage is "An apple a day keeps the doctor away" not a banana a day.

6-TASTES MAGIC MUFFINS

Use All 6-Tastes to Maintain Healthy Balance ~

Sweet	Oats
Sour	Raisins
Salty	Salt
Bitter	Almonds
Pungent	Cinnamon
Astringent	Apples

RECIPE

Mix Together

1 ½ c Quaker Oats
(not instant and not steel cut)
1 ½ c oat bran
1 c whole wheat flour or coconut flour
½ c brown sugar
4 t baking powder
1 t salt
2 t cinnamon

In a Separate Bowl

½ c skim milk
(or coconut milk or almond milk)
1 c apple juice
2 eggs
4 T sunflower oil or ghee
4 T honey (¼ c)
2 c diced apples

Blend both mixtures separately. Then combine together and mix again.
Add 2 large diced apples (about 2 cups). Do not forget the apples, as they are a large part of the moisture. Diced not mushy.

Optional Additions (try any or all ingredients)
1 c raisins, 1 c cranberries, 1 c dates, 1 c coconut flakes and/or 1 c chopped nuts
Since the coconut and dates have sugar, you may choose to reduce the brown sugar by half.

Ladle mixture into greased muffin tins, use muffin papers or silicone muffin pan. Bake at 400°
for 25-30 minutes. Enjoy warm from the oven, or slice, toast and serve warm with cream cheese, butter or preserves. Makes 24 muffins.

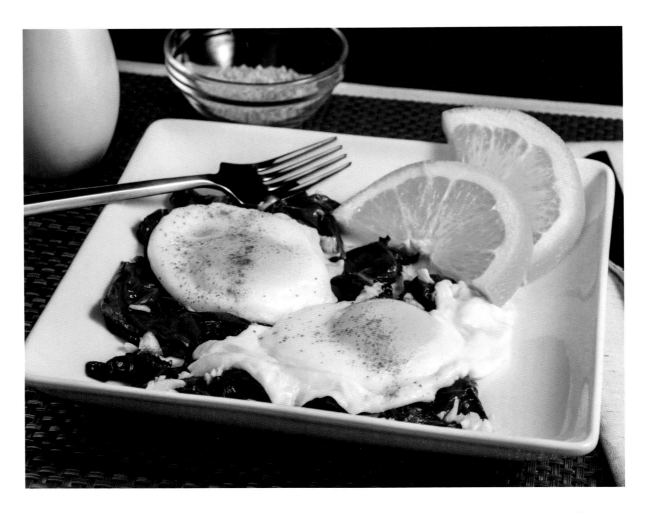

QUICK 6 BREAKFAST: EGGS & SPINACH

The goodness of eggs includes protein, B2, B12, zinc, iron, copper and selenium. Lecithin, found in the yolk, reduces cholesterol and symptoms of memory disorders. This quick morning breakfast gets the day started right. If you're trying to lose weight, do not eat bread or carbs at breakfast time. Cook the eggs anyway you like with sautéed garlic spinach and orange slice garnish to complete the 6-tastes. Slices not juice.

QUICK 6 BREAKFAST: EGGS & SPINACH

Use all 6-Tastes to Maintain Healthy Balance ~

Sweet	Eggs, Ghee
Sour	Orange Slices
Salty	Salt
Bitter	Spinach, Garlic, Rosemary, Turmeric
Pungent	Garlic, Rosemary, Turmeric, Black Pepper
Astringent	Garlic, Turmeric

RECIPE

2 eggs
2 c raw spinach
2 T ghee or oil
1 t garlic
Additional spices as desired
½ t black pepper
½ t turmeric
½ t rosemary

Warm 1 T ghee or 1 T dosha-specific oil (sesame oil for *vata*, olive oil for *pitta*, sunflower for *kapha*). Then add garlic and/or other spices to spark their medicinal powers. (No need to add all four spices to one dish. Choose 2 different spices each time you make this dish.)

Add spinach and sauté for 5 minutes until wilted. Don't over cook as the spices can burn and lose healing property, and the spinach will turn soggy losing its nutritional value.

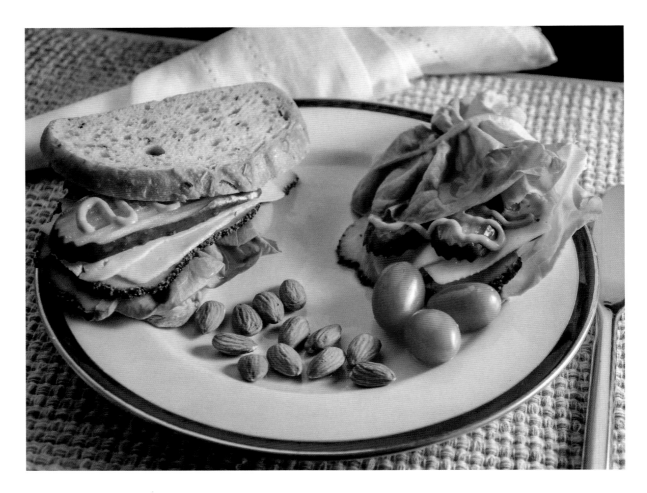

HEARTY OR LITE
TURKEY & CHEESE DELIGHT

Turkey contains zinc, calcium, vitamins D, K, B-6, B-12 and phosphorus. Most celebrated for its tryptophan that boosts serotonin, balancing your mood and even reducing sadness. High in protein and low in fat, turkey increases the metabolism while satisfying your appetite. Sandwiches are a common meal available almost anywhere, and turkey is the best choice of the processed meats. Select freshly baked artisan or gluten-free bread when possible, or lettuce hand wrap for those who are losing weight. Lettuce and tomatoes contain fiber, improve digestion and reduce plaque in arteries. Rich in vitamins, minerals and potassium, tomatoes provide the antioxidant lycopene that reduces risk of disease and improves overall health.

HEARTY OR LITE
TURKEY & CHEESE DELIGHT

Use All 6-Tastes to Maintain Healthy Balance ~

Sweet	Turkey, Bread
Sour	Cheese, Tomatoes, Pickle, Mustard
Salty	Salt
Bitter	Almonds, Lettuce
Pungent	Mustard, Pepper
Astringent	Lettuce

RECIPE

Hearty	**Lite**
1-2 slices of bread	1-2 large pieces of bibb lettuce
2-3 slices of turkey	2-3 slices of turkey
1 slice of cheese	1 slice of cheese
1-2 T mustard	1-2 T mustard
1 pickle	1 pickle
3 tomatoes	3 tomatoes
1 large leaf of lettuce	

Choose thin-sliced and/or sprouted bread stacked with peppered turkey. A fold-over sandwich at noon and another one at 2pm can be quite satisfying without the afternoon energy level dip. Feta, goat or blue cheeses are more pungent and healthier but not commonly found in sandwich shops. Select havarti, munster or jack over American or cheddar. Skip the cheese periodically, especially if trying to lose weight. Cheese is delicious but contains sugar & fat, and can cause extra mucus in the organs that can lead to weight gain and/or sinus infections. Do not eat dairy products while sick! Choose mustard over mayonnaise and crunchy nuts or celery sticks instead of chips when possible. There are many flavors of baked bean chips or nutcrackers available today that are healthier than fried corn chips or potato chips.

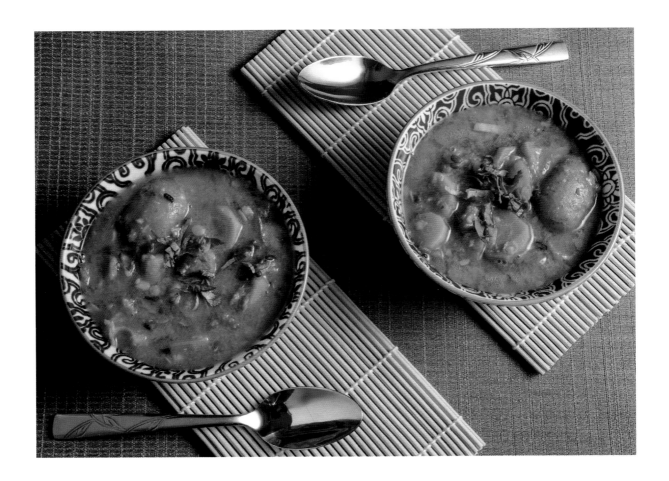

ROBUST LENTIL SOUP CROCKPOT

Lentils fall into the legume family and cover two tastes–sweet and astringent. Lentils are a great source of vegetarian protein, fiber and folate, low in fat, high in potassium, iron and magnesium. Lentils improve digestion, reduce cholesterol, increase healthy gut bacteria and decrease blood sugar levels and insulin. This is a quality meal for everyone, especially Diabetics. Lentils are a delicious warm family meal and easy to microwave at the office the following day.

ROBUST LENTIL SOUP CROCKPOT

Use all 6-Tastes to Maintain Healthy Balance ~

Sweet	Carrots, Bell Peppers
Sour	Garlic, Oregano, Lime Wedge
Salty	Salt, Celery
Bitter	Spinach, Onion, Squash
Pungent	Garlic, Black Pepper, Paprika, Turmeric, Cayenne, Cumin
Astringent	Lentils, Bell Peppers, Cilantro

RECIPE

Veggies

1-2 c fresh spinach (remove stems)
1-2 c celery
1-2 c carrots
1-2 c yellow squash
½ medium sized onion chopped
1 c small potatoes (optional)
1 c bell peppers

Spice Mix

2 T fresh garlic
2 T cumin
1 T turmeric
1 T salt
1 t paprika
1 t black pepper
1 t cilantro garnish

Add to Crockpot 2 cups dry lentils and 7 cups water (or vegetable broth for more flavor). Add 2 Tablespoons coconut oil.

Add 1-2 cups raw coarsely chopped fresh veggies (choose 4-7 different kinds).

In a skillet, prime the spices. Lightly sauté the garlic in a skillet with 3-4 T hot dosha-specific oil (sesame oil for *vata*, olive oil for *pitta*, sunflower for *kapha* & ghee is good for all doshas). Once garlic releases its fragrant aroma, then add dry spice mix for 2-3 minutes. Add the heated spice mix to the Crockpot. Also, rinse spice pan with a small amount of water to clean it and add that water to the Crockpot. Cook for 6-8 hours. Sample the soup and flavor to taste with additional salt or spices. You may need to add 1-2 cups extra water to maintain the soupy goodness.

Consider quinoa, rice or couscous for a hearty meal. If you're trying to lose weight, skip the carbohydrates and spice it up by increasing the paprika or pepper.

Serve in bowl with lime and/or cilantro garnish. Fresh limejuice reduces heats and spikes flavor.

Leftover Option: Remove 2 c and freeze for leftovers. When ready to eat, boil with 1 c vegetable broth for about 20-minutes.

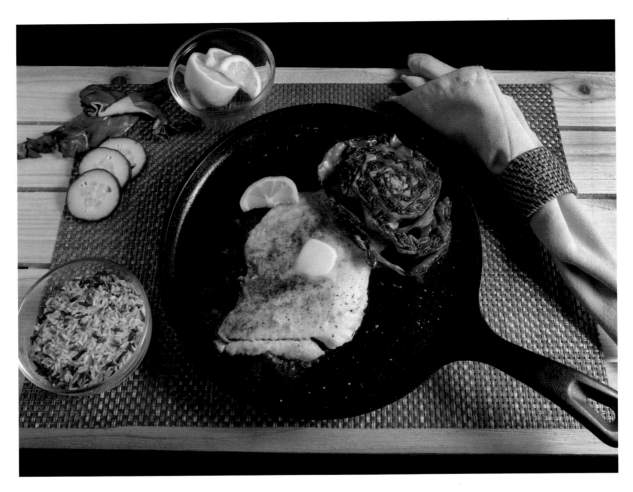

FRESH FLOUNDER AND CABBAGE FLOWER

Baked or grilled flounder is ideal for losing or maintaining weight. Fresh flounder has a delicate sweet taste, high in protein, low in fat and no carbohydrates. All fish have some mercury, and it is recommended to only eat fish about 2-3 times per week. The beautiful purple cabbage flower took the longest to cook (about an hour). Cabbage is rich in nutrients, Vitamin C and K, improves digestion and helps reduce weight, but too much cabbage can lead to flatulence. Add tri-color multigrain rice to finish the dish or, if trying to lose weight, include squash (astringent) or bok choy (bitter) as a secondary vegetable.

FRESH FLOUNDER AND CABBAGE FLOWER

Use all 6-Tastes to Maintain Healthy Balance ~

Sweet	Cucumber, Rice
Sour	Lemon Wedges
Salty	Flounder, Salt
Bitter	Black Pepper, Garlic, Ginger, Turmeric
Pungent	Garlic, Ginger
Astringent	Cabbage, Garlic, Ginger

RECIPE

1 large piece flounder
1 large purple cabbage
½ t salt
½ t black pepper
½ t turmeric

Lightly coat 1-2 large slices of purple cabbage with ghee or dosha-specific oil (sesame oil for *vata*, coconut oil for *pitta*, sunflower for *kapha*). Sprinkle with 3 spices listed above. Cook cabbage at 400° for 50 minutes or until soft. Outside edges may cook quicker and you can remove those from the oven at 35-40 minutes. Keep the center cabbage flower intact.

Steam 1 cup wild rice in 1½ cups filtered water. Follow directions on rice container.

Fish Spice Mix
Lightly dust fish with salt and pepper.
½ t garlic and/or ½ t salt
½ t ginger ½ t pepper

During the final 10 minutes of cabbage and rice cooking, dust flounder with fish spice mix and place flounder on hot griddle. Gently flip at 3 minutes. Be careful flipping, as fish is delicate and can easily break apart.

Serve with lemon and cucumber garnish.

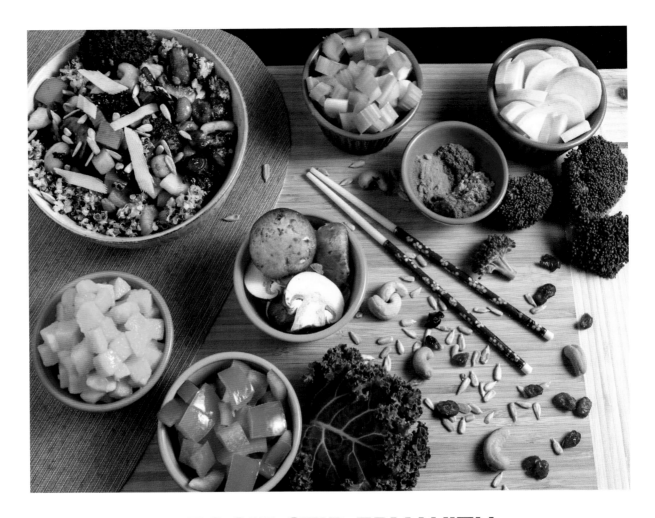

VEGGIE STIR FRY WITH TRICOLOR QUINOA

Benefits of this dish are many because of the variety of colorful vegetables you can choose. Quinoa is a gluten-free sprouted grain and packs a lot of nutrients into each bite. It's a quality carbohydrate for everyone, easily digested with a low-glycemic index and increases metabolism. High in protein, iron, potassium, magnesium and fiber, quinoa also contains healthy omega fats.

VEGGIE STIR FRY WITH TRICOLOR QUINOA

Use all 6-Tastes to Maintain Healthy Balance ~

Sweet	Mushrooms, Celery, Bell Peppers, Seeds, Raw Cashews
Sour	Dried Cranberries
Salty	Salt, Celery, Coconut Aminos
Bitter	Yellow Squash, Kale
Pungent	Rosemary, Cumin, Garlic, Ginger (spices are typically pungent)
Astringent	Broccoli, Butternut Squash, Red Bell Peppers, Sunflower Seeds

RECIPE

1 c broccoli
1 c celery
1 c butternut squash
1 c yellow squash
1 c red bell peppers
1 c sliced mushrooms
¾ c raw cashews
2 T sunflower seeds
½ c dried cranberries

Spice Mix
½ T rosemary
½ T cumin
1 T fresh garlic
½ T ginger

Cook quinoa as directed on the box. Soak 1 cup quinoa in 2 cups water for 2 minutes. Drain then combine 1 cup grain to 2 cups water with a dash of salt. It usually takes about 20 minutes to cook. Start that first.

Next, combine the spice mix into one small bowl. Devein the kale and use only the flowery leaves. In a Wok, heat ½ of the spice mix for 2 minutes with 2 Tablespoons of ghee or dosha-specific oil (sesame oil for *vata*, olive oil for *pitta*, sunflower for *kapha*). Hear it sizzle. Then add kale, broccoli and celery and cook for 6 minutes. Add the remaining ingredients (veggies, nuts, seeds and cranberries) and remainder spice mix for another 5 minutes. Those with delicate digestion should skip the seeds.

Serve the vegetables over the quinoa in a bowl. Salt to taste or use ½ T coconut aminos for a low-sodium delicious salty alternative.

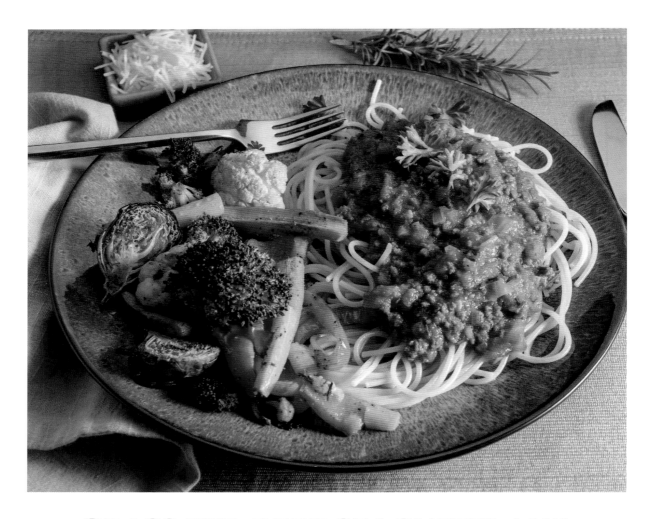

GRASS-FED BEEF SPAGHETTI AND ROASTED VEGGIES

Grass-fed beef has less fat, lower cholesterol, higher levels of antioxidants, vitamin E and A and usually fewer hormones and antibiotics than regular beef. Roasted vegetables are anti-inflammatory and the source of many healthy nutrients including fiber, folic acid, vitamins, and potassium. Spaghetti squash, instead of regular pasta, reduces calories and carbs while still satisfying the appetite. This colorful dish is a tasty beauty for dinner and a quick reheat at lunch the following day. Of course, you can make your own spaghetti sauce or purchase a quality jar of your favorite at the health food store.

GRASS-FED BEEF SPAGHETTI AND ROASTED VEGGIES

Use all 6-Tastes to Maintain Healthy Balance ~

Sweet	Beef, Carrots
Sour	Diced Tomatoes, Oregano
Salty	Salt
Bitter	Onion, Garlic, Broccoli, Rosemary, Spaghetti Squash
Pungent	Garlic, Red Pepper Flakes, Black Pepper, Worcestershire Sauce
Astringent	Parsley, Oregano, Garlic, Brussel Sprouts, Bell Peppers, Snap Peas

Vegetable medley can be comprised of 3-5 different veggies. Choose your favorites, no potatoes.

RECIPE

1 pound grass-fed ground beef
1 medium sized onion
1 jar quality pasta sauce
1 c broccoli
1 medium sized bell pepper (any color)
1 c carrots
1 c snap peas
1 c brussel sprouts
1 spaghetti squash

Vegetable Spice Mix
½ T Rosemary
Sprinkle salt & pepper to taste

Beef Spice Mix
1 T parsley
2 T garlic
½ T red pepper flakes
1 T Worcestershire sauce

Rough cut the vegetables, cover with 2 tablespoons dosha-specific oil (sesame oil for *vata*, olive oil for *pitta*, sunflower for *kapha*, ghee is great for all doshas) and dust with vegetable spice mix. Place on tray and cook at 400° for 50 minutes.

Delicious Pasta Substitute ~ Spaghetti squash is a large yellow vegetable usually only provided at grocery stores during the warm seasons. Cut in half long ways, remove seeds, sprinkle with salt and pepper and turn upside down onto the tray. Fork the back of the squash skin about 8 times for better steaming. Cook at 400° for 40-60 minutes (less for al dente spaghetti or one-hour for softer morsels). Cool for 10-15 minutes. Use a fork to scrape the strands inside creating a spaghetti style appearance. Otherwise, boil your favorite style of pasta in separate pot and follow cooking directions on the spaghetti package. If trying to lose or maintain weight eat beef sauce with spaghetti squash, roasted vegetables, or try gluten-free pasta or quinoa pasta. Keep angel hair pasta nearby in case you don't like the pasta substitutes. Angel hair pasta cooks in about 5 minutes.

Next, heat the beef spices. Hear it sizzle! Add the beef and onions and brown with beef spice mix. Add your choice pasta sauce to beef and meld together for 20 minutes. Voilá!

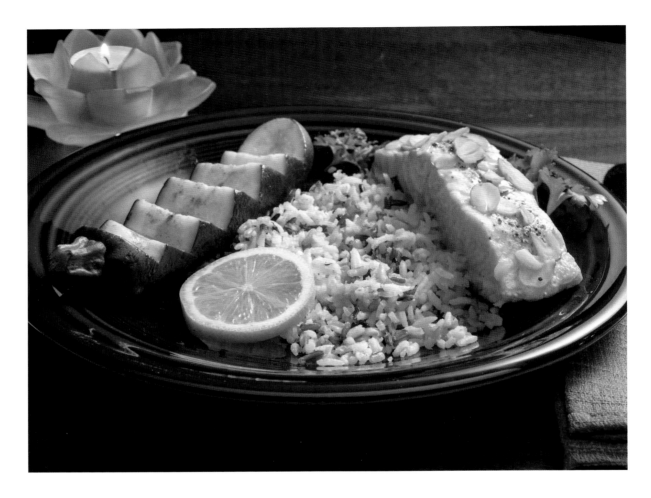

FRESH SALMON AND
ZESTFUL ZUCCHINI BOAT

Baked or grilled salmon is high in B vitamins, potassium, selenium, a great source of protein with the heart-healthy omega-3 fatty acids. Great for weight control, promotes brain health, improves bone density and is anti-inflammatory. All fish have some mercury, and it is recommended to only eat fish about 2-3 times per week. Zucchini improves eyes, thyroid and adrenal functioning, and boosts energy and circulation. Choose organic when possible. Add wild rice to finish the dish or, if trying to lose weight, include a secondary vegetable like asparagus (bitter) or broccoli (astringent).

FRESH SALMON AND ZESTFUL ZUCCHINI BOAT

Use all 6-Tastes to Maintain Healthy Balance ~

Sweet	Nuts, Almond Slivers
Sour	Lemon Wedges
Salty	Salt, Fresh Salmon
Bitter	Garlic
Pungent	Paprika, Black Pepper, Garlic
Astringent	Zucchini, Parsley

RECIPE

1 large piece salmon
1 large organic zucchini
2-4 T almond slivers

Fish Spice Mix
½ t salt and ½ t pepper
½ t garlic and/or
½ t ginger

Veggie Spice Mix
½ t salt
½ t black pepper
½ t paprika

Start with steaming 1 c wild rice in 1 ½ c filtered water. Follow directions on rice container. Dust salmon with fish spice mix and place on baking tray for 20 minutes at 400°. Add almond slivers in the final 3 minutes.

Cut zucchini decoratively or slice down middle. Lightly coat 1-2 large slices of zucchini with ghee or dosha-specific oil (sesame oil for *vata*, coconut oil for *pitta*, sunflower for *kapha*). Sprinkle with veggie spice mix and bake at 400° for 15 minutes or until soft. Once fish has cooked 5 minutes, add the zucchini and bake both together.

Serve with lemon wedges and antioxidant-rich parsley garnish. Both are great for detoxifying.

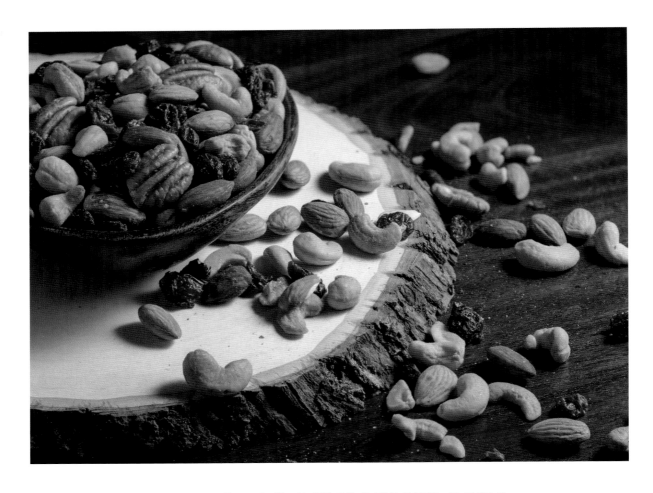

6-TASTES MUNCHIE MIX

Nuts contain quality nutrients and antioxidants that improve overall health. They are high in protein and good fats and low in carbohydrates. Nuts can even reduce symptoms of Type 2 Diabetes. Almonds are great brain food and are high in calcium. Walnuts reduce cholesterol and even depression. Cashews are rich in magnesium and iron. Hazelnuts contain Vitamins B and E and improve digestive health. Pecans are heart healthy and contain beta-sitisterol that boosts the immune system and reduces enlarged prostate. Health food grocers supply bulk nuts that are typically more economical. This is a snack not a meal. Only eat about 2 small handfuls at a time. When you avoid getting hungry through the day you're less likely to eat too much at your next meal. Cravings are an indication that you need a certain taste and frequently don't know which one. When you eat all six tastes at each meal, or at least each day, you will crave less and naturally reduce your weight.

6-TASTES MUNCHIE MIX

Use all 6-Tastes to Maintain Healthy Balance ~

Sweet	All Nuts (pick 3-4 favorites)
Sour	Dried Raisins
Salty	Salt, Salted Nuts
Bitter	Raw Almonds, Cocoa, Cumin
Pungent	Cayenne, Cinnamon
Astringent	Nutmeg, Dried Cranberries

RECIPE

Spicy Mix
1-2 c almonds
½ t cumin
½ t cayenne
½ t salt
1 T sesame oil

Sweet Mix
1-2 c almonds
½ t cinnamon
½ t nutmeg
1 T coconut oil

Place nuts in container with oil to evenly distribute then add seasonings. Roast 1 cup nuts in the selected seasonings (almonds in this example). Do not roast all the nuts in the seasonings. Keep some nuts, or most nuts, raw. Adjust amounts to suit your tastes.

Roast seasoned nuts on cookie sheet at 400° for 10-12 minutes (depends on oven). Wait for the aroma of toasted nuts to fill the air.

While the nuts are roasting, add ½-1 cup each of your 3-4 favorite kinds of nuts to the container. Choose a variety of nuts to suit your taste. Consider using different nuts each time you make the Munchie Mix. Dried fruit is better than a candy bar but still has a lot of sugar so don't overdo the fruit and/or dark chocolate. Choose 4 cups nuts to ¾ cup fruit.

Additional Options

Sour	Dried Apricots, Dried Mango Chunks, Dried Pineapple Chunks, Dried Papaya
Bitter	Dark Chocolate Chips
Pungent	Rosemary, Paprika
Astringent	Dried Cherries, Bananas Chips, Raw Pecans, Macadamia, Hazelnut, Pinenuts, Seeds

If choosing dark chocolate chips, wait until nuts completely cool before adding or the chips will melt.

BEVERAGES

If the screaming kids, honking horns and office back-biters got you down, what ya gonna do? When the yoga, meditation and journaling just ain't working, then consider a KiTini. Create your favorite ritual while enjoying a relaxing cocktail or mocktail. Consider this affirmation with each sip… "I am happy and peaceful NOW!"

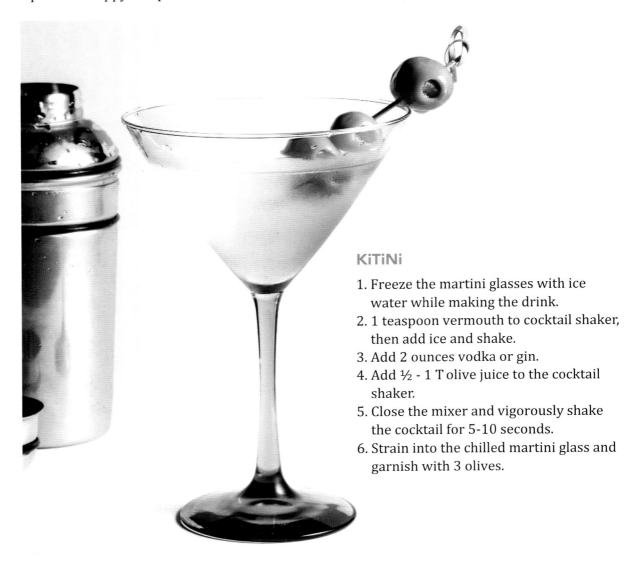

KiTiNi

1. Freeze the martini glasses with ice water while making the drink.
2. 1 teaspoon vermouth to cocktail shaker, then add ice and shake.
3. Add 2 ounces vodka or gin.
4. Add ½ - 1 T olive juice to the cocktail shaker.
5. Close the mixer and vigorously shake the cocktail for 5-10 seconds.
6. Strain into the chilled martini glass and garnish with 3 olives.

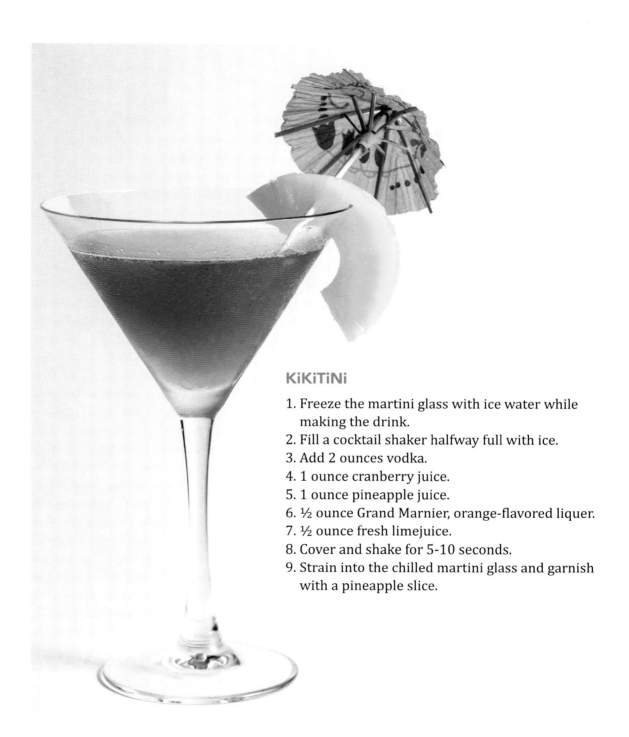

KiKiTiNi

1. Freeze the martini glass with ice water while making the drink.
2. Fill a cocktail shaker halfway full with ice.
3. Add 2 ounces vodka.
4. 1 ounce cranberry juice.
5. 1 ounce pineapple juice.
6. ½ ounce Grand Marnier, orange-flavored liquer.
7. ½ ounce fresh limejuice.
8. Cover and shake for 5-10 seconds.
9. Strain into the chilled martini glass and garnish with a pineapple slice.

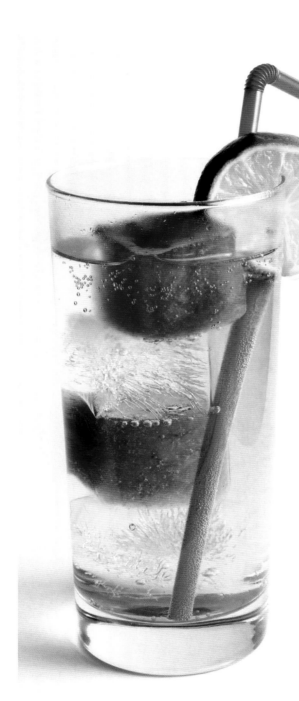

CRANBERRY MOCKTiNi

1. Freeze 50/50 cranberry juice into ice cubes.
   Add 2-4 cubes to a tall glass.
2. Fill with plain or flavored club soda.
   Lime flavored in this recipe.
3. Add lime squeeze and watch the ice cubes melt.

SLEEPYTiNi

1. Warm 2 cups almond, pecan, cashew or coconut milk (no dairy before bedtime).
2. Add 1 T turmeric and ½ tsp cinnamon.
3. Small piece of fresh peeled ginger root or ¼ tsp ginger powder.
4. 1 t to 1 T honey or maple syrup.
5. Serve warm in a coffee mug and head to bed.

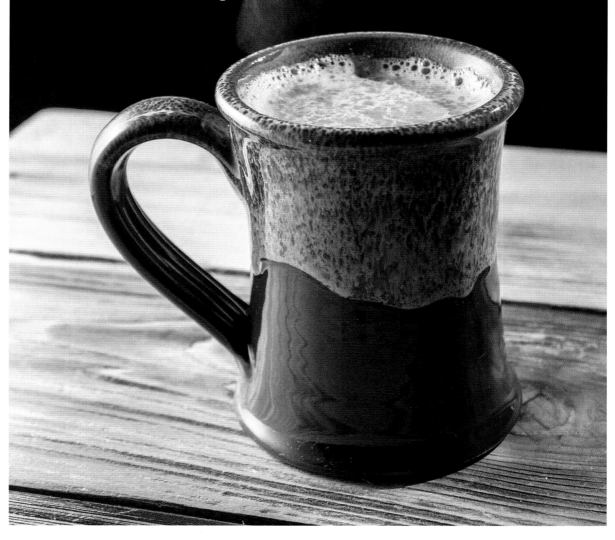

SPIRITUALIZING YOUR FOOD

Purify your meal by holding an attitude of gratitude while preparing the food or waiting for its delivery to your table. Ask God's power and protection over the body to increase effectiveness of the nutrients in the delicious food so that your body and mind collaborate efficiently. Keep it simple. Repeating "thank you" is an easy way to meditate while you cook or wait for your food. Reciting a prayer is also a wonderful way to shift gears and pay attention to the food preparation process. Offering a vocal or silent prayer of appreciation to the Creator for the people who prepared and presented the food or delivered it to your grocery store, as well as the nutrients themselves, offers a mindful practice that has been lost by many. Occasionally, think back to the farmer who originally harvested the commodity and all the hands that touched the product on its way to your mouth. Feel that connection to all that is with a bite or each bite. Elevating your consciousness around food sets the tone for a reverent and joyful dining experience. Think only kind and loving thoughts while preparing your food. You can recite prayers, sing hymns or chant during food preparation, either silently or vocally, and infuse the food with your loving vibrations. Intermingle cooking with spiritual devotion. Reinforcing a higher vibration through prayer and chanting transforms your kitchen into a spiritual nutritious altar.

We frequently eat with our eyes, so take a moment and look at your meal. During this time, notice that you're salivating and excited to eat that appetizing meal. Raising your hands over your food and giving Reiki to your meal enhances it with divine life force. (See Spiritual Section for more information on Reiki.) The simple act of charging your food with positive intent makes a significant difference in the way you digest and metabolize it. You can do this visibly or in your mind's eye. Prayer is about intent and others do not need to witness your acts of reverence for their delivery to Great Spirit.

Marvel that your body knows exactly how to build the appropriate cellular structure to maintain health from the food you eat. Give thanks and gratitude to your body for brilliantly knowing how to transform the flavorful food into your cellular structure of bone, tissue, hair and blood. The body offers us a unique place to experience all the senses and a multitude of encounters throughout a lifetime. Mistakenly, your body doesn't produce wrist cells at your ankle or an extra ear on your abdomen. Your miraculous physical form converts the nutrients for cellular rejuvenation and maintains proper functioning. Consciously feel gratitude for your food and body, and notice how your digestion improves in all seven tissues (plasma, blood, muscle, fat, bone, grey matter and reproductive tissues).

Maintain a pleasant conversation during mealtime or eat in silence. Providing a comfortable environment at mealtime can strengthen the family unit and activate a higher consciousness while eating. Avoid technology during meals but if you must, choose positive upbeat shows and eliminate watching violence, especially while eating. Even if you forgot all the ritual with food preparation and started eating anyway, you can still take a moment at any time during a meal, silently or vocally, to say a word of gratitude. Purposing a simple toast at any time during a meal like "to a wonderful meal with wonderful people" can casually bless it without being too ceremonial. Thoughtfulness toward your food and during the dining experience opens the door to creating better health and happiness.

ZENERGY BOOST TO SPIRITUALIZE YOUR DINING EXPERIENCE
Listen to calming ambient music, chants or hymns while cooking next time. Pray for better digestion and nutrient absorption and notice your health improve.

DETOXING

DO YOU NEED TO DETOX?

Today we have countless magazines and TV networks dedicated entirely to food, not to mention the all-you-can-eat banquet-style buffet restaurants that encourage binging and gorging. "Don't forget your ice cream on the way out the door, Ma'am." America will ultimately starve in its lavish lifestyle. When you look at the basic Western diet, you come to realize why poor health is so common now. Granted, some people can eat junk food and not feel the toxins flowing through their blood stream, but what does true vitality actually feel like? If you've been eating fast food since elementary school then you might not realize just how toxic your body is. How can you compare your current poor health to your potential good health? When you have too many toxins in the body, the liver cannot produce enough enzymes to metabolize proteins, fats and carbohydrates properly. The kidneys fill with debris causing strain on the filtering system. The intestines pack with rancid food that putrefies and sits in the center of your body slowing or even stopping the elimination process. If you don't go to the bathroom daily, then food is rotting in your gut. You might not notice it this month or year but over time that corrosive food clogging your organs will cause all types of diseases. Being fat, belching, farting, constipation, sinus infections, colds, bodily aches and leg cramps are a few symptoms of imbalance that can easily be improved with a detox.

Alopathic Medicine or Western Medicine is entirely focused on the symptoms of poor health and not resolving the root cause. Toxic overload affects every area of your health, and most of us totally ignore it. Talk to any Naturopathic or Functional Medicine Doctor, and they will tell you to detox first or you will not heal. Think about it, fish cannot live in toxic water, no matter how well you feed them! Daily exposure to pollutants in the air, water, foods and even personal care and cleaning products impact your health. Frequently, a 1-day to 10-day detox can be very useful.

Signs you need to Detox
• Coated Tongue and/or Bad Breath
• Allergies, Congestion or Sinus Infection
• Lowered Immune Function
• Weight Gain
• Cravings
• Headaches
• Skin Problems/Acne

- Yeast Infections
- Impotency
- Digestive Problems or Abdominal Bloating
- Inflammation
- Joint Pain
- Gallbladder Issues or You Had it Removed
- Insomnia
- Recurring Acid Reflux

Try One of these Simple Detoxes for 1-10 days

1. **Eat all the vegetables that you want.** Pig Out! Steam or lightly sauté your choice of vegetables in sesame oil. While detoxing it is preferred to eat food that is not raw but also not overcooked. Limit only one large baked potato for the entire 10 days. 2 pats butter or 2 T of coconut oil is acceptable. Otherwise, skip potatoes.
2. **Eliminate Dairy** as it can create excess mucus in the body.
3. **Eliminate Bread, Pasta and Rice.** The body slows down while digesting refined carbs. Replace grains with quinoa, steel cut oats or buckwheat or eat one-half sandwich with gluten-free bread.
4. **Eat Smaller Meals Throughout the Day.** If you eat every 2-3 hours then you will stop gorging. The body can digest a small meal quicker providing more energy and efficiency to the system. Eating half a meal at noon and the other half at 2:00p can provide the vitality you need to finish the workday with zest and vigor. Eat your largest meal between 10am-2pm.
5. **Apple Diet.** Eat as many apples as you want for 3 days. On the evening of the third night ingest a big dose of quality olive oil (2 teaspoons up to 6 tablespoons). Stay near a toilet that evening and the next day for ultimate elimination. Red and Golden Delicious brand was most recommended by Edgar Cayce. Choose apples grown as close to you as possible and preferably organic. Drink plenty of water and relax over the weekend. Visit *www.EdgarCayce.org* for more details.

During a detox, drink only 1 cup of coffee each day, preferably without any condiments. Drink only warm filtered water. You can add lemon or fresh ginger to the water, as desired.

Detoxing is intended to eliminate build-up of waste. Some people experience mild discomfort like nausea, diarrhea or headaches during a cleanse. Also, you're more likely to move slower or be introverted, so give yourself time to be alone and get to bed early. If reactions occur that are too unpleasant, then discontinue the cleanse. If necessary, consult a physician. Take your measurements in advance. You may not notice a decrease on the scale, but you will see a change in your physique.

Benefits of Detoxing

1. Lowered Inflammation
2. Decrease in Inches (maybe not pounds)
3. Weight Management
4. Better Digestion
5. Improved Sleep
6. More Vitality
7. Balanced Blood Sugars (especially for Diabetics)
8. Shinier Hair
9. Become more Patient and Forgiving
10. Better Sex

If you haven't achieved physiological improvements from your pharmaceuticals within three-six months, consider talking to your doctor about your prescription. You may need to reassess the current line of treatment. Remember, many doctors get a kick-back or a "reimbursement" (sometimes up to 6%) for prescribing certain medicines, including chemotherapy ("The Quest for the Cure," video by Ty Bolinger, 2015). Occasionally, a disease diagnosis is inaccurate. Research your symptoms to learn more about the potential causes. Double check the information provided regarding the side effects of your current pharmaceuticals to see if your symptoms (or new symptoms) are drug related.

When you have true vitality it's easy to walk a block or a flight of stairs. Your libido increases and you can enjoy sex without huffing & puffing (until the end). You regain your curiosity for new ideas and activities. A toxic body can lead to toxic thoughts. You communicate more effectively when you are less toxic. Don't waste another month on that typical mainstream diet. You deserve a better future.

Additional Ways to Detox

1. Ask the representative at your health food store for detox supplements.
2. Juicing ~ room temperature raw vegetable & fruit juice ~ not recommended for those with IBS or similar illnesses. Fruits are not recommended for Diabetics.
3. Drink More Water ~ drink up to one gallon slowly throughout the day. The kidneys can accommodate about ½ cup of water per ½ hour.
4. Change your cook wear ~ discard aluminum or Teflon pots & pans.
5. Lymphatic Massage ~ light healing touch (discussed in Integrative Therapies chapter).
6. Practice Gentle or Restorative Yoga or Yoga Nidra.

CASTOR OIL PACKS FOR DETOXING

Edgar Cayce (1877-1945) is considered the Father of Holistic Medicine. His contributions to humanity are far-reaching in many areas of mind, body and spirit. He offered remarkable remedies for health, healing, diet, dreams and spirituality. In the 1920s, 30s and 40s, Mr. Cayce entered periods of self-induced sleep-like trance in which he diagnosed illness and prescribed medical treatments for many people whom he never met. Initially through a photo and later just through a name, he could aid those who frequently were condemned as "hopeless" with remedies that he himself had never studied. Edgar Cayce is one of the most documented American Psychics in the 20th Century, and his 14,000 readings are cross-referenced and available for public review today at the Association for Research and Enlightenment in Virginia Beach, Virginia. Well before his time, many of Cayce's teachings concur with modern schools of thought such as The Law of Attraction popularized now in *The Secret*. See *EdgarCayce.org* to learn more details about castor oil packs and the plethora of Edgar Cayce natural remedies.

Castor oil packs were recommended for just about every organ and have a medical effect on the autonomic nervous system. Highly effective and messy to use, the packs provide a soothing effect wherever placed. Recommended for liver, stomach and intestinal detoxification, constipation, ringworm, skin conditions, arthritis, tumors, breast sensitivity, lymph stimulation, reproduction of hair, sciatic relief and more. Tens of thousands of people have tried this natural remedy with wonderful success.

Materials Needed for Castor Oil Pack
1. White wool flannel pack (unbleached wool)
2. 2 Plastic sheets (big trash bag will suffice)
3. Hot water bottle or heating pad
4. 1-2 Towels

Place a towel on the bed and cover with a plastic sheet or big trash bag where you will recline for one hour. Saturate flannel in cold-pressed castor oil. Pre-warm the oil, if possible. Place oil-soaked flannel directly on skin at treated area. Cover body with another plastic wrap and a towel. A cut plastic bag wrapped around entire body and a towel on the outside prevents soiling the bed. Lie down on the bed for one hour. Use a heat source to drive the oil into the skin. A heat lamp, or hot water bottle, provides a safe source for heating the pack. A heating pad will suffice but is not suggested because of the electromagnetic field it produces. Shower and cleanse skin afterwards with warm water and baking soda. Packs can be reused if flannel is not stained or dark afterwards. If soiled, acquire a new pack. Do not share packs. It is recommended to apply castor oil pack once a day for 20-60 minutes for three days in a row at the same hour.

DETOXIFYING THE SKIN

What goes ON the skin goes IN the skin. Your skin is the largest organ of your body. "Many cheap lotions and cosmetics include parabens, a synthesized preservative. Certain pharmaceutical products also contain chemicals. While the 'jury is still out' regarding the safety of parabens in America, "cumulative exposure to the chemicals from several different products could be overloading our bodies and contributing to a wide range of health problems. 'Of greatest concern is that parabens are known to disrupt hormone function, an effect that is linked to increased risk of breast cancer and reproductive toxicity,' reports the non-profit Campaign for Safe Cosmetics (CSC). Parabens mimic estrogen by binding to estrogen receptors on cells. Research has shown that the perceived influx of estrogen beyond normal levels can in some cases trigger reactions such as increasing breast cell division and the growth of tumors" (*Scientific American*, Should People Be Concerns About Parabens in Beauty Products).

According to the NIH, "Disruption of the endocrine homoeostasis might lead to multidirectional implications causing disruption of fitness and functions of the body and produce adverse developmental, reproductive, neurological, and immune effects in both humans and wildlife" (National Institute of Environmental Health Sciences). The chemicals in most lotions extend the shelf life of the product, not yours. By law, American companies are not obligated to disclose what ingredients incorporate their product's "fragrance," and the term is used to describe over 3,000 chemical ingredients. Additionally, mineral oil is a byproduct of petroleum refinement and is commonly used in baby lotion. Detoxifying the skin by reducing or eliminating cheap lotions not only can improve your skin but also your overall health. What you apply to your skin is almost like drinking it. Be mindful when purchasing personal care items, and choose healthier products in the future. Visit *ewg.org* for a list of clean products.

Drinking plenty of water is an effective way to detoxify the entire body and especially the skin. Drink one large glass of warm water upon awakening in the morning (about 10-12 oz) and continue throughout the day drinking approximately ½ cup per ½ hour. Don't underestimate the power of bathing in clean clear water. The skin will absorb some of the water through the pores and this helps to purify the cellular structure. Do not add bubbles or Epsom salt, just soak in clean plain water once a week.

Dry brushes have been around for decades and are making a comeback. As the Natural Healthcare Industry expands, more people are learning about the benefits of dry brushing. It's a natural exfoliator, cleans all the pores and increases lymphatic drainage. The soft natural hair and long wooden handle make it easy to brush the entire body. Some report it even reduces cellulite (*WellnessMama.com*, April, 2018). Stroke or brush the skin from the bottom up or outside in.

Begin brushing from the feet and ankles upward toward the heart and from the fingertips to the shoulders toward the heart. Move in long strokes to assist the circulation of lymph back toward the heart for cleansing and purification. Be sure to brush under the armpits. Lymph glands are located throughout the body, mainly in the armpits, shoulders, neck and groin. The lymph fluid contains infection-fighting white blood cells and rids the body of toxins, and dry brushing cleans the skin, improving overall vitality (*MayoClinic.com*).

Quality Oils, Nature's Skin Moisturizer
Sesame oil seems to be the fail-safe for almost all skin types ~ dry, sensitive or moist. The Chopra Center recommends it for all doshas and all orifices. **Grape seed oil** can help strengthen and repair damaged or broken capillaries and blood vessels and has a high amount of Vitamin E and not much of an odor. Aromatic oils like **coconut and olive** stimulate the olfactory system and nourish the liver and potentially reduce the risk for breast cancer in contrast to other vegetable oils. Studies on individuals with dry skin show that **coconut oil** can improve the moisture and lipid content. Integrative Medicine Medical Leader Dr. Andrew Weil recommends evening **primrose oil, black currant oil** and **borage oil** as good sources of GLA (gamma-linolenic acid), which promote healthy growth of skin, hair and nails. If you have oily or acne-prone skin, consider using mud clay masks to dry the skin naturally. Cooked and cooled oatmeal packs provide a useful mask for both inflamed skin and oily skin.

ZENERGY BOOST FOR DETOXING
Daily *abyanga*, self-massage, is recommended with dosha-specific oil. In the morning, briskly stroke your skin and firmly massage your muscles to increase circulation, lubricate joints and awaken the body. In the evening, use slow gentle stokes to calm the nerves, move lymph for detoxifying and prepare the body for rest. Stroke from extremities inward toward heart.

TOP DIGESTION STRESSORS

Many people eat when they are stressed with little or no awareness of what they are popping into their mouths. If you have general aches and discomfort or don't digest your food easily, consider eliminating one or two of the following stressors to detoxify your body.

1. **Bad Fats** ~ avoid anything fried.
2. **Overeating** ~ too much of a good thing makes it a bad thing. You can eat it all, just not on the same day. Your stomach can comfortably hold only one plate of food not two or three. Slow down and push away from the buffet. Get a to-go box.
3. **Eating When Stressed,** or more specifically eating when you're crying, can cause acid reflux and other digestion stressors.
4. **Ingesting ice cold drinks** with meals challenges digestion.
5. **Dairy** can cause constipation and excess mucus. Sprinkle it through your weekly nutrition. Don't eat daily.
6. **Alcohol** by itself can cause digestion discomfort and the hangovers also cause a tendency to overeat and drink more the next day. Limit consumption and/or only drink on weekends.
7. **Sugar** ~ refined white sugar is highly addictive, like cocaine. If you have a sweet tooth eat more fruit.
8. **Refined Carbohydrates** ~ white flour, cheap white bread, pastries, cookies and processed grains clog the intestinal track.
9. **Caffeine** ~ drink only 1-2 cups daily.
10. **Red meat**, processed meats, pickled pigs feet, spam, and other questionable meats, take days to digest fully. Eat sparingly or not at all.

DIRTY DOZEN AND CLEAN FIFTEEN

Over the last decade agricultural farmers increased their pesticides by more than 20X, but the increase in pesticide usage has been growing exponentially each decade. No wonder you feel toxic. The Environmental Working Group delivers its "Dirty Dozen" annual report highlighting the most pesticide-laden fruits and vegetables. Nearly two-thirds of America's produce is covered with pesticide residues and many of those are carcinogenic. The American people are asking for organic food but until the government stops subsidizing established corporations and foreign governments and starts focusing on feeding the citizens, we may just remain the proverbial guinea pig until we die a short life.

USDA economists reported that organic produce sales spiked from $5.4 billion in 2005 to $15 billion in 2014. USDA's Economic Research Service estimates that the organically produced food sector, though just 4 percent of all U.S. food sales, has enjoyed double-digit growth in recent years. The trend is predominantly strong for sales of organic fruits and vegetables, which is the primary portion of all organic food sales. Also, it's good to know that with all the laws the U.S. lawmakers enforce they have no special rules for pesticide residues in baby food. If you want real change, vote with your pocketbook. Buy organic, even if its only one item each time you visit the grocery store.

It is recommended that you avoid the dirty dozen or only buy that type of produce organically grown. The clean fifteen indicates the fruits and vegetables that are safely produced by conventional methods; however, please wash all your produce well, soak in diluted apple cider vinegar, or even shave the skin when appropriate. This list is modified annually.

Dirty Dozen/Avoid or Buy Organic
1. Apples
2. Celery
3. Nectarines
4. Strawberries
5. Grapes
6. Peaches
7. Spinach
8. Sweet Bell Peppers
9. Cucumbers
10. Cherry Tomatoes
11. Cherries
12. Potatoes

Clean Fifteen
1. Avocadoes
2. Sweet Corn
3. Pineapples
4. Cabbage
5. Sweet Peas
6. Onions
7. Asparagus
8. Mangoes
9. Papaya
10. Kiwi
11. Eggplant
12. Grapefruit
13. Cantaloupe
14. Cauliflower
15. Honeydew Melons

Learn more about your fruits and vegetables and how to cause change in your community. Check out the Environmental Working Group's website at *www.ewg.org*.

NUTRITIONAL TIPS

- Aquire bags of fruits and veggies from your bulk grocer. Having fresh fruit around the house is a great way to satisfy your sweet tooth without the guilt.
- Fruit and nuts are a good combination.
- Fruit smoothies are a great way to satisfy the sweet tooth. You can add some nut butter as well to reduce the glycemic index.
- Frozen grapes are delicious for the hot summer afternoons.
- Cut veggies and leave them in small containers in the refrigerator for food-on-the-go. Grab a few bags on your way out the door.
- Eat organic when possible.
- Provide bowls of fresh raw almonds around the house and in the refrigerator. Almonds offer brain-boosting healthy fats, especially helpful when sitting in day seminars, conferences or other types of meetings.
- Cook a platter of chicken breasts or legs and cut into small strips. Leave in the refrigerator as ready-to-eat snacks.
- Choose red wine over white wine.
- Beer has a lot of calories, carbohydrates and makes you fat fast; try vodka and drink less.
- Water down your juices and Gatorade if you must drink them at all. They have high sugar and carbohydrate content.
- Try the 50% less sugar or low sodium items when available.
- Boil a dozen eggs. Peel them and leave in the refrigerator. Quick and easy protein when on-the-go.
- Place a glass of water by your bedside at night (8-10 oz) and drink it first thing in the morning. It's room temperature (the warmer, the better) and therefore easy for the body to assimilate.
- Instead of showering, take a bath once a week. Sitting in plain water is good for the body. No oils or bubbles. Your skin is soluble and will absorb some of the water.
- For pain management, consider taking an Epsom Salt Soak once a week.
- Use oils as a skin moisturizer instead of lotions. The skin is soluble. What goes on the skin goes in the skin. Many lotions are filled with petroleum, formaldehyde, MSG and other artificial fillers that steal water from your skin, the largest organ in your body. Consider grapeseed, sesame or coconut oils.
- Eat your water! Eat watermelons, cantaloupe, honey melons, cucumbers and celery. They're loaded with water and fiber. Great for the digestive track.
- Exchange coffee for tea periodically.

HOW TO LOSE 10 POUNDS FAST

- Eat Less and Exercise More.
- Only eat when you're hungry. Stop when you're full. Sit down to eat.
- Pray that your body uses the food for its highest good. Spiritualize your food.
- If you're not hungry for breakfast, then eat around 10a.
- Fasting is rarely recommended, but it can be useful to shrink the stomach initially. 12-14 hour fasts are easier if you're sleeping for most of that time.
- Skip one meal once a week; fast one-full day once a month or once a quarter.
- Drink more water ~ ½ - 1 gallon daily.
- Exchange sandwich bread with sprouted tortillas or, better yet, lettuce wraps.
- Sip warm water or tea during meals or skip beverages entirely. Reduce diluting digestive acids.
- Eat less salt and salty foods.
- 2 hours before bedtime, drink 1 oz apple cider vinegar diluted with 1 cup water and add 1 T raw local honey.
- Try an organic vegetable juice fast for one meal or one day or a week.
- Take your vitamins.
- Floss and brush your teeth more often.
- Stop eating mints and candy after each meal. Try fennel seeds instead.
- Take the stairs instead of the elevator, especially after a meal.
- Park at the far end of the parking lot. Exchange your 'parking space angels' with 'fat fighting angels.'
- Have a walkie-talkie with friends or colleagues. Instead of meeting for a meal, meet at the park for a walk. Instead of sitting in the office, meet in the fitness center on treadmills side by side. Record your notes with voice activation device on your phone instead of writing them down.
- Visualize yourself thin.
- Create a vision board with images of the body that you want then place a photo of your face on top. Truly SEE yourself thin.
- Place sticky notes on your mirrors and affirm you're ideal weight daily. (i.e., "I love weighing 150 pounds.")
- Try hypnosis for weight loss. It has proven results.
- Reduce or eliminate mayonnaise. Use more mustard, hummus or avocado.
- Reduce or eliminate butter. Use oils ~ sesame, coconut, olive and grapeseed.
- Reduce or eliminate sugar. Exchange it with stevia, xlylotol, honey or fresh fruit.
- Reduce or eliminate ice-cold beverages and foods. Just have tea, don't add the ice. Usually it's cool enough anyway.
- Eat all 6-Tastes at every meal or at least every day.

INTEGRATIVE AND NATURAL THERAPIES

MIND-BODY INTEGRATION

Millions of people will see a doctor or medical professional this year for symptoms that diagnostic equipment cannot identify. For many, the cause of the illness is stress. The symptoms are real and may occur anywhere in the body, but the origin is unknown. Psychosomatics was introduced during the Greek Era (1200-800 BCE and attention on it waxed and waned over the centuries. The word caught hold again around 1938 and was applied to physical disorders with psychological causes (like anorexia nervosa and this philosophy continues today but with little media attention.

Dr. John Sarno wrote several books introducing his groundbreaking research on TMS (Tension Myoneural Syndrome) and his bestselling book *Healing Back Pain: The Mind-Body Connection* (1991) sold millions of copies mostly through word of mouth. Tens of thousands assert to have been cured of back pain (and generalized pain) just by reading his books and the books of his famed patient, Steven Ozanich.

Dr. Sarno's movie, *All the Rage* (2017 explains that 100 million Americans suffer from pain and many are on pharmaceutical drugs, steroid injections, and implantable drug delivery systems or had surgery, and none of the current treatments prevent chronic pain. We spend more on pain management than cancer, diabetes and heart disease. Chronic pain costs exploded from $56 billion in 1986 to $210 billion in 2001 and $636 billion in 2012. Why are we getting worse if we are spending that much money on medical care? Dr. Sarno upheld that most non-traumatic occurrences of chronic pain, including back pain, gastrointestinal disorders, headaches and fibromyalgia, are a physical expression of underlying psychological anxieties. Dr. Sarno aided millions in getting to the bottom line of their issues. It's not just "in your head" and therefore the pain isn't real. Oh no, that is real pain, but the real question is, "What is the origination of that pain?" Go to the source of your concerns to dissolve the discomfort. Dr. Sarno proved that by becoming aware of your internal dialogue of life's daily challenges you can alleviate many aches and pains, regardless of how long you've had them. The mind-body connection is real.

Quantum Physicist, Researcher and Author Dr. Joe Dispenza also documented natural healing and spontaneous remissions in his most recent book *Becoming Supernatural: How Common People are doing the Uncommon* (2017. In fact, tens of thousands will experience a spontaneous remission each year, but many won't report it except to their friends and the doctor's account is that the patient stopped coming. The acclaimed Quantum Physicist educates about the quantum field of pure potential and if you can imagine being healthy then you can achieve it. All possibilities exist right now and are available to us right now. We just keep choosing the thoughts that don't support the healthy outcomes we really want. Choosing cynicism and reaffirming day after day that you feel awful not only generates biochemistry to support your thoughts but the corresponding aches and pains. Consequently, you may have a good day but miss it because your pessimism outweighs what great feelings you actually have. Dr. Dispenza teaches meditation techniques to transcend a health crisis, even those lasting years. Thousands report health and healing from reading his books, attending his retreats and practicing his meditation methods. He lays the groundwork for believing that your thinking is contributing to, if not outright causing, your pain, and then gives a new plan of action to transform your future.

Founder of Hay House Publishing Louise Hay wrote the health classic *You Can Heal Your Life* (1984) and millions purchased her book over the past decades. Ms. Hay has a simple and systematic approach to healing the mind and body through the use of affirmations. She provides a simple body-mind-emotion dictionary for easy reference. A basic example is that the back is associated with support and feeling supported in life. Specifically, low back pain is connected with financial fear and not feeling supported in life. She recommends countering the negative thoughts associated with finances by affirming, "I trust the process of life. All I need is always taken care of. I am safe." Her main philosophy is "Every thought we think is creating our future and releasing resentments will dissolve even cancer." She healed herself of cervical cancer that she contracted after being raped as a young woman.

The Adverse Childhood Experience Study came out in 1999. Dr. David Clarke headed the study and his clinic performed 18,000 routine checkups over 20 years. Patients were asked about Adverse Childhood Experiences (ACEs), which included the following:
1. Physical Abuse
2. Emotional Abuse
3. Sexual Abuse
4. Physical Neglect
5. Emotional Neglect
6. Substance Abuse
7. Parental Divorce
8. Mental Illness
9. Mother was Abused
10. Incarcerated Relative

Those patients who had four or more of these ACEs, compared to those who had none, found that they were three times more likely to suffer from multiple bodily symptoms, twice as likely to be obese, have emphysema and on the average died 20 years younger, yet they were decades removed from childhood stress. With appropriate attention to excavating the wounded inner child, you can overcome the physical issues or diseases you may be experiencing which may have originated when you were a child. Founder of the Arizona Center for Integrative Medicine Dr. Andrew Weil states, "Mind-body practices are low cost and low-tech interventions. You can spend an hour a day exercising or 20 minutes a day relaxing or 10 seconds taking a pill which doesn't work, weakens your organs and quite likely will give you other symptoms (side effects)."

I invite you to read some of the above-mentioned books to gain a comprehensive understanding on this topic. These are just a few examples of established authors and doctors who are strong proponents of "thoughts are things." We can heal the body by healing the mind. Just a simple statement like "I am worthy of peace and health," even if you don't believe that you deserve it, will begin to transform your outlook. Continuously making that statement to yourself hundreds of times each day will ultimately lead you to the belief of being worthy of health and healing, not hope but belief. Belief is stronger. You start to see evidence of peaceful moments when you start appreciating your body exactly how it is today. Wisdom and a positive outlook open the door to your ultimate vitality!

PLACEBO EFFECT

Your mind is more powerful than you think. Have you ever worried yourself sick? Many of us have spent all night imagining the worst-case scenario initiating a stress cold or tummy ache. Thank goodness most of those erroneous thoughts never came to pass. The opposite is true too. You can think yourself well. According to *MedicineNet.com*, "the Placebo effect is a remarkable phenomenon in which a fake treatment, an inactive substance like sugar, distilled water, or saline solution, can sometimes improve a patient's condition simply because the person has the expectation that it will be helpful." For hundreds of years, doctors have known that when a patient with a health condition expects their symptoms to improve, they often do.

Every experimental medical treatment includes a placebo as an additional measurement for the drug, therapy or remedy. It has been found in countless experiments that your mind can deliver the same effect as a pill. With a mind like that, wouldn't you want to explore it? You come equipped with your own pharmaceutical store in your brain. Albeit, not every brain can manufacture every drug known to mankind but, according to the American Cancer Society, 1 in 3 people experience a positive change in symptoms after the consumption of a placebo. About 33% feel better just by thinking a positive thought. Your brain is an amazing free pharmaceutical center. "An injection of saline, for example, that has been described as a drug not only will reduce symptoms of Parkinson's Disease (PD), but also can help a patient produce more of the dopamine that the disease destroys," stated Professor of Medicine at Harvard Medical School, Researcher and Acupuncturist Ted Kaptchuk (2011). Results like those provide scientists with chemical evidence of something they long suspected: simply believing in a treatment can be as effective as the treatment itself. In several recent studies, placebos performed as well as the drugs that Americans spend millions of dollar on each year ("The Power of Nothing," *The New Yorker*, December 12, 2011).

The biomedical model of the day—that the mind and the body operate on separate tracks—is incorrect. The belief that "the only way to get sick is through the introduction of a pathogen, and the only way to get well is to get rid of it, are off-base" says Dr. Barbara Langer, a psychology researcher since the 50s and the longest-serving Professor of Psychology at Harvard. Your brain has infinite abilities and researching your own personal power can make an impressive impact upon your psychology and biology.

While rivals like Pfizer and GlaxoSmithKline produced some of the best-selling pharmaceuticals in the world, Merck Pharmaceutical Corporation fell behind in the antidepressant market. "To remain dominant in the future," Merck's Research Director, Edward Scolnick told Forbes, "we need to dominate the central nervous system." In the clinical studies, many test subjects treated with the Merck medication felt their hopelessness and anxiety decrease, but so did almost the same amount that took a placebo. The fact that taking a faux drug can impressively increase some subject's health has long been considered an embarrassment to the serious practice of pharmacology. ("Placebo Effect", *Wired*, 2009). Belief can be so strong that pharmaceutical companies use double-and triple-blind randomized studies to try to exclude the power of the mind over the body when evaluating new drugs, and even then they still cannot explain away the placebo effect.

Today, we know that patients who are given empty injections or pills can experience an improvement in a wide range of health conditions if they only believe in the medicine. Belief is more valuable than hope. If you are aware of what you're thinking, then you can utilize your full chemistry for maximum benefit. For instance, if a Diabetic patient believes they are receiving insulin, their glucose levels drop just from taking a saline pill. I'm not saying this would be true for everyone, but there are many people (about 33% of us) who can experience benefits just by sheer optimism and many others just need training on how to think positively.

How about the opposite? What if your doctor gives an inaccurate diagnosis? This happens to approximately 12 million Americans every year according to CBS Newscaster Jessica Firger, (April

17, 2014). After being misdiagnosed with a fatal illness, if you believe the doctor, your body will begin to shut down and prepare for death. Many pre-med students report that while reading all the signs of certain diseases, some develop a few symptoms, rightly named the *nocebo effect*. If you believe that you have a disease or genetic condition, you can start generating the symptoms and ultimately the disease (which you didn't have previously). Just because your parents or a sibling have Alzheimer's or Parkinson's Disease doesn't mean you're automatically going to get it. Spouses and family members frequently don't get the disease; so it's neither contagious nor genetic.

Dr. Ellen Langer, in her Harvard Research Center, also recruited a number of healthy test subjects in 2010 and gave them the mission to make themselves unwell. The subjects watched videos of people coughing and sneezing. There were tissues around and those in the experimental group were encouraged to act as if they did have a cold. No deception was involved: The subjects were not misled, for example, into thinking they were being put into a germ chamber or anything like that. This was explicitly a test to see if they could voluntarily change their immune system in measurable ways. In the study, which is ongoing, 40% of the experimental group reported cold symptoms following the experiment, while 10% of those in control group did. Do you think that the advertisers and manufacturers of cold and allergy medicine know this data when they broadcast "cold and flu season" commercials in October? (What if Age Is Nothing but a Mind-Set? Bruce Griersonoct, *The New York Times*, 2014,)

Dr. Bruce Lipton, author of *The Biology of Belief* (2005), encourages us to rethink the gene theory altogether. Stanford Professor and Researcher completed his investigation on epigenetics in 1992; however, the Human Genome Project (genetic mapping research) occurred about the same time, 1990-2003, and Dr. Lipton's research dropped like a submarine. 23andMe launched a multi-million dollar marketing campaign and began mapping the individual genome of millions of people. "Our goal is to connect you to the 23 paired volumes of your own genetic blueprint...bringing you personal insight into ancestry, genealogy, and inherited traits," found on the company's website. Dr. Lipton proved epigenetics (that the gene doesn't decide disease, the environment of the cell does), before the genome project gained public recognition. It's great to know your genes alone do not determine your biological future, influence yes, but not certain determination. It's your day-to-day lifestyle that impacts your cellular structure. According to Dr. Lipton and Dr. John Sarno, 90% of doctor's visits are caused by stress alone.

Dr. Lipton continues, "The human body is made out of approximately 100,000 protein blocks, like a giant lego kit. The innate intelligence of the body assembles the proteins to make a brain, bone or finger. It's a blueprint. The blueprint isn't the problem. The contractor who reads the blueprint is really the one who brings the building into reality." That's you. How you live, whether you like your body or not, what you think, and the habitual behavior you express daily is what causes

168

disease or vitality. Dr. Lipton continues, "Seven major diseases are connected to one gene, but cancer is linked to at least 12-14 genes, and then you have to sit in a cesspool of cortisol for cancer to actually ignite." Remember, people have spontaneous remissions daily. What's unlocking the door for that?

Dr. Joe Dispenza, author of *You Are the Placebo* (2014), encourages us to link how we feel with what we are thinking. Dr. Dispenza shares several documented cases of spontaneous remissions (those who reversed cancer, heart disease, depression, crippling arthritis, and even the tremors of Parkinson's Disease) by believing in a placebo. Holding a heightened level of emotion, like enthusiasm, inspiration or love, can transform the mind-body connection. In the field of infinite possibilities you can begin to create a new body and a new life. The placebo effect works since your brain contributes immensely to how healthy you are. It's not all biology or genetics.

When we act emotionally we are altered chemically. When you allow an emotion to linger over days and weeks it will take its toll on your health. For example, let's say you almost have a car wreck on the way to work. Certainly you may be startled initially, but how long do you stay anxious or irritated by the situation? How many people do you need to tell to validate the experience? Are you looking for an "appropriate" response from your listeners? Repeating the story keeps that same emotional state spinning, and there is a direct connection between what you are thinking and how you are feeling. So you could prolong the anxiety or irritation for the rest of the day or week over something that didn't happen just by discussing it or thinking about it obsessively.

Why not obsess about something fantastic or the possibility of something awesome on its way to you, like perfect health? Knowing that thoughts are things and that your thoughts are influencing your life can offer sweeping improvements immediately. Consider the innovative approach of the Law of Attraction that has been around hundreds of years. It is now gaining more popularity through the book and docudrama *The Secret* by Rhonda Byrne (2006). You can radically alter your life by updating your thinking. Abraham Hicks, based in San Antonio, is a world-renowned speaker and teacher, who encourages the simple (and not so simple) act of thinking positively to increase your vibrational frequency and ultimately attract exactly what you want. If you want to be healthy but continuously focus on aches and pains, you can't shift your mind and uplift your frequency; however, if you start to notice the parts of your body that do not ache or that which is working properly, then you open the door to a higher level of consciousness and a higher frequency. When you feel victimized by your body and dwell in uncertainty your frequency is lower than when you are joyously excited about life. You create your outlook, and therefore your reality. So if you don't like the reality you're living today, then shift your thinking. Obsess about what is working and watch your mind, body, spirit transform. Remember belief is more valuable than hope, but hope is better than despair.

Take charge of your body and brain right now. Begin with PMA–Positive Mental Attitude. Affirm your greatest good physically, mentally, financially, spiritually, in your relationships and at work. You have the power! Affirmations are effective, free and available to you right now; I also discuss other ways to transform your life later in this book. Here are a few suggested affirmations to get you started. Silently declare these statements hundreds of times each day.

I am healthy, wealthy and wise.
I have vibrant health.
I am worthy of receiving health & healing.
I deserve to be healthy.
I am financially stable.
I am abundant.
I am smart. I know what to do.
I am loved and loving.

EAST MEETS WEST

Just 30 years ago, alternative medicine was gaining steam and integrative medicine wasn't even a common word yet. Truly, in many parts of America, you couldn't find a chiropractor, acupuncturist or massage therapist, but now cumulatively it's a multibillion dollar industry. The next generation of doctors are available to train and sustain integrative medicine bridging Eastern and Western medical practices. In this brief introduction, you will learn about the benefits of natural therapy and you probably have several of these types of doctors in your hometown or nearby. You can learn a lot about your body and your health just by reading these techniques; you don't have to try them. If you've already talked to your doctor about your medical condition and that route hasn't yielded the outcome you desire, then consider other professional opinions from quality therapists.

CHIROPRACTIC CARE

Chiropractic care was discovered in 1895. According to Random House Dictionary, chiro comes from the Greek word "kheir" meaning "hand." *Practic* comes from the Greek word "pracktikós" meaning practice. Literally it's a hands-on method of healing, and Chiropractic care is the second largest healing system in America. The philosophy of Chiropractic is based on the nervous system. It has been proven that our nervous system is the most important system of the human body because it controls and coordinates all function and healing. Our nervous system consists of the brain and spinal cord. Chiropractors believe the most important structure of the body is the spine, because the spine surrounds and protects the nervous system also known as the "spinal cord." Your spine consists of 33 moveable bones called vertebrae and each vertebra should move in approximately 7 different directions. The only way your body knows how to function and heal is by way of your brain transmitting life. Your brain communicates down your spinal cord and across the peripheral nerves into the body, basically sending life throughout the body. When your vertebrae are out of alignment, this interferes with that communication, and chiropractors refer to this interference as a subluxation. Chiropractors specialize in the detection and correction of spinal subluxations. Chiropractors believe that a spinal manipulation will remove nerve interference and restore normal function and health to the body. Your limbic system contains three key functions with the emotions, memories and arousal (or stimulation). The thalamus is located within the brainstem and is part of the pathway of information into the cerebrum, which is the section of the brain that is responsible for thinking and movement. The communication flows through your central nervous system that resides along the spinal column and throughout the entire body. When your spine is out of alignment, communication between your brain and body can be impeded.

Your miraculous brain naturally wants to heal and repair the body efficiently. Your body has an inherent method to maintain metabolic balance called homeostasis. The chiropractic motto is "the innate wisdom that created the body can heal the body." For example, if you cut your arm, blood will coagulate, create a scab and begin the healing process to repair the skin. In a few days or weeks, the cut or scab will have disappeared leaving no trace of an injury. The body is magnificent in this way. This same type of mysterious healing occurs constantly between the brain, spine and organs. Your arm doesn't mistakenly grow a toenail and your liver doesn't accidently duplicate. The brilliance of your physical form is due to the mind-body communication along the spinal column. When the spine is out of alignment the interaction is limited between the brain and the organs associated with each vertebra, and that's when illness and disease can begin. A spinal adjustment once or twice a month can keep your body in alignment allowing the central nervous system to function in a healthy manner. A chiropractor can adjust every bone in your body. Sometimes the fingers, toes or elbows get out of whack, and a simple adjustment can dissolve neuropathy and restore your vitality quickly. I find yoga and chiropractic care go hand-in-hand but nothing compares to having a skilled doctor with expert dexterity adjust your spine.

Spinal Regenerative Specialist Dr. Chris Centeno states, "The number of fusion surgeries are up about 600-700% since 2000. The costs of the surgeries have almost tripled due to the expensive hardware being implanted. In addition, about half of the surgeries are considered unnecessary." Chiropractic benefits include naturally reducing or eliminating back and neck pain and aide in surgical prevention. It worked for me more than once!

Sadly, it has been noted that after millions of carpal tunnel surgeries, (approximately 230,000 annually) many people actually needed just a simple chiropractic adjustment in the wrist, elbow, shoulder, neck or jaw. That manual manipulation could have saved many people from further surgical damage and long term physical therapy, most of which is not covered by insurance companies (Bureau of Labor and Statistics and the National Institute for Occupational Safety and Health, NIOSH).

An adjustment can improve mental clarity, alleviate headaches, sinus and ear infections, reduce PMS and menopausal symptoms and improve healthy organ functioning. I've had several of my clients receive chiropractic adjustments to alleviate the painful symptoms associated with shingles. Specifically adjusting the vertebrae located near the lesions (or the painful area prior to the onset of lesions) restored the virus to its dormant stage in just two or three visits. Additionally, many chiropractic educational programs incorporate an entire year of PhD-level advanced nutrition training making them a go-to doctor for improved immune system functioning, circulation and elimination. Please visit a chiropractor before you schedule surgery.

ACUPUNCTURE

Millions have been restored to health from all types of ailments through the application of acupuncture and oriental medicine. It's remarkable how placing a tiny needle in the skin can transform your entire biological system. Many people have experienced impressive improvement from migraines, back pain, constipation, Attention Deficit Disorder (ADD), Attention Deficit and Hyperactivity Disorder (ADHD), menstrual cramps, menopause concerns and even cancer. Almost every major city in America has an acupuncturist now and many medical centers consider this a complimentary healing modality, although not all insurance companies cover the therapy now.

Acupuncture promotes and restores the balance of energy by positioning needles at certain meridian pathways throughout the body. These energy channels provide access to your body's natural pain suppressants and increase blood flow. Life force flows through meridians like a river revitalizing every cell and organ, the entire body and the seven tissues mentioned in the Ayurveda chapter (plasma, blood, muscle, fat, bone, grey matter and reproductive tissues). The Doctor of Oriental Medicine effectively evaluates stagnation in the body through your pulse and tongue examination and proceeds to restore Qi (pronounced "chee") or Chi or life force energy throughout your system. The breadth of benefits from acupuncture treatments can expand from emotional concerns like anxiety and depression, to digestive disorders like irritable bowel syndrome and nausea. It can also be useful in treating neurological problems like Parkinson's Disease and even assist in recovery from a stroke. Relief from respiratory conditions, including sinusitis, asthma and seasonal allergies, are also common.

The holistic approach to health and wellbeing provides countless ways to transform your body, mind and spirit without surgery. Frequently, the doctor will prescribe Chinese herbal remedies. Cooking the raw herbs and drinking them can sometimes cure you overnight. These natural formulas can assist with energy and endurance, elimination and purification, environmental allergies, hormonal imbalances, and other common grievances. Herbal formulas, and their effects on the body in connection with the immune system and the internal organs, are the mainstay to Chinese medicine.

The oldest known book on Chinese medicine is the *Neiching*, also known as *The Yellow Emperor's Classic of Internal Medicine*. It was written in the form of a dialogue between the Yellow Emperor Huang Ti and Chi Po, a Taoist teacher and physician. It is believed that the Yellow Emperor lived around 2700 BC, but acupuncture was widely practiced by oral tradition in China much before that time.

I had a rare opportunity to spend three weeks in Egypt. It was an exhilarating experience, but I left with walking pneumonia. When I landed in Singapore I was blessed that my hostel was walking distance from a Chinese Acupuncture Clinic. I ploddered to the healing center, the Doctors of Oriental Medicine looked at my tongue and gasped. Some doctors know how to inspect the tongue to determine the functioning ability of the organs. The doctors would elbow each other and suggest an additional inspection of my tongue. I must have stuck my tongue out about 10 times. Each clinician squinting with furrowed brow and conferring together (in Chinese, of course) and ultimately deciding I needed moxa. I didn't know what it was, but I knew I needed help. On a prayer, we began the lung treatment. I could barely feel the 10 or so needles when first inserted. Upon the top of the needles the doctor applied a small amount of moxa, an Artemesia herbal formula. Then the Chinese doctor illuminated the moxa. She fired it up and my chest smoked for 20 minutes. I laughed and cried simultaneously. I knew I needed to get well and wasn't sure what to do. I deeply believed it would work. I returned daily for two weeks until I was able to continue my travels onto Thailand where I fasted and cleansed for another month for ultimate recovery. Despite the obvious travails, it was a gift to travel the world.

DRY NEEDLING

Dry needling was also described in the Yellow Emperor's Inner Classic. Mainly utilized by acupuncturists, now physical therapists are beginning to include dry needling in their treatments. Also known as myofascial trigger point, this drugless therapy treats pain and dysfunction of the neuromusculoskeletal system. Simply described, dry needling involves inserting an acupuncture needle into a tender point (like a muscle spasm) or trigger point and then appropriately manipulating it (rotating and/or pistoning) for therapeutic purposes. The needle allows a therapist to target tissues not manually palpable with the hand as in acupressure. This treatment accelerates the patient's return to active rehabilitation and improves movement repatterning. Depending on the location and duration of the injury, positioning the needle is felt only momentarily. When the needle is inserted deeply into the tight muscle, blood, water and oxygen begin to recirculate throughout the injured area. Albeit, it can be temporarily painful (depending on the location), I found it extremely beneficial. I do not recommend doing this type of treatment with a beginner therapist. The certification course is only 27 hours and does not impart the full understanding of Oriental Medicine. It has been a point of contention (pun intended) between Licensed Acupuncturists and Physical Therapists, but the treatment offers amazingly fast results with a seasoned professional.

MASSAGE THERAPY

Once associated with massage parlors and prostitutes, massage is now considered a professional therapeutic approach to nonsurgical healing. You don't even have to disrobe. Chair massage is an effective way to destress and today many corporations are periodically providing this gift of wellness to their staff, instead of cholesterol-laden, diabetic enhancing donuts.

Registered Massage Therapists use their thumbs, hands and elbows to focus on muscular relaxation. The therapist transforms your body in just a few minutes. If you hobble around with sciatica pain and/or countless other muscle aches, see a Registered Massage Therapist for natural healing. You'd be surprised how much better you feel in just one hour.

There are many therapeutic styles. Consider what type you want in advance.
• **Swedish Massage** uses light touch and is ideal for stress management and insomnia. It reduces adrenalin overload due to tension or trauma, and enhances a sense of inner peace. The therapist incorporates candles and aromatherapy for a soothing ambiance. Great for *vata* dosha.
• **Deep Tissue/Sports Massage** is the opposite, using hands and elbows with long strokes and circular movements, kneading or karate chopping and targeting pressure points. Beneficial for recreational and professional athletes to release the lactic acid congestion in muscles after intense exercise. Ideal for pitta dosha.
• **Thai Yoga Massage** is an ancient healing system combining acupressure, Indian Ayurvedic principles and assisted yoga postures. It is very active for both the therapist and the patient. This style of massage introduces new movement to the body, increasing the mind-body

communication. You stay fully clothed, and the therapist moves you through many yoga positions on the floor for effective muscular release. Very helpful for *kapha* dosha.

- **Shiatsu Massage** means "finger pressure" like acupressure. The therapist uses their thumbs like needles. It releases spasmed muscles, improves joint flexibility and increases overall circulation. If you find acupuncture or dry needling unsettling, try this method for those with chronic muscular cramps and spasms. The abdominal protocol is effective for those with constipation.

- **Lymphatic Massage** is a gentle, hands-on therapy performed to stimulate the flow of lymph, a colorless fluid that transports large proteins, foreign bodies, pathogenic substances (germs, toxins, etc). The body contains 500-600 lymph nodes connected by capillaries and vessels throughout the body, which act like little filters breaking down and destroying particles eventually eliminated from the body through natural channels of the bladder and rectum. The mother nodes enhance the lymph flow, like a vacuum, of the entire body located in the neck, armpits and near the groin. The lymphatic system can become compromised due to surgery, trauma, burns, infections, stress, age or disease. Lymphatic massage improves organ functioning, and the immune system and naturally eliminates toxins. Everybody can benefit from a lymph massage. It's very gentle and usually you fall asleep during the treatment. To promote a healthy lymph system you can dry brush starting at the feet and fingers moving toward the heart. Also using a washcloth when bathing gently stimulates the lymph. Again, stroke from the outer extremities moving inward toward the heart.

- **Neural Manipulation** as described by Jean Pierre Barral is a gentle massage technique that releases restrictions throughout the nervous system. The ability to free up trapped or impinged nerves decreases pain, restores function and softens connective tissue enhancing mobility. When nerves cannot glide properly through the skeletal system, they can become fixed, causing discomfort leading to chronic pain (sometimes misdiagnosed as arthritis). Neural manipulation restores circulation to the tissue around the restricted areas. It's additionally useful around the organs where emotions can get stored causing congestion in internal functioning that can lead to disease. I used this type of therapy for a frozen thumb (which some misdiagnosed as carpal tunnel or arthritis) and restored perfect health to my hands in less than three months without surgery. I discuss it briefly in "Yoga on a Peg" at the end of the Body Section. I highly recommend this method prior to any surgical consideration. You can release years, even decades, of dysfunctional physiological patterns through neural manipulation.

There are many different styles of massage well worthy of investigation. Sitting in a chair all day is dreadful for your low back. Most people do not have the muscular strength to sit up straight and therefore the lumbar region of the spine is forced to round in the opposite direction of the natural curve. Even if you spend $1000 on an ergonomic chair you still have to sit properly. Whether it's an office chair, airplane seat or a recliner, you need to stretch the spine, and a massage is a great way to regain overall circulation.

HYPNOSIS WORKS!

Deemed a medical tool in 1958 by the American Medical Association, Hypnosis is a powerful means that helps you create change in your life in a short period of time. Likened to daydreaming or meditating, hypnosis can be a useful method to improve your outlook and develop healthy behaviors quickly. Hypnosis is a trancelike state using the alpha-theta brainwave. It's a "do-with" process not a "do-to" process. When the therapist says, "Take a deep breath" you must follow directions, or you won't benefit from the treatment. It has nothing to do with intelligence or gullibility. You simply relax and follow the therapist to a calmer state of consciousness where you can transform your mind. It's not about surrendering; it is about reorganizing your internal dialogue.

Although drug and alcohol addiction are commonly more involved than smoking cessation or weight loss, Hypnosis can help you in a multitude of ways. You can desensitize triggers, diminish cravings and manage underlying emotional distress, while improving your discipline and self-confidence. Addiction can be deeply rooted as it forms part of the internal picture and dialogue you hold of yourself. Hypnosis offers a way of touching and transforming these underlying pictures and feelings. Positive suggestions stated by the therapist reduce interest in the bad habit and open the mind to creating new healthy practices.

During hypnotherapy sessions you recall the source of any feelings of fear, anger, anxiety, sadness and even buried emotions. This enables you to recall the origination of those emotions and the behaviors associated with them. By going back to the source of these feelings, you recognize and express them with greater clarity, thus releasing emotional or physical pain. Unconscious fears and feelings can stunt growth but the problem is, they are unknown. Hypnosis opens the door for considerable awareness and can be quite empowering.

Hypnosis has a proven track record for pain management. Millions are affected by chronic pain annually and pain medication has diminishing benefits. Hypnosis reduces the need for anesthesia during some surgeries and speeds post-operative healing as well. Hypnosis, or hypno-birthing, has supported many mothers who opted out of epidurals and other medication during the delivery process. This drugless therapy has numerous benefits and no side effects.

After several hypnotherapy sessions, you will most likely experience less tension, more rejuvenating sleep and improved memory. Hypnosis can make you feel better, creating a sense of overall health and wholeness. It produces enhanced rational responses, reduces cravings, eliminates test anxiety, improves self-efficacy and increases productivity. The success rate depends on your hypnotizability, motivation and disorder. The longer you've had a certain concern and your attachment to it may require extra treatments, but for many 2-10 sessions can resolve most problems.

In closing, I invite you to always get a second, third and fourth opinion and discuss your situation with a natural therapist or integrative physician. Consider a combination of approaches to find the best relief. If you sample a few chiropractic adjustments or dry needling sessions and they don't work for you, then you haven't really lost much. You had a few different experiences. Once you start surgical procedures it's difficult to backtrack if they are unsuccessful. I strongly recommend finding a quality therapist. No beginners. If you visit a student practitioner at the school who is still learning, and they injure you more, then you're contributing further to your problems. Think about the cost of surgery ~ $20,000, $50,000, $100,000 ~ include downtime, trouble sleeping, inability to drive and the value of each workday missed. Contemplate how much you are willing to pay for routine treatments of natural healthcare, like massage therapy treatments or hypnosis, over the course of one year. Paying $1,000, $2,000 or $3000 is cheaper than surgery, and it may be all you need.

Health is a state of complete physical, mental and social wellbeing and not merely the absence of disease or infirmity.
World Health Organization (WHO)

ESSENTIAL OILS

Essential oils have been around for thousands of years. They contain spices, herbs, roots, flowers, resins and leaves. Oils are the essence of the plant obtained through a steam or water distillation process or cold-pressing. The all natural aromatic liquids stimulate the sense of smell, energize the body and increase cellular vitality. The small molecular size and the carbon based similarities between humans and plants make them so compatible with our physiology. They can be absorbed directly into the bloodstream making them indispensable. Quality oils are certified organic or wild crafted, and indicate where they sourced their botanicals. If you cannot ingest them, they probably have parabens, or other substandard oil as a base, or were commonly created in a chemical process. Those are not considered true essential oils. Doterra® and Young Living® provide the highest quality oils available today.

Oils are referenced repeatedly in the *Bible*, and the offering to Baby Jesus of frankincense and myrrh, natural resins, clearly indicate valued properties of the time (*KJV*, Matthew 2:11). Today, we know that frankincense has proven benefits for those with tumors or cancer. Since cancer cells are not foreign invaders but actually live dormantly within us all, some natural elixirs, like frankincense, can prevent infection, eradicate harmful bacteria and combat pain and swelling while still maintaining healthy gene expression (*HealthLine, 2018*). A recent study found that burning frankincense and myrrh incense reduced airborne bacterial by 68% (*NIH*, June 2018). Frankincense is the dried sap of trees in the boswellia genus, and the boswellia supplement is rising in popularity for those with inflammation (which is anyone with any disease). Results vary, like with medications.

You can absorb the herbal medicine in concentrated form by inhaling (diffuser), soaking or ingesting it. Diffusers disburse oils into the air, and breathing the essence throughout the night or day can open the sinus cavity or uproot congestion in the lungs, strengthen the immune system or provide deep relaxation throughout the night. Taking a whiff directly from the bottle can shift your outlook quickly. If you get anxious while driving, keep a bottle in your car and spritz the air with the exquisite fragrance before you embark on your next journey. Placing a drop or two on the impacted area or receiving a full body massage can move the oil's healing properties into the skin topically. Soaking in a bath with several drops can reduce aches and pains, rejuvenate the body and relax your mood. Adding a few drops into your drinking water can aid as an antiseptic, or placing it directly under the tongue are other ways to ingest the oils to reduce inflammation, improve digestion and increase elimination. Essential oils work best with a drop or two on the hour. Less is better, just do it more often.

You don't need an extensive set of oils to get started. One or two will suffice for you to become a citizen scientist and prove to yourself that it's working. Chart your symptoms daily and measure your progress over the course of one to three months. How long are you willing to ingest a pharmaceutical before you expect results? Use the elixir that long. Your ailment determines which one to try. The following are a few popular aromas, and *The Complete Aromatherapy Handbook* provides details on exact formulas.

• **Lavender** has received more than it's fair share of positive press over the years mainly because it pacifies the central nervous system, reduces anxiety, diminishes insomnia, and can relieve sun burnt skin. It received some bad press as it mimics the estrogen gene and is contraindicated for those with breast cancer, or possibly any type of active cancer.
• **Lemon** oil is a powerful antibacterial, astringent, and antiseptic agent.
• **Clary Sage** can balance hormones and may have antidepressant properties.
• **Rosemary** decreases cortisol and diminishes respiratory infections.

The Essential Life suggests the following (5th Edition, 2018):

Basil	Adrenal fatigue, mental fatigue and focus
Cardamom	Congestion, stomach ache, constipation
Clove	Liver and brain support
Frankincense	Cancer, tumors, seizures and trauma weight
Grapefruit	Loss and obesity
Peppermint	Allergies, headaches, hangovers and sinusitis
Red Mandarin	Acne, stretch marks
Ylang Ylang	Low libido, impotence, infertility

Doterra research shows remarkable results with many physiological problems. Oils are preventative medicine but also can aid where mainstream medicine may have failed. All pharmaceuticals began at one point from a botanical, and you may need to return to the roots to find the remedy you desire. If your colleagues or family members are coughing and sneezing, begin administering essential oils immediately. Start the oils in the first hour or certainly the first day if you begin to feel weak or tired. Using antibiotics sparingly and supplementing with quality oils can positively impact your vitality. Blend Eastern and Western treatments for a wholistic approach to wellness.

BENEFITS OF CBD, CANNABIDIOL

CBD oil is rich in plant based chemicals called cannabinoids derived from the cannabis plant. The most known cannabinoid is tetrahydrocannabinol (THC), which produces a "high" feeling experienced after using marijuana. CBD doesn't produce an elated feeling, but it can reduce symptoms of pain and discomfort, specifically for those receiving cancer treatments. It's not what you feel; it's what you don't feel. The nausea associated with chemical treatments or the tension caused from anxiety reduces dramatically for most people when they ingest CBD oil. You can eat it, cook with it or apply it topically to the skin. CBD cream alleviates achy hands, hips and knees. Cannabidiol additionally offers therapeutic effects on several conditions, including Parkinson's disease, Alzheimer's disease, cerebral ischemia, diabetes, rheumatoid arthritis, other inflammatory diseases, nausea and cancer (*Medical Marijuana*, July 2019).

According to Medical Marijuana ProCon, "33 states legalized medical marijuana, and the remaining 17 states have all passed laws allowing the use of CBD extract, usually in oil form, with minimal tetrahydrocannabinol (THC), and often for the treatment of epilepsy or seizures in seriously ill children. CBD, one of the 400+ ingredients found in marijuana, is not psychoactive." You do not experience an altered feeling from CBD like from opioids (oxycodone, OxyContin®, hydrocodone, Vicodin®, codeine and morphine).

In July 2018, Medical News Today indicated CBD provided a wide range of applications including:
• Smoking cessation and drug withdrawal assistance
• Treating seizures with Parkinsons Disease and epilepsy
• Antipsychotic effects on people with schizophrenia
• Combating acne and aiding arthritis
• Balancing type 1 diabetes and even cancer
• Reducing blood pressure and preventing heart damage

Given the popularity, consider being a citizen scientist and perform your own investigation. You can find CBD almost anywhere now. According to Industry Analyst Motley Fool, "Major companies like

Walgreens, Rite Aid, CVS, Ulta Beauty, and most tattoo shops are selling it now" (June 2019). Even JuiceLand provides CBD shots in smoothies (for an additional fee, of course). You might consider giving it a shot if you've received no relief from other treatments and, with no side effects, what have you got to lose?

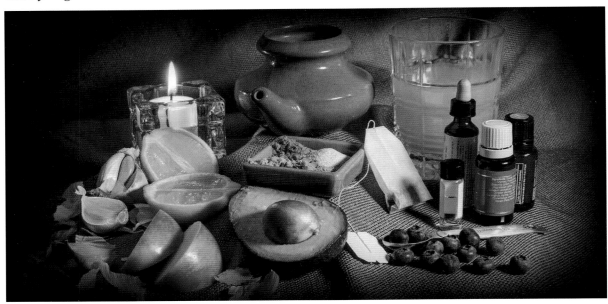

NATURAL REMEDIES

Native Americans and other ancient civilizations traditionally used natural remedies for hundreds of years. Our Ancestors of just one or two generations ago, your grandparents and great-grandparents were using botanicals and spices on a regular basis to maintain good health. My grandmother said if you went to the hospital in the 40s, 50s and 60s they frequently gave an enema to gently remove any toxic fecal matter that was influencing the body negatively. Much of that simple wholistic wisdom is not practiced today. There are many natural products at your local health food store, and you may even have some in your cupboards already. These remedies have been in the domain of the common people for centuries. Many have heard, "You are what you eat," and what goes into your body is creating your future cellular structure. Many medications and over-the-counter products have negative side effects and detoxifying may simply mean switching to a natural remedy for a week or two. Check with your healthcare provider to see if your prescription drugs will have a negative effect on the natural remedy. Frequently, these holistic tonics might be just what the doctor ordered. This chart is intended for informational purposes only. I intentionally omitted the formula. You can "DIY" (do it yourself) and conduct your own online research at Dr. Google, or contact a representative at your natural grocer to learn more about the exact formula for your specific concern.

Acid Reflux	Apple Cider Vinegar, Baking Soda, Ginger Tea, Marshmallow
Acne	Zinc, Vitamin E, Aloe Vera, Frankincense
Anti-Inflammatory	Epsom Salt Soaks, Turmeric, White Willow Bark
Anxiety	Lavender or Bergamot Oil, Rescue Remedy, Kava, Valerian Root
Appetite Suppressant	Apple Cider Vinegar, Spirulina
Arthritis	Rosemary Root, Eucalyptus or Copaiba Essential Oil, Epsom Salt Soak, Fish Oils, Eliminate Bread, Remove Acrylic Nails
Asthma	Eucalyptus Oil, Rosemary Oil, Lobelia, Eliminate Dairy
Bad Breath	Tea Tree Oil, Oil Pulling with Coconut Oil, HCl (hydrochloric acid capsules), Brush & Floss Daily
Bronchitis	Eucalyptus Oil, Fennel or Ocean Pine Oil, Drink more Water, Use Humidifier, Eliminate Dairy
Boils	Burdock Root, Turmeric, Tea Tree Oil, Chamomile Oil
Canker Sores	GlycoThymaline Mouth Rinse, Eat less Spicy, Salty & Acidic Foods
Constipation	Castor Oil Packs on the intestines, Senna, Eat less Dairy, HCl (hydrochloric acid capsules), Enema/Colonic
Cough/Sore Throat	Marshmallow, Ginger, Warm Honey-Lemon Water
Intestinal Cramps	Slippery Elm, Hossup Tea, Massage for Circulation
Dehydration	Electrolytes, Drink more Water, Soak in a Plain Warm Bath for One Hour
Diabetes	Ginseng, Eat more Veggies, specifically beets, Consume Less Sugar and Bread
Diarrhea	Drink More Water, Electrolytes, Neroli or Sandalwood Oil, Slippery Elm, BRAT (bananas, rice, applesauce, toast)
Digestion	Enzymes, Pineapple, Apple Cider Vinegar, Angelica Oil, Tarragon Spice, Ginger Root, Eat Bitter Greens like Kale and Spinach
Fungal Infection	Black Walnut, Apple Cider Vinegar, Aloe Vera
Gallbladder	Peppermint Tea, Turmeric, Apple Cider Vinegar, Eat Bitter Greens like Kale and Spinach
Gastritis	Eliminate Gluten, Chamomile Tea, Sandalwood Oil, GlycoThymoline Mouthrinse
Hangover	Co Q 10, Milk Thistle, Hair of the Dog, More Sleep
Headaches	White Willow Bark, Lavender Oil, Ginger Root Tea
High Cholesterol	Red Yeast Rice, Eliminate Fried Foods
Immune Builder	Echinacea, Golden Seal, Garlic, Oregano, Astragulus, Frankincense, Melaleuca
Impotence	Saw Palmetto, Neroli Essential Oil, Ginseng
In-Grown Toe Nails	Soak Foot in Epsom Salt or Apple Cider Vinegar

Insomnia	Rose or Lavender Oil, Kava, Valerian Root, Melatonin
Kidneys	Parsley Juice, CranActin Cranberry Concentrate Tablets, Distilled Water, Avoid Sugar, Eliminate Grapefruit
Liver	Castor Oil Packs, Rosemary Oil, Lavender Oil, Milk Thistle
Low Testerone	Saw Palmetto Berries, Ashwaganda, Ginger, DHEA
Menopause	Black Cohosh, Ginsing, Geranium Oil, Kava, Fennel Essential Oil
Menstruation Cramps	Vitamin E, B1, Bergamot Oil, Have Sex
Muscle Cramps	Magnesium, ½ Banana, Epsom Salt Soaks, Rosemary Root Oil
Osteoarthritis	Eat More Green Leafy Veggies, Broccoli, Avocados, Garlic, Green Tea, Juniper Oil, Exercise Daily on Land
Pneumonia	Lobelia can make you vomit and that can eliminate mucus in the lungs, Peppermint Tea or Oil, Fenugreek Tea
Pre-Diabetic	Reduce Carbohydrates and Sugars, Eat More Veggies
Pre-Hypertensive	Reduce Sodium, Reduce Red Meat, Eat More Veggies
Psoriasis	Milk Thistle, Aloe Vera Gel, Castor Oil, Bergamot Oil, Rockrose Oil, Cooked and Cooled Oatmeal salve
Sadness	St. John's Wort, Rescue Remedy, Happy Camper, Bergamot Oil, Kava, Lemon Water, Lemon Oil
Sinus Infection	Neti Pot with Saltwater, Frankincense Oil, Eliminate Dairy
Stings or Bites	Black Ointment Salve, Melaleuca
Stress	Bergamot Oil, Fennel Root, Valerian Root, Exercise
Tumors	Frankincense Oil, Black Ointment Salve
Ulcers	Burdock Root, Eliminate Dairy, Meditate Daily
Urinary Tract Infections	CranActin Concentrated Cranberry tablets, Yin Vaginal Care, Reduce Sex for a Week or Two, Use Only Cotton Pads (no tampons)
Vision	Ginko Biloba, Fennel Root, Carrots, Eye Exercises–slowly rotate eyes in wide circle 5-10 x each direction daily
Vomiting	Mint Tea, Angelica Oil, Wrist Bands for Motion Sickness
Yeast Infection	Vaginal Tea Tree Suppositories, Yin Vaginal Care, Eliminate Sugar, Use only Cotton Pads (no tampons)

LET'S TALK ABOUT SEX

It's all over the magazine covers, multitudes of books have been published on the topic, and *50 Shades of Gray* hit the silver screen in 2015. We talk about it a lot, but how many people are experiencing intimacy? Intimacy and sexuality impact every other area of life.

Check out these 2017 Stats from Life Science
Sex toys are a $15 billion industry in America alone.
22% surveyed say they enjoy being friends with benefits.
75% of men and 29% of women achieve orgasm each time.

More American Sexual Behavior Stats from Statista
65% of women surveyed own a sex toy.
58% of American Adults has a one-night stand.
51% of American Adults had unprotected sex.
Approximately 40% of high school students have sex.
67% of American Adults stated homosexuality should be accepted by society.
Almost 5% surveyed identify as LBGTQIA.
About 85% of men and women enjoyed oral sex.

Think of an orgasm as a reset button. Drop the guilt, and push, pull, stroke or stimulate to reboot your body...ahhh. For many, just releasing the guilt of this biological pleasure could transform your romantic partnership immediately. Think of relationships with yin and yang energy. Yin energy is internal, receptive, passive, feeling or feminine. Yang energy is active, external, expanding, manifesting or masculine. Even though you may have male bits you might have more yin energy or vice versa having female bits but associating with yang energy. All relationships have one who is more yin and one who is more yang, and I invite you to interpret the suggestions below depending on your gender and not only by physiological anatomy.

Many want to have better sex but better doesn't mean longer. Sex really starts outside the bedroom through the many ways we communicate, verbally and non-verbally. What are you doing to turn on your partner? Are you just thinking about yourself or do you actually take into account your lover's desires? You might already be the perfect partner and maybe you're spinning circles trying to be someone else to please your partner. Find out the truth by asking honest questions. Dim the lights, toast a glass of courageous cabernet, turn on some romantic music and let the seduction begin. If you're consenting adults, then start the dialogue. It's ok to giggle. Try not to "finish" the conversation. Keep it open for times in the future. Maybe tomorrow.

Ask your partner some or all of the following questions:
1. What do you like most about sex (beyond the obvious orgasm)?
2. What's your favorite body part (beyond the obvious genitalia)?
3. Do you enjoy having sex with the lights on or off?
4. Do you like oral sex?
5. What turns you on? What could I do to turn you on tonight?
6. Do you prefer monogamy or being polyamorous?
7. Do you prefer to shower before making love?
8. Do you like lingerie, thongs or Tarzan outfits? Will you wear one for me?
9. What is your sexual fantasy?
10. Would you like to have sex in an airplane (or other naughty locations)?
11. Would you like to have sex with me? Be sure to ask the main question.
12. The list goes on and on....

Ask your partner all types of questions about sex. Be bold! Be explicit about what you like sexually. So much goes unsaid. What, when, where, how long, etc. Be specific about it. "I'd like to have sex for 30-minutes near the pool in the backyard at 10pm when no one is watching." Keep it real. Most men prefer this type of clear instruction; however, many women prefer to be romanced first with flowers, wine and intimate conversation. Kiss, touch and allure women sensually into thinking about sex before undressing. The small and large ways we encourage and support each other can be a big turn-on.

Women, ask for what you want. Do you know what you want? Many women need 10 minutes a week or 10 minutes a day getting to know their body. The clitoris has 8,000 nerve endings, and the upper left quadrant of the clitoris is the most sensitive. The penis has 4,000 nerve endings, and touching the rim around the tip is very pleasing. Spend some time alone in self-pleasure, and then you can instruct your lover how to intimately touch you. If you don't feel comfortable with self-pleasure how can you expect to relax and orgasm with your partner? He wants you to have a good experience because he wants to do it daily or near daily. Be direct about your desire and don't expect your partner to know when you're ready, especially if you've declined a few times or for a few weeks.

Female orgasms are as varied as women themselves. Clitoral, G-spot or anal orgasms heighten pleasure and build sexual interest. The more a man is willing to explore a woman's naturally changing pathway to orgasm, the more comfort she will have in the bedroom. We all enjoy varied experiences and knowing that a woman's heightened sexual pleasure evolves over time allows the man to continue his natural desire for a chase. Knowing in advance that the same sexual technique is not going to work every time, encourages a man to investigate new ways to pursue his partner's ecstasy. A man's body creates semen approximately every 20 minutes. A woman's body creates one egg one time per month, and none after menopause. Men and women have higher and lower arousal rates respectively based on their physiological differences. That one-to-three day period during ovulation is when a woman's arousal levels can match a man's interest. Ladies, imagine being that aroused on a daily basis. Now, you know why you're man is always ready for love. The male anatomy is external, and the penis pursues what it desires. The vagina is inside and receptive, waiting for pursuit. That's not to say women don't pursue men, but generally speaking, women are more sensitive to being approached. The long, sticky and stringy discharge is a sign that a woman is ovulating. That is usually when women are most aroused and will risk the effort of pursuit. Men, be mindful, if a woman is pursuing you, she is most likely hormonally ripe for pregnancy.

Dr. John Gray's most celebrated book is *Men are From Mars, Women are From Venus* (1992). He identifies that if men want their women to get the Big O, then they need to add a 0 (zero) to how long it takes them to cum. It typically takes a man about 2-5 minutes to cum (less than 10 minutes). If you want your woman to cum, you should spend about 20-50 minutes focused solely on her erogenous zones (or choose an amount of time to prime her pumps). Find them all, explore them, and both of you will be so happy you did. Men typically fall asleep after orgasm but women frequently get uplifted. After a fun frolic, allow your Rocketman to take a nap while you hit the gym or garden for 30 minutes. Don't expect to have the same type of experience as your partner. Let them enjoy their reset button benefits in their physiologically unique way. I highly recommend Dr. Gray's series, especially *Mars and Venus in the Bedroom* (1995).

Viewing soft eroticism is intended to guide you to that romantic vibe. Looking at sexy videos or photos and thinking about sex puts you in the mood. You might not be aroused when you start the video, but it will move your attention in that direction. Masturbation is important for rebalancing hormones and adjusting the genital fluids. Many porn videos today are all about the bump and grind and the ultimate cum shot, and many women have absolutely no interest in it. It's unfortunate that *erotica with instruction* is less available because many men have watched thousands of hours of porn and have absolutely no idea how to enchant a woman. The focus on what men want sexually leaves us all undereducated about how to have better sex together. Addiction to porn does not make you a better lover. Likely, the person you choose will not perform like a porn star leaving you both to feel a bit disappointed. Also, porn addicts frequently get distracted or awkward when interacting with women on a basic day-to-day social level. Those who are offended by porn require more poetry, foot rubs, Frank Sinatra and late night seaside strolls.

The internationally acclaimed singer and performer Sting promoted Tantric Sex for decades. Ancient texts on Tantric Sex and the *Kama Sutra* have been modernized and explain the importance of building tension before the orgasmic release. Just because you can cum, doesn't mean jump off the deep end. The ancient Indian text encourages men to pull back, let the blood and body build two or three times. You will feel a dynamic ejaculation like never before. Women should do the opposite. Women should cum as often as possible, and as quickly as possible. Sometimes women can orgasm two, three or four times in one love making session. The human body releases oxytocin, the pleasure hormone, with each climax. Oxytocin not only makes us feel good, but also deepens the commitment to that partner. Psychology professor at Florida State Andrea Meltzer asserts, "We know from past studies that there are biological changes after sex, such as increases in dopamine, oxytocin, and vasopressin" and the afterglow can continue for 48-hours. Let it rip! On the other hand, if you're trying to break-up and decide some Friday night mattress dancing might be delicious, think again! You are only intensifying your connection through the sexual hormonal release making it more difficult to ultimately move onward and, sadly, that's when some couples get pregnant.

Lowered libido can be caused by many things, like the side effects of antidepressants, antianxiety and other pharmaceuticals. Decreased hormonal levels and a loss of vaginal lubrication during menopause frequently reduce libido in older women. Natural lubricants and organic sesame oil can improve sexual satisfaction. Overall, a decrease in female sexual responsiveness is due to many different things like a loss of intimacy or trust, inability to connect outside of the bedroom, stress, trying to be super woman and performance anxiety. Many commercials leave women feeling like their natural odors and monthly process is dirty or abnormal causing many women to dismiss their biological urges. Most men do not agree with those commercials and enjoy a woman's musky sent; however, unpleasant odors, overgrowth of yeast or colored discharge are an indication that the pH is imbalanced. A quality probiotic can restore the natural flora in the intestines and vagina. Ask your partner what will increase interest in sex. Couples massage or simply cuddling for a night or two can restore trust and evoke a woman's sexual interest again. Also, exercise increases libido. When you exercise on a regular basis you have more interest and stamina for sex. Exercise increases endorphins, lowers cortisol (the stress hormone) and can stimulate arousal. According to *Men's Journal*, "swimming builds endurance, boosts blood flow, improves flexibility and strength, and slashes stress." Give yourself a few weeks before you see that endurance in the bedroom. Get your heart, core muscles and low back in shape prior to your next robust romp!

If you're trying to lose weight, ask your partner about oral sex. I mean really, it's clear that you're orally fixated. Ask your partner about low-calorie chow time and munch away. Semen only has about 5-25 calories per load, and a clitoris orgasm has no calories at all! Hang out for 10-30 minutes and feel what happens. She doesn't have to swallow to benefit from working the tongue and jaw; plus, he'll love it. Also, she doesn't have to orgasm every time to enjoy the attention, and it sets the tone for another romantic interlude soon. Dr. Gray points out, a woman's orgasm is like the moon, sometimes waning, sometimes waxing and sometimes in full bloom. Don't pressure yourself or your partner to orgasm just enjoy the delightful attention. Showering prior to sex is a common Tantric step toward greater elation. It will make you feel more comfortable and refreshed before someone heads south for some sensuous dining. Skip a meal and give it a try.

Sex and Aging
Since we are no longer in the procreation phase of life we enjoy companionship in different forms. Slowing down intercourse and increasing affectionate glances, light touches and pecks, maintains the endearing feelings of intimacy between long term partners. Dancing, cuddling, spooning, snuggling, licking ears (and other body parts) are highly seductive, and you don't have to go all the way. Touching, teasing and massaging are great ways to connect without intercourse and reminds your partner that they are desirable. Feeling desired is very important for both partners even if you're not having intercourse. Pretend that you're in high school again and make-out on the couch for one or two minutes once or twice a week. You can be intimate without expecting an orgasm, and never force yourself on your partner. Consider affection like a dance   sometimes a fast salsa, sometimes a romantic waltz, other times a sashay in the park.

Shifting sexual routines, adding toys or lotions can enhance sexual exploration. Sexual pharmaceuticals can be very helpful for men's erections and improve circulation in the penis. According to the *Journal of Sexual Medicine*, "L-arginine is an amino acid that your body turns into nitric oxide. Studies showed about one third of men who took 5 grams per day for 6 weeks had improved erections. Propionyl-L-carnitine used in combination with sildenafil (Viagra) is more effective for men with diabetes and erectile dysfunction. For those men who tried sildenafil at least eight times with no luck, experienced results when they added 2 grams of propionyl-L-carnitine per day to their nutritional plan." Research the best formula for you, as there can be some side effects with supplements and pharmaceuticals (August 2011).

The pelvic floor includes muscles, tendons and ligaments at the base of the spine creating a hammock lifting the pelvis. It's common to cue "lift the pelvic floor" during Yoga and Pilates as it helps with maintaining the energy level inward and upward. Lifting the perineum improves the genital muscles, increases circulation and sensation in the vaginal and penis area, and can increase vaginal lubrication. Also known as Kegels, these exercises improve erectile dysfunction, increase ejaculatory control and maintain bladder muscles. Locate the proper muscles by stopping urination midstream. Lift, squeeze and hold for one deep breath (or three seconds) and then release back to neutral. Practice lifting the perineum and engaging the abdominal muscles for 3-5 seconds, or one long deep breath, then release. Slowly perform 10 repetitions daily. Best of all you can do it virtually anywhere, and no one will know what you're doing.

Cum Hither ~

Woodsy-smelling **sandalwood** essential oil or incense are natural aphrodisiacs known to raise libidos and increase sexual desire while reducing inhibitions. **Ginseng**, the age old natural Viagra, increases sexual hormones, improves desire, facilitates penile erection, and relaxes the clitoral muscles improving female sexual function. **Ashwagandha**, also known as the "strength of the stallion," doesn't disappoint in the bedroom. It's been used for centuries as an aphrodisiac and stress reliever. **Zinc**, also a stress reliever and libido increaser, is easy to obtain in naturally high protein animal foods like lamb, grass-fed beef and chicken, as well as chickpeas, yogurt and cashews. Other traditional sultry food choices include **oysters, ginger** and **dark chocolate**. **Niacin**, a **B3 vitamin**, known to improve orgasm, raises your good cholesterol, lowers the effects of aging, augments circulation and fosters relaxation. If you're feeling a little listless, supplement your diet with vitamin B12. The National Institute of Health published one study in 2011 indicating that men with high cholesterol and moderate to severe erectile dysfunction who took 1,500 milligrams of niacin for 12 weeks saw improvements. **Black cohosh** and **chasteberry** have been known to assist with vaginal dryness and hormonal rebalance respectively to lift sexual interest. Numerous online companies make investigating which supplements work best for you quite easy today.

Remember, we all have insecurities, especially when we're naked. No need to prance around nude. You would be pleasantly surprised how even a basic towel with a provocative voice or alluring look can invite sensual delight. Dim the lights, create the ambiance and encourage your partner without expectation. Enjoy some aromatherapy, silky sheets and a feather tickler. You and your partner feel affection for each other and want to share erotic sensation. Affirm silently and out loud phrases like, "I love you. You're hot. I want you. You're my dream partner. You turn me on." Whatever is true for you. Let those soft meaningful words flow freely from your luscious lips (in and out of the bedroom). Lovers unite in healing pleasures of sensual touch, and after years of marriage many couples have mature sex. They just ask the question, "Do you want me to take a pill?" or "Do you want to take a pill?" Some sex pills can cost $20 or more each, and it's an unfortunate waste of money if you're both not in the mood because sometimes you're hot and sometimes your not. When a gentle decline is offered because it's just not the right time for either partner, convene for some good spooning and movie watching on the couch. Create intimacy in and out of the bedroom for lifelong companionship and joyous lovemaking.

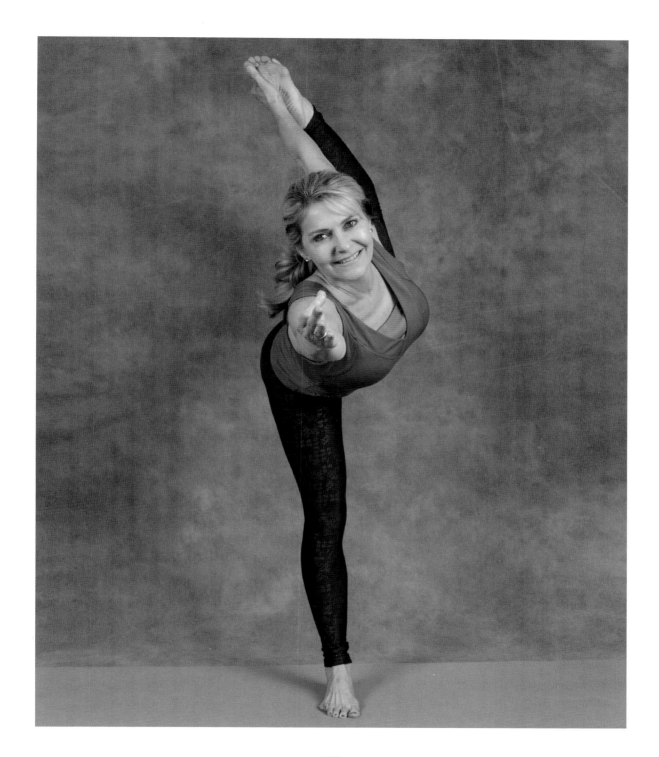

YOGA TABLE OF CONTENTS

1. EXERCISE WITH MINDFUL AWARENESS

2. KEEP MOVING

3. BENEFITS OF YOGA AND EXERCISE

4. REFRAMING EXERCISE

5. SUN SALUTATION

6. SPINAL HEALTH YOGA SEQUENCE

Strengthen your spine when feeling healthy.
Gently stretch your spine when in pain.
Level 1 in the chair, Level 2 near the chair, Level 3 on the mat

a.	Cat & Cow	6 DIRECTIONS
b.	Side Bends	OF THE
c.	Seated Twists	SPINE
d.	Forward Fold	
e.	Pyramid Pose	

—ON THE MAT—

f. Low Cobra
g. Super Woman/ Super Man
h. Swan
i. Seated Twists on the Mat

7. SCIATICA RELEASE YOGA SEQUENCE

When you're in pain, practice the first two postures in your bed.
a. Double Knees to Chest
b. Reclined & Seated Pigeon on the Mat
c. Happy Baby
d. Reclined Twists
e. Cat & Cow
f. Seated Squat
g. Seated Pigeon in a Chair

8. YOGA FOR WEIGHT MANAGEMENT & STRENGTH
Eat less and drink more water and practice yoga 30-60 minutes daily.
a. Downward Facing Dog
b. Down Dog Lift
c. Lower Plank
d. Side Plank – L1, L2, L3
e. Warrior Trilogy
      1. Warrior II
      2. Side Angle Lunge
      3. Triangle

9. YOGA FOR DIGESTION
a. Relaxation Pose
b. Extended Child Pose
c. Cat & Cow on the Mat
d. Lateral Turns
e. Double Knees to Chest
f. Happy Baby
g. Reclined Pigeon
h. Reclined Twists
i. Seated Twists
j. Side Angle Lunge

10. POSTURES FOR BALANCE & POISE
a. Mountain Pose
b. Tree Pose – L1, L2, L3
b. Quad Stretch
c. Dancer Pose
d. Airplane

11. ADVANCED YOGA ASANAS
a. Bound Exalted Warrior
b. Half Moon, Bound Half Moon
c. Bound Prayer Twist

12. YOGA ON A PEG ~ A Yogi recounts her harrowing motorcycle adventure through the Andes

EXERCISE WITH MINDFUL AWARENESS

Please consult your doctor prior to beginning any exercise program as some of these postures may be contraindicated (not recommended). Work within your own range of movement and abilities. Strength train and build muscles when you feel strong and vibrant. Practice gentle yoga or simply stroll through the neighborhood for 15 minutes when you're fatigued or injured. Commit to some sort of movement or exercise on a daily or near daily basis and don't over-train. Listen to your body and move accordingly. Don't force your body to athletically perform on the days when you just need gentle stretches.

Practicing any yoga postures with the support of a chair, desk, countertop or wall can build confidence. Find a focal point on the floor, wall or ceiling and feel your eyes move into a soft gaze. Feel the micro movements in the knee, ankle and foot during each posture. Stay grounded. Relax your jaw and soften your face. Hold each posture for 5-10 deep breaths approximately 30-60 seconds. Counting your breaths keeps you focused on your breathing style. Watching the clock allows the mind to drift-off. Consider counting to four on the inhale and four on the exhale, at least attempt to keep your inhale and exhale the same length.

One side is shown in the photos, but be sure to practice both sides equally. These postures have numerous benefits, strengthen the spine and can aide with weight reduction. Those with neck injuries or current neck pain should gaze straight ahead with both sides of neck evenly extended. Practice 30-60 minutes daily. Start with the chair postures and add new ones in upcoming weeks. It's good to have small goals at the beginning, like 15 minutes twice weekly, so that you feel successful. Build your daily practice making it part of your permanent lifestyle.

KEEP MOVING

What I know for sure is it's easier to maintain what you have than to lose it and start over. A little bit of consistent activity can make all the difference over the weeks and years to come. Even if you're 100 pounds over weight or 100 years old, it's easier to do gentle yoga postures to sustain what you have instead of doing nothing and gaining another 20 pounds. Imagine if you had a broken arm, hip replacement or heart surgery. The health you have right now may very well be better than any of those conditions. Even a small paper cut can irritate and distract you. So be thankful for what you have right now and maintain it.

I am a Registered Yoga Teacher with the Yoga Alliance. I trained with many internationally recognized yoga masters like Manju Jois of the Astanga Yoga Institute, BNS Iyengar in Mysore, India, and American Icons Rod Stryker, Shiva Rea, Rodney Yee and Bryan Kest. Additionally, I traveled extensively around the world visiting over 30-countries studying yoga and meditation in a variety of different studios. I took the opportunity to tour India for six-months and visited the top three yoga villages in Mysore, Goa and Rishikesh. I trained with some of the oldest living yogis in the world in yoga studios, Ashrams, sacred sites and caves. Furthermore, I am a Certified Strength Trainer and Fitness Over Fifty Specialist with a focus on Parkinson's Disease (PD). Upon my return to America, I began teaching in 2002 with Dr. Kenneth Cooper at the Cooper Aerobics Center, Tom Landry Fitness Center, Premier Athletic Club and Telos Performance Center in Dallas, Texas. Currently, I teach power yoga and strength training in Austin, Texas, and gentle yoga to vibrant older adults at Sun City Retirement Village in Georgetown, Texas.

I've found the integrative approach of yoga is what makes it a superior form of exercise for just about anyone. Bridging exercise with stress management so you feel the difference immediately makes each hour on the mat or in a chair valuable, and it's ideal for all ages at most any stage of physical fitness development. This understanding gives you more presence not just bigger muscles. Yes, you can become slim and sleek, build muscles, get toned and also gain clarity of mind, grace in movements and a new respect for your body. Your body will become your sacred temple. Let's polish it up like your favorite vehicle and refine the fluency of your physical movements.

Patanjali is credited with bringing yoga to the world thousands of years ago. Yoga means union between body, mind and breath. The sun salutation is 12-postures linked together and the combination of these positions uses all the major muscles, stimulates the joints, and increases circulation of blood, water and oxygen throughout the body. A gentle routine or an intensely athletic practice can be achieved with just those 12-postures giving you balance, strength, stamina, extended range of motion, mental focus and inner peace. When your body is agile it affects your overall outlook. When you feel emotionally balanced and optimistic, you are naturally kind to yourself and others, and can rise above the stress of daily living.

Yoga can be a simple exercise program or a life path for spiritual development. The 8-Limbs of Yoga are steps, or guidelines, to achieve total vibrancy of mind-body-spirit.

8-LIMBS OF YOGA

1. Yama: Universal Morality
    a. Ahimsa–Compassion For All Living Things; Nonviolence
    b. Satya–Commitment to Truthfulness
    c. Asteya–Non-stealing
    d. Brahmacharya–Sense Control
    e. Aparigraha–Neutralizing the Desire to Acquire and Hoard Wealth
2. Niyama: Personal Observances
    a. Purity or Cleanliness
    b. Samtosa–Contentment
    c. Tapas–Disciplined Use of Energy
    d. Svadhyaya–Self Study of Sacred Scriptures
    e. Isvara pranidhana–Surrender to God's Wisdom
3. Asanas: Body Postures (this is what most people call "Yoga")
4. Pranayama: Breathing Exercises, Control of Prana, Life Force Energy
5. Pratyahara: Control of the Senses
6. Dharana: Concentration and Cultivating Inner Perceptual Awareness
7. Dhyana: Devotion, Meditation on the Divine
8. Samadhi: Union with the Divine

It's basically 16 Commandments. Yoga is a complete life path and worthy of at least a quick review. Contemplate any one limb for a day or two, and consider its application into your life.

I teach simple, down-to-earth yoga postures that you can practice in a chair, with the support of a chair or on the floor. You don't need a new outfit, new shoes or even a yoga mat. Right now just notice the quality of your breath. Feel the body breathing on its own while you're reading. Once you notice your breath you'll probably change your rhythm or even breathe deeper. That's good. Think about the **six directions of the lungs**. The rib cage expands left and right, the collarbones lift as the diaphragm drops down, and the chest and back expand outward away from each other creating the six directions of the lungs. Maintain that awareness of your lungs expanding while practicing the postures on the following pages.

BENEFITS OF YOGA AND EXERCISE

- Reduces inflammation which is the root cause to all disease
- Increases flexibility, agility and balance
- Develops muscular strength, tone and endurance
- Reduces weight and improves athletic performance
- Improves immune system and invigorates health
- Lowers blood pressure and improves heart functioning
- Lessens pain from new and old injuries
- Teens become less impulsive and test anxiety reduces
- Decreases PMS symptoms, balances pregnancy & menopause hormones
- Reduces anxiety, panic and depressive symptoms
- Decreases attention disorders, improves memory and cognitive abilities
- Calms you down to regain mental clarity
- Increases the happy hormone, serotonin and dopamine
- Decreases the stress hormone, cortisol
- Normalizes melatonin levels in the brain and improves sleeping patterns
- No side effects and a multitude of health benefits

REFRAMING EXERCISE

I don't like to sweat.
Practice gentle yoga in an air-conditioned room, like your living room.

I don't have time to exercise.
Start with 10 minutes twice a week. Slowly building a solid routine assures your longterm success.

I'm exhausted.
Exercise gives you the energy you're missing. Spend 10-15 minutes walking around the building on your lunch break and notice the additional energy you have for the second half of the day. Allow two to three weeks to acclimate to new activity.

I'm injured.
After physical therapy, start slowly and develop necessary muscles to exercise. Attend a class with an instructor or hire a personal trainer to make sure you're exercising properly.

I'd rather watch TV.
While watching TV, do some sit-ups or hatha yoga. Simple stretches make a big difference in your overall abilities. Practicing 30-60 second postures, about the length of a commercial, is a natural stopwatch. Almost anyone can do it, and your pets may join you.

195

I'm lazy/depressed.	Exercise gives you endorphins that elevate your serotonin and dopamine levels. When you feel the worst, walk around the block for five minutes and notice how your mood improves quickly. Even washing your car or gardening are forms of activity that can break the habit of lethargy.
I'm frustrated & angry.	Blood, sweat and tears. Take your aggression out on the treadmill or punching bag. Get some oxygen! The perfect time for a kickboxing class is when you're mad, irritated or feel over-powered by another. Shift disempowerment and rebuild your inner confidence through intense activity.

When you are healthy, you have more energy to do the things you love; you are more thoughtful, energetic, peaceful, sexy, creative, productive, polite, patient, expressive, relaxed, kind, compassionate, and you sleep better which gives you energy for the following day to be curious, attentive, dynamic, resilient and industrious.

SUN SALUTATION ~ *SURYA NAMASKAR*

The sun salutation is a complete workout. Surya Namaskar, annunciated SUR-yuh nah-ma-SKAR-uh, means *to bow to the sun*. The sun salutation consists of 12 basic postures linked together with the breath rhythmically flowing from one pose to the next. This classic sequence of yoga postures heats up the body, activates the muscles, joints and tendons, increases circulation through the organs and improves overall conditioning. You work and rest each muscle in the entire body while moving through the sun salute. The sun salutation improves posture, increases spinal mobility, expands range of motion, alleviates stress and reduces potential injuries by heating the body from the inside out. You can slowly practice two or four rounds in a few minutes, or flow quickly through the same sequence of postures for 10, 20 or 30-minutes. It becomes a moving meditation and calms the mind.

Alignment and the breath go hand-in-hand. In the 15th Century Classic *Hatha Yoga Pradipika*, Swami Svatmarama states, "the mind is lord of the body, and *prana*, or life force, is lord of the mind" (Chapter 11, verses 29-30). Orchestrate your movements with your breath. Consciously breathing in and out as directed in the chapters to follow will assist you in cultivating a richer vocabulary with your body. When you're breathing properly, accurate alignment is easier. When you maintain proper alignment, it's natural to breathe deeply. Inhale when you expand and reach, exhale when you contract or fold. Even if you get the breathing wrong the first few times, maintain focus on your breathing while exercising.

Feeling your feet on the ground is the basis of all postures. There are four points on each foot, two in the pads and two points in the heel (inner and outer edge). Ground through the four points of your feet and lengthen through the toes to gain and maintain balance. Biomechanically, the feet either roll out (supinate), roll in (pronate), and the toes flex (dorsiflexion) or point (plantarflexion). All balance and imbalance begins as a result of the interaction of these four movements. The spine is the structural core of all movement and maintaining correct alignment over the four-points of the feet leaves you feeling grounded, stable and strong during your practice and throughout the day.

Practice the positions, learning the names of the postures and the sequence. This creates the neurological awareness for the movements. Muscular acuity and flexibility follow. Don't expect it all to happen at once. Practicing the asanas is not about being flexible. Flexibility is an outcome of practicing, but you don't have to be flexible to gain a strong supple body. Some of the postures over the next several pages could take you a decade to achieve so don't compare yourself to my flexibility. Modify as needed, go at your own pace and continue practicing daily. Over the course of the next few weeks and months, you will gain a new level of awareness of your body and that, in turn, will encourage you to practice other healthy methods. Consistent practice makes permanent.

SUN SALUTATION

Surya Namaskar

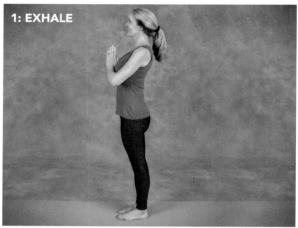

1: EXHALE

Prayer Pose ~ *Pranamasana*
Stand tall, feet hip width apart. Keep top of thighs over heels. Spine long, sternum lifted and shoulders broad.

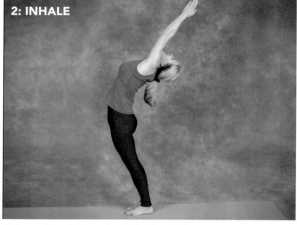

2: INHALE

Micro Backbend ~ *Hasta Uttansana*
Extend arms out & up with arms overhead. Elongate the spine and neck. Look up and bend backward slightly.

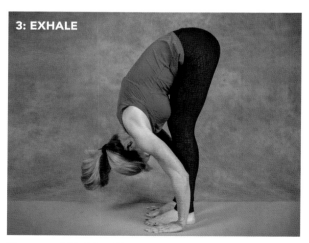

3: EXHALE

Forward Fold ~ *Uttanasana*
Reach for your knees, ankles or toes and elongate neck toward mat. Bend knees slightly for those with tight hamstrings.

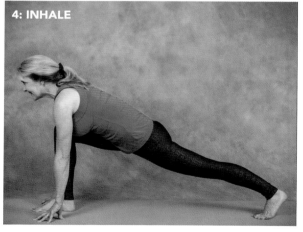

4: INHALE

Runners Lunge ~ *Ashwa Sanchalanasana*
Left leg moves backward as hands meet the mat. Keep right shin straight while extending left leg. Touch back knee to mat for support.

SUN SALUTATION
Surya Namaskar

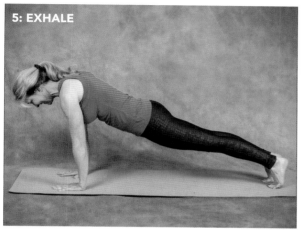

Upper Plank ~ *Kumbhakasana*
Extend both feet back to upper pushup with hands directly under shoulders. Engage abs and remain on toes.

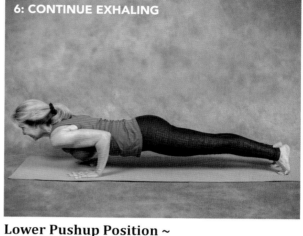

Lower Pushup Position ~ *Chaturanga Dandasana*
Lower to mat skimming ribcage with elbows. Keep abs engaged to protect core.

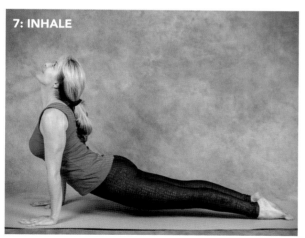

Up Dog ~ *Vrdva Mukha Svanasana*
Roll over your toes moving forward. Keep shoulders directly over the palms. Sternum out, elbows straight without slouching forward. Knees on the mat for Level 1.

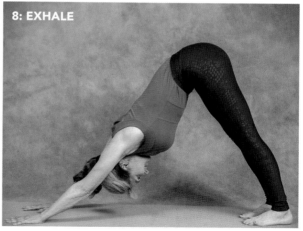

Down Dog ~ *Adho Mukha Svanasana*
Push back while lifting hips high and walk feet in one step. Lower head toward mat. Keep palms flat, elbows straight. Lengthen legs & heels toward floor.

SUN SALUTATION
Surya Namaskar

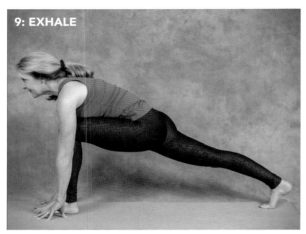

Runners Lunge ~ *Ashwa Sanchalanasana*
Left leg moves forward. Keep left shin straight and right leg long. Touch back knee to mat for support.

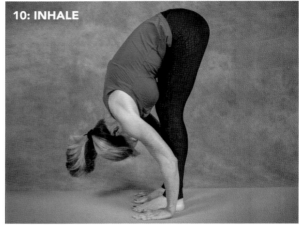

Forward Fold ~ Uttanasana
Walk forward with right leg. Hinge forward and reach for your knees, ankles or toes. Lower crown of head toward the mat. Bend knees slightly for those with tight hamstrings.

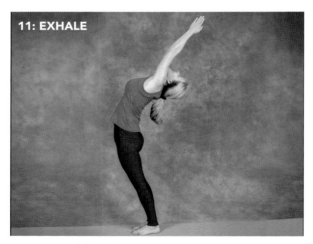

Micro Backbend ~ *Hasta Uttansana*
Reverse swan dive sweeping arms out and up. Return to micro backbend and look upward.

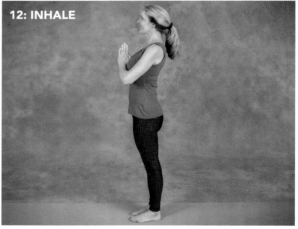

Prayer Pose ~ *Pranamasana*
Return hands to Namaste Position. Stand tall, feet hip width apart. Keep weight evenly distributed over the four points of each foot.

SPINAL HEALTH YOGA SEQUENCE

6 Directions of the Spine
Contraindicated for those with chronic spinal injuries.

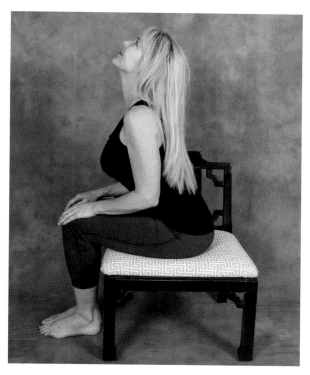 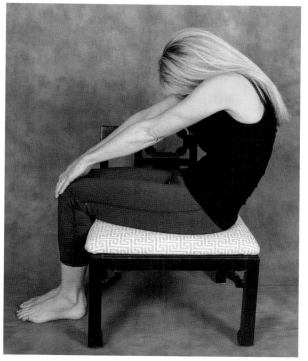

Seated Cow ~ *Bitilasana*
- Inhale deeply lift the chin.
- Arch the spine from the low back to crown of head.
- Retract the shoulders back and down the spine.

Seated Cat ~ *Marjaryasana*
- Exhale and round the spine (like a cat hissing).
- Tuck the neck, chin to chest.
- Keep hands on lap.

Benefits
- Increases circulation to vertebrae.
- Improves spinal flexibility.
- Invigorates life force energy.

Contraindicated for those with neck injuries. Keep neck in alignment with spine. Only move mid to lower back. Otherwise, move freely and slowly with your breath.

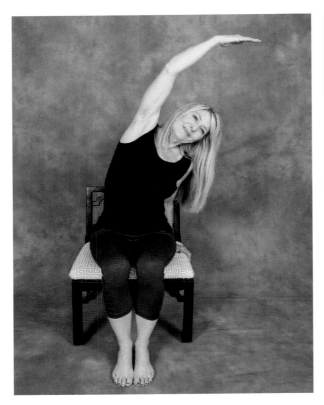
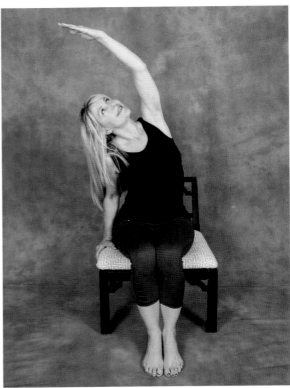

Seated Side Bends ~ *Parsva Sukhasana*

• Press hips down while reaching to each side.

• Elongate through the side body and arm.

• Keep neck on the diagonal.

• Move your awareness inward from side body to rib cage to the spine on the tilt.

Benefits

• Improves core flexibility.

• Increases awareness and
  concentration.

Contraindicated for those with very low blood pressure, dizziness, headaches, or diarrhea.

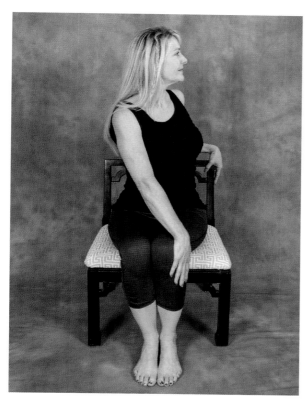 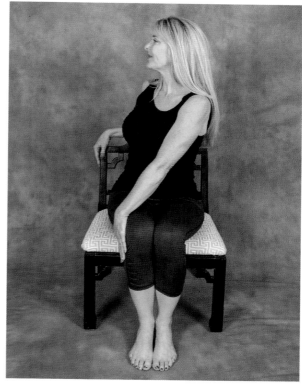

Seated Twists ~ *Ardha Matsyendrasana*
• Press buttocks to the chair while turning right and left.
• Turn slowly and deliberately. Do not crank into your deepest twist.
• On each additional turn, twist just a little bit more & look over shoulder.

Benefits
• Keeps the spine supple.
• Gently releases sciatica and low back tension
• Aids digestion.
• Detoxifying.

Contraindicated for those with chronic spinal injuries.

Practice the 6 Directions of the Spine at least once a day.

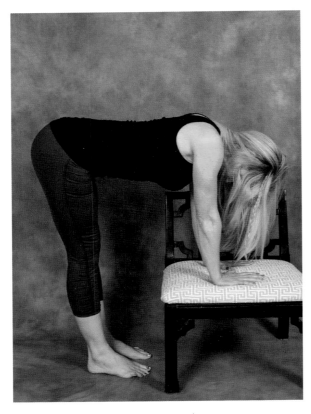 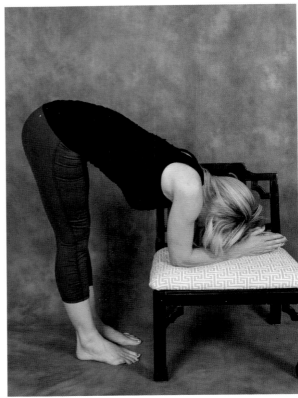

Forward Fold ~ *Uttanasana*
Level 1
- Stand to the side of chair with both feet facing the chair.
- Feel the four points of your feet as you hinge forward from the hips.
- Keep top of thighs over heels & rest hands on the chair.
- Keep knees as straight as you can without locking them (soft knees).

Level 2
- For those who have more flexibility, lean on the elbows.
- Relax the neck & look at your knees.
- Keep knees straight and soft.
- Don't round your upper back.

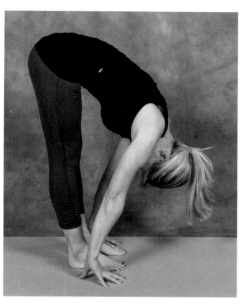

Level 3
- If you desire more intensity, reach for the floor.
- Keep knees straight and soft. If you need to bend your knees, return to Level 2.
- Align fingertips with toes.
- Relax neck & jaw. Look at your knees or navel.

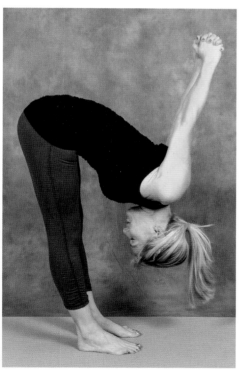

Level 4
- Great posture if you've been sitting for hours in a chair, car or airplane seat.
- Once in forward fold, interlock fingers behind back or hold wrists.
- Elongate neck toward floor and relax jaw.
- Hold neck erect if you get dizzy.

Benefits
- Elongates hamstrings and calves.
- Tight hamstrings can lead to low back tension. Improves both areas.
- Strengthens thighs and knees.
- Inversions diminish mental activity and anxiety.

Contraindicated for those with sciatica, or bend knees to decrease intensity. Avoid if you've had a recent or chronic injury to the legs, hips or back. Level 4 is not intended for anyone with vertigo, heart disease or cataracts.

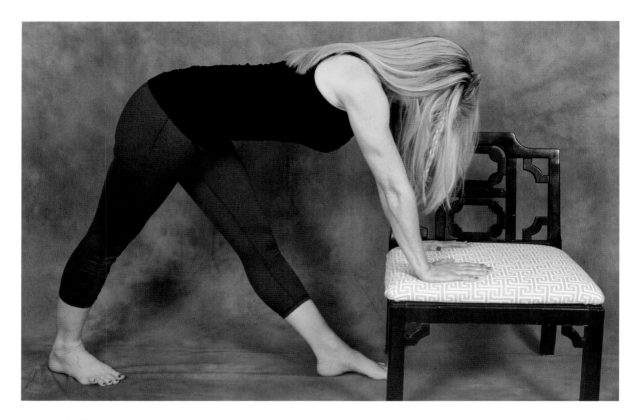

Pyramid Pose ~ *Parsvottanasana*
• Leaning on the chair, take one leg forward.
• Keep knees straight but not locked.
• Press to the ground through back heel. Tailbone reaching downward.
• Wrap your back hip forward (right hip in this picture).
• Hold hips square to the chair and both feet facing the chair.
• Keep spine straight & parallel to the floor.

Benefits
• Lengthens hamstrings and calves.
• Stretches low back.
• Increases circulation.
• Preventative stretch for sciatica tension.

Contraindicated for those with hamstring injury. Keep knees slightly bent.

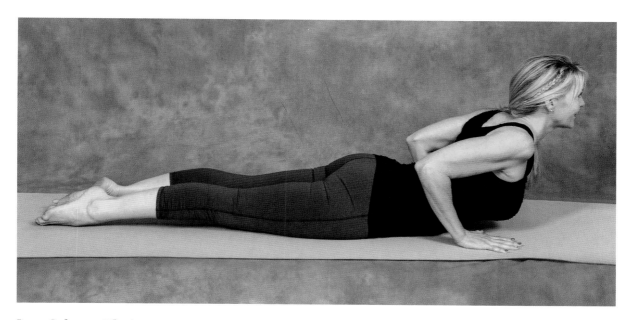

Low Cobra ~ *Bhujangasana*

Stretch your back-body to alleviate pressure and strengthen your spine to prevent future back tension. Practice low cobra & super woman on days when you don't ache.

• Lie in a prone position on your stomach.
• Bend elbows and rest fingertips under shoulders.
• Glide the tops of your shoulders away from ears while elbows skim the ribcage.
• Inhale and lift chest slightly off floor.
• Distribute the length of the arc evenly through entire spine.
• Lift up and down a few times. Lift up with an inhale; lower on the exhale.
• Don't squeeze your buttox.

Benefits
• Develops strength and suppleness in spine.
• Stretches and strengthens chest, shoulders, arms, legs, and glutes.
• Maintains spinal flexibility.
• Improves circulation.
• Rejuvenating.

Contraindicated for those with chronic spinal injuries.

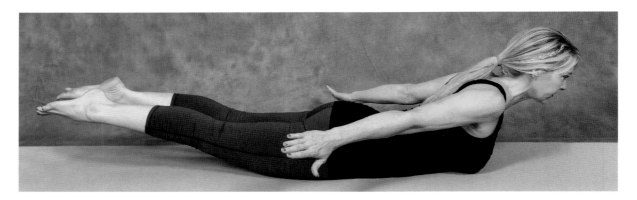

Super Woman/Cobra Variation ~ *Viparita Shalabhasana*
• Lie on your stomach with your toes flat on the floor & rest chin on the mat.
• Hold legs close together with feet lightly touching each other.
• Extend arms down the ribcage. Activate the back-body.
• Inhale deeply and lift chest, arms, legs and thighs off the floor.
• Exhale as you gently lower and relax on mat.
• Variation: Lift only upper body or lift only lower body.

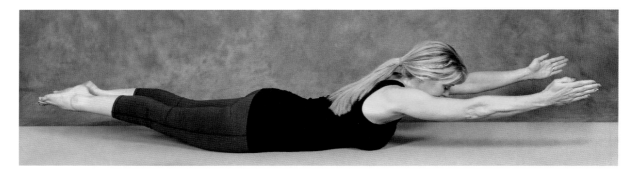

Super Man/Cobra Variation
• Advancing the posture, extend arms forward.
• Reaching arms in a "V" position is easier than lengthening arms near ears.
• Vigorously extend arms forward away from hips.
• Lift thighs off the floor moving to pelvic bone.
• Variation: Lift only upper body or lift only lower body.

Benefits
• Increases strength in spine.
• Develops shoulders, arms, legs and glutes.
• Maintains spinal muscles.
• Improves circulation.

Contraindicated for those with chronic spinal injuries.

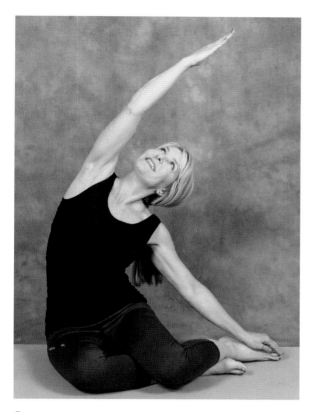 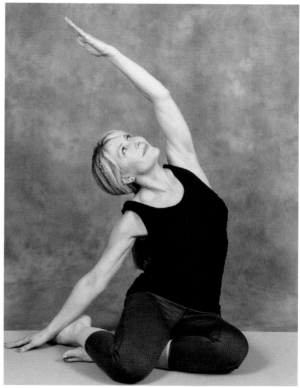

Swan
- Sit on the right hip and wave your legs to the left.
- The classic position maintains the left ankle to right arch (modify hips and knees if you have injuries or lack flexibility).
- Inhale and reach your right hand up and over the head.
- Look at your hand if you have flexibility in the neck.
- Reach in opposite direction too.

Benefits
- Elongation through side body.
- Deep stretch in low back and hips.
- Decreases compression from standing.
- Opens shoulder girdle.
- Increases lung capacity.

Contraindicated for those with chronic lumbar, hip or knee injuries.

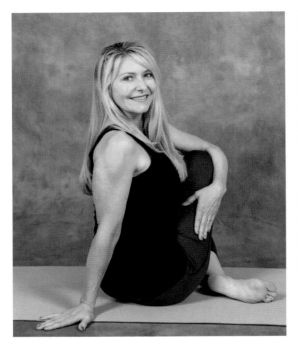

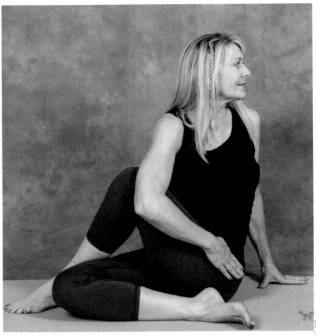

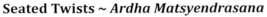

Seated Twists ~ *Ardha Matsyendrasana*

- Sit on mat and bend right knee.
- Cross left foot under right knee or extend straight with ankle to mat.
- Keep both sit bones on the mat. Pelvis needs to be square first, then twist the spine.
- Inhale and elongate spine, exhale and twist.
- Twist smoothly from the tailbone to the crown of the head.
- If the right knee is up, place the right hand on the floor behind you. Turn and gently look to the right.
- If the left knee is up, place the left hand on floor behind you. Turn and gently look to the left.
- Never crank into your deepest twist.

Benefits

- Restores suppleness to spine.
- Improves digestion, detoxifying for organs.
- Stretches hip and low back.
- Increases synovial fluid along spinal column.
- Twisting aids peristalsis.

Contraindicated for those who are pregnant or with chronic spinal injuries. If your sit bones are not equally touching the mat when you begin benefits are reduced.

SCIATICA RELEASE YOGA SEQUENCE

The sciatic nerve is located in the low back & buttocks area, branches down each leg and delivers nerve signals to the feet. Compression is commonly caused by a herniated disc or protruding vertebrae in the low back, spinal tumors or injury. Some have a congenital effect in the spine causing a narrowing of the nerve root passageway called stenosis. This can get worse with age. The piriformis muscle wraps around the sciatic nerve. A tight periformis muscle can cause a pinching, tingling or burning sensation down the leg. Inflammation in the piriformis can also lead to pain in the low back and buttocks. You might have low back pain, but it could be due to tension in the piriformis. Sometimes the pressure can be intolerable making it difficult to sit for long periods and equally difficult to stand for long periods. Typically, pressure will build mainly in one leg.

Pigeon is the primary pose to release the piriformis. Try it in your bed, a chair, on the mat or reclining on the floor. Practice all four positions to experience the varied sensations. Be mindful of your knees and hips while doing these postures or avoid if you have chronic injuries. Also, the Warrior Trilogy sequence (shown in the Yoga for Weight Management Sequence) is very effective for strengthening and stretching the low back and hamstrings.

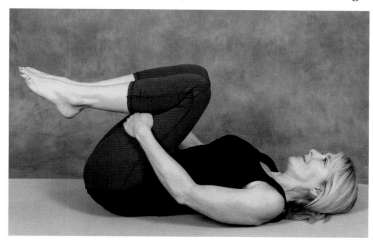

Reclined Double Knees to Chest on Floor or in your Bed ~ *Apanasana*
- Recline on the floor or in bed & squeeze both knees to chest.
- Hold back of your legs (hamstrings).
- Rest head, neck and shoulders to mat (don't hunch).
- Also try this with just one leg at a time.
- Start with right leg first to assist the ascending colon.

Benefits
- Releases low back and kidney band.
- Increases circulation to lower abdomen, hips and hamstrings.
- Increases peristalsis.

Contraindicated for those who are pregnant or with lumbar or knee injuries. Do not squeeze your knees. Hold the hamstrings.

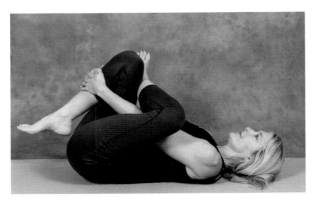
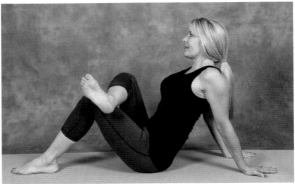

Reclined Pigeon on the Floor or in your Bed/Eye of the Needle ~ *Sucirandhrasana*
- Lie on your back, and bend knees with both feet on the mat.
- Cross left ankle to lower right thigh.
- Reach through the triangle of the legs and hold the back of right thigh or shin.
- Relax head, neck and shoulders to the surface beneath you. Don't hunch.
- Flex the left foot angling toes toward knee.
- Ground spine down to the mat from the back of your head to your tailbone.
- Hold for 10 breaths & slowly release to other leg.

Seated Pigeon on the Mat
- Sit on the floor with knees bent.
- Elongate spine and retract shoulders from the ears.
- Place hands behind your hips on the floor for stability.
- Cross right ankle to lower left thigh.
- Flex your right foot and externally rotate right thigh away from chest.
- Alternate direction of fingers on the floor behind your hips (fingers facing hips and pointing away ~ externally rotating the shoulders).

Benefits
- Releases piriformis.
- Stretches hips and hamstrings.
- Relieves tension in buttocks & lower back.
- Improves circulation through legs, hips and back.

Contraindicated for those who are pregnant or with a recent or chronic injury to knees, hips, low back or spine. Work within your own range of limits and abilities.

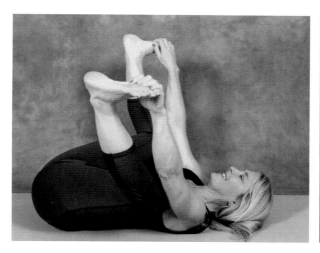

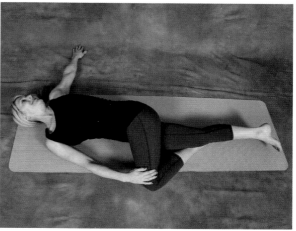

Happy Baby ~ *Ananda Balasana*
- Recline on spine on the floor or in bed, hold feet, ankles or hamstrings.
- Take legs out wider than the torso & press feet flat as if to walk on the ceiling.
- Release low back and tailbone down. Relax head, neck & shoulders (don't hunch).

Benefits
- Stretches inner thigh, groin and hamstrings.
- Relief from low back discomfort.
- Calms the mind.

Contraindicated for those who are pregnant beyond the second trimester. If you have knee or ankle injury, hold hamstrings instead of feet.

Practice Cat and Cow to alleviate sciatica. Shown in a chair in the Spinal Health Sequence. Shown on the mat in Digestion Sequence.

Reclined Twists ~ *Supta Matsyendrasana*
- Recline on your back with extended arms from shoulders.
- Bend the left knee, place left foot across right knee & keep other leg straight.
- Exhale and twist toward the right.
- Move the bent knee toward the chest to release sciatica.
- Get comfortable with the twist to the right before reaching and looking to the left.

Benefits
- Realigns spine.
- Releases tension in the spine.
- Restores equilibrium in the nervous system.
- Massages the stomach and decreases gastritis.

Contraindicated for those with recent or chronic injury to the knees, hips or spine. Do not twist if you have severe spinal injuries or are pregnant.

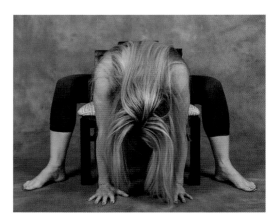

Seated Squat in a Chair

- Sit on a chair and take your legs wider than the chair.
- Fold the torso forward, relax the neck down & reach hands to the floor.
- If you have hip or low back injuries, rest elbows on your thighs.

Benefits

- Superb hip opener with less gravity to joint.
- Releases low back.
- Lowering head below heart is calming for the mind.

Contraindicated for those with chronic injuries to hips, low back or spine. Reduce stretch by keeping legs closer. Lowering head below heart can cause dizziness.

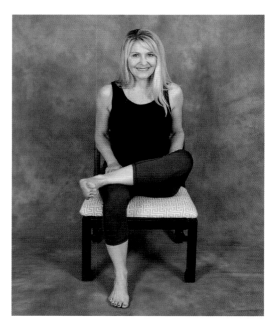

Seated Pigeon in a Chair

- Relax your back and cross the left ankle to lower right thigh.
- Flex the left foot & press thigh down toward floor for an external rotation of the left femur.
- Level 1 relaxed, rounded spine.
- Level 2 sitting up straight.
- Level 3, lean forward nose toward toes with straight spine.
- Hold for 5-10 deep breaths.

Benefits

- Releases piriformis.
- Stretches hips and hamstrings.
- Relieves tension in buttocks, lower back & leg.
- Improves circulation through legs, hips and back.

Contraindicated for those with a recent or chronic injury to knees, hips, low back or spine. Work within your own range of limits and abilities.

YOGA FOR WEIGHT MANAGEMENT & STRENGTH

Downward Facing Dog ~ *Adho Mukha Svanasana*

Considered one of the best yoga poses as it energizes and rejuvenates the entire body. It deeply stretches the legs, calves and even arches while strengthening the arms and shoulders. Inversions offer preventative relief from fatigue, headaches, insomnia and mild depression.

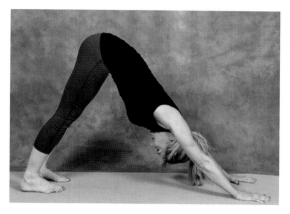

- Begin on all fours, tabletop position.
- Hands under the shoulders; knees under hips and feet aligned with knees.
- Exhale and straighten legs. Never lock your knees.
- Lift hips high creating an A-Frame position.
- Externally rotate biceps with palms flat.
- Inwardly rotate femurs.
- Softly release neck and jaw.
- Engage abs lifting stomach to spine & press heels toward the ground.

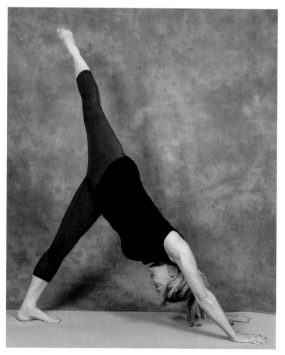

One-Leg Down Dog Lift ~
Eka Pada Adho Mukha Svanasana

- From Down Dog extend one leg to the sky.
- Inhale deeply and elongate through the side body.
- Continue pressing other heel to the floor.
- Be mindful to safely stretch inner thigh and groin.

Benefits

- Strengthens upper body, stretches back and opens chest.
- Lengthens hamstrings and calves.
- Flattens palms & increases circulation in hands.
- Inversions are ideal for natural cervical traction.
- Helps prevent osteoporosis.
- Increases blood flow to brain & relieves stress.

Contraindicated for those with carpel tunnel, high blood pressure, eye or inner ear infections or those in late-term pregnancy. It's preventative for headaches; not recommended if you currently have one.

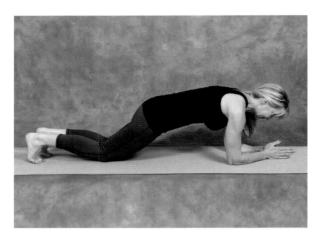
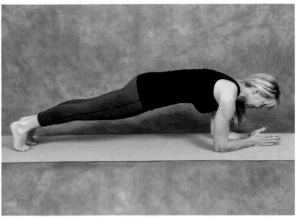

Lower Plank ~ *Chaturanga Dandasana*
• Recline on stomach in a prone position.
• Place elbows underneath shoulders.
• Maintain neck in alignment with spine.
• Hold hips at same height as shoulders.
• Do not lift your hips up high (that's easier).
• Keep knees on mat and press through toes to modify for Level 1.
• Flex feet and extend through heels.

Lower Plank – Level 2
• Lift knees.
• Maintain shoulders over elbows.
• Hold for 10 breaths or longer.

Benefits
• Builds core strength.
• Builds leg muscles.
• Increases strength in shoulders.
• Develops spinal health.

Contraindicated for those with neck, shoulder or elbow injuries.

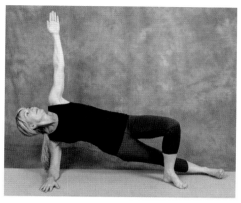

Side Plank ~ Level 1 ~ *Vasisthasana*
- Recline on side.
- Align lower elbow (right one in this photo) directly under shoulder.
- Separate shoulder blades and stretch through arms.
- Extend legs straight from spine.
- Place one foot in front of the other knee.
- Push on front foot (left) to assist shoulder.
- Feel in deltoid not armpit.
- Hold for 5-10 breaths or longer.

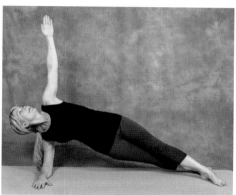

Side Plank ~ Level 2
- Elongate both legs and extend feet to the mat.
- Position top foot in front of lower foot (left in front).
- Maintain alignment of elbow and shoulder.
- If you are out of alignment you will feel it in armpit (weakens rotator cuff).
- Lift hips up and engage abs.
- Hold for 5-10 breaths or longer.

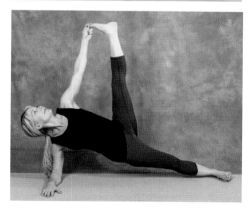

Side Plank ~ Level 3
- Bind hand to foot on top leg (left).
- Maintain perpendicular alignment of arm to floor.
- Keep neck long and look up or forward.
- Soften your jaw and deepen your breath.
- Maintain enough energy to complete both sides.
- Hold for 5-10 breaths or longer.

Benefits
- Builds core strength quickly.
- Increases leg muscles & strength in shoulders.
- Develops spinal health.
- Stretches hamstring and inner thigh.

Contraindicated for those with neck, shoulder or elbow injuries.

Warrior Trilogy ~ *"Lunging, Leaning & Straightening"*
Warming up is recommended prior to any fitness activity. This sequence activates the main muscle groups in the legs, torso and arms. Practice Warrior II on each side once or twice; then lean into Side Angle Lunge on each side a time or two; finish with Triangle Pose. If you like to walk, jog, run, golf, bike, swim, basically any activity, then try the Warrior Trilogy 1-5 minutes just before and immediately following your activity.

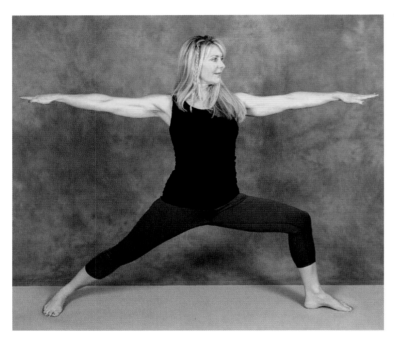

Warrior II ~ Lunging ~
Virabhadrasana II
- Place feet about 4' apart or underneath your hands of extended arms.
- Bend front knee (left knee) directly over left heel.
- Align front knee with second toe & feel the weight balanced throughout the foot, not just in the toes.
- Keep back leg (right) straight & strong with the toes aimed toward the long edge of the mat. Press hip to heel, flex buttocks & keep back leg active.
- Sink into the legs and hips while elongating your torso upward.
- Hold arms parallel to the earth and reach through the collarbones.
- Look forward or align chin with shoulder and gaze at left hand.
- Hold 5-10 breaths or longer.

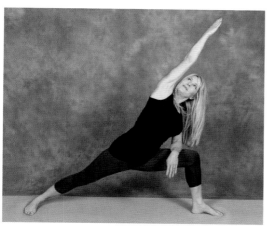

Side Angle Lunge ~ Leaning ~ *Utthita Parsvakonasana*

- Moving onward from Warrior II
- Keep the back leg (right) straight and strong.
- Place left elbow to left thigh (not knee) & extend right arm high.
- Elbow to thigh, opposite hand to the sky.
- Some may be able to touch the floor with right hand for Level 2.
- Elongate through right side of body reaching hand away from heel over the ear.
- Look at your left palm or look forward.
- Hold 5-10 breaths or longer.

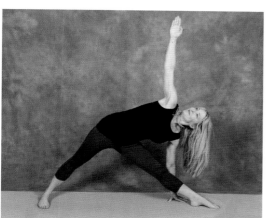

Triangle ~ Straightening ~ *Utthita Trikonasana*

- Straighten legs, activate front of thighs (quadriceps) by slightly lifting kneecaps.
- Retract weight to the back leg (right) while reaching for the left ankle.
- Reach the left rib cage off the left thigh.
- Align right shoulder over left knee while hinging to the side.
- Slide hand down shin or to the floor. Do not arch low back.
- Extend arms outward and look up toward the sky at the top palm.
- Hold 5-10 breaths or longer.
- Bend left knee, lift torso up, and pivot feet to aim at other end of mat. Lunge with right leg to proceed to other side. You can do each posture two or three times, and then blend the sequence.

Benefits
- Stretches & strengthens legs and torso.
- Opens hips and chest.
- Improves circulation and respiration.
- Spinal alignment energizes the entire body.

Contraindicated if you have severe injuries to hips, knees or shoulders. Those with very low blood pressure, dizziness, headaches, or diarrhea should avoid side bends. Extend neck evenly and look forward if you have a neck injury.

YOGA FOR DIGESTION

If you experience gas or constipation try gentle yoga movements and moderate twisting to alleviate tension in the intestines. Even a self-massage can assist circulation in the bowels. Massage with light pressure in a clockwise direction around navel. Many natural digestion cures are available at the local drugstore now. If you purchase laxatives, BeanO, antacids or other medicinal treatments consider adding natural remedies to your cart also. Senna is an herbal laxative now found at most grocery stores. Apple cider vinegar offers natural relief to a wide variety of digestive ailments. The recipe of one tablespoon vinegar in one cup of water quickly relieves acid reflux and heartburn. Do not twist if you have acid reflux. See Natural Remedies on page 181.

Relaxation Pose ~ *Savasana* is frequently overlooked when we feel imbalanced. Lying in bed or on the floor, place a pillow under legs raising them above the head and heart. This can calm the entire body in 10-15 minutes. Silently sing your sacred mantra.

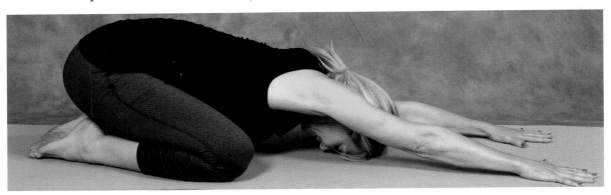

Extended Child Pose ~ *Utthita Balasana*
• Kneel on the floor on all fours in Tabletop Position.
• Push hips back to heels.
• Rest the weight of the body on the heels.
• Widen knees as you fold forward if you are pregnant.
• Keep knees together pressing abdomen to thighs.
• Keep arms long lengthening the torso. Rest forehead on the mat or hands.

Benefits
• Stretches low back.
• Prone positions reduce mind chatter.
• Gentle massage for abdomen by pressing belly to knees.
• Expect to emit gas.

Contraindicated for those with knee injuries. You may need to keep hips up in the air while pressing forehead to forearm.

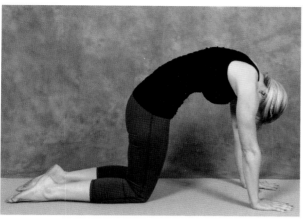

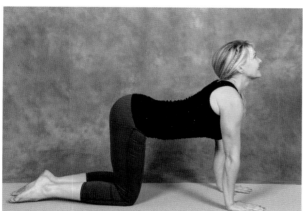

Cat & Cow on the Mat ~
Marjaryasana & Bitilasana
- Start on the hands and knees in a Tabletop Position.
- Place hands directly under the shoulders.
- Knees under the hips (not touching).
- Engage your core muscles and lift upward.
- Move spine from a rounded position (flexion) to an arched one (extension).
- It might feel like your sticking your tummy out when you lift the tailbone.
- Elongate the neck and look up at the end of Cow.
- Move the chin toward the chest on the exhale returning back to Cat.
- Flow between these two with the breath ~ inhale into Cow, exhale into Cat (like a cat hissing).

Lateral Turns (no photo)
Lateral turns are simple and helpful for low back pain and may result in a low back adjustment. Maintain the Tabletop Position and look back toward your hip, then glance at the other hip. Inhale to one side and exhale to the other side. You'll feel the lengthening of the side body as you take these lateral moves.

Benefits
- Increases circulation throughout entire spine.
- Stretches supporting muscles along spinal column.
- Gentle massage for the abdomen.

Contraindicated for those with neck or wrist injuries. Keep neck in alignment with spine. Only move mid to lower back. Press on knuckles if wrists are injured, using a non-violent fist.

ALSO SEE YOGA POSES PRESENTED IN OTHER SECTIONS ~

Double Knees to Chest (See Sciatic Release Yoga Sequence)
• Also practice with just one leg at a time.
• Start with right leg first to assist the ascending colon.

Happy Baby (See Sciatic Release Yoga Sequence)
• Rock a bit from side to side to massage the low back.

Reclined Pigeon on the Floor (See Sciatica Release Sequence)
• Stretching the low back, hips and hamstrings improves circulation to intestinal track.

Reclined Twists (See Sciatica Release Yoga Sequence)
• Twisting reduces constipation.
• Do not practice twists if you have acid reflux or heartburn. Drink apple cider vinegar (1 T vinegar in 1 c water).

Seated Twists (See Spinal Health Yoga Sequence)
• Twisting aids peristalsis.

Side Angle Lunge (See Warrior Trilogy in Weight Management Sequence)
• Unlocking the low back can improve digestion quickly.
• Depending on the discomfort, you could start with these postures.

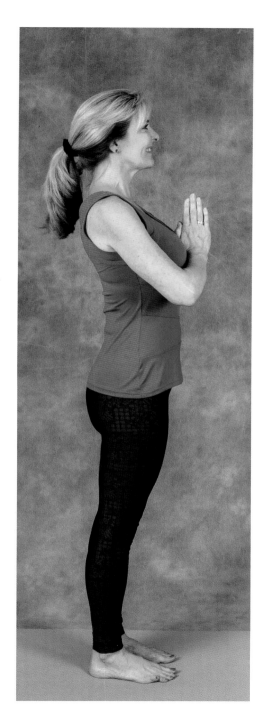

POSTURES FOR BALANCE & POISE

While practicing balancing postures you will feel a little sway and that's fine. Over time you will become more comfortable with your natural sway. It resembles the feeling of falling. If you're familiar with that feeling from doing balancing postures in a controlled setting, then if you ever have a slip & fall (which is quite common) you might be able to save yourself prior to hitting the floor. If you lose your footing you'll be less surprised. That's a slip & catch!

Mountain Pose, *Tadasana*, is simply standing upright. Standing tall and strong like a mountain is fundamental to all balancing postures. It's something you can practice all day, every day, and no one would know you're doing yoga. Looking around can cause you to lose balance, but finding a focal point, or *dristi*, helps reduce swaying. You may feel more stable on one leg over the other for a variety of reasons. Injuries or even emotional imbalances can throw us off kilter periodically.

- Find a focal point while standing in Mountain Pose.
- Stand tall with the crown of your head over the tailbone.
- Feel the four points of the feet on the floor.
- Lean back slightly & move the top of the thighs over your heels.
- Notice the soft inward rotation of the femurs.
- Drop the tailbone, engage the abs, elongate your spine and retract the shoulders.
- Keep the backside active.
- Feel the broadening of the collarbones as you lift the sternum.
- Draw the neck upward yet keep the chin parallel to the floor.
- Stand confidently and breathe comfortably.

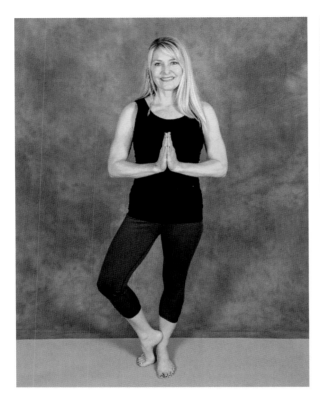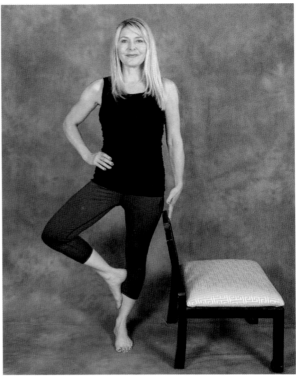

Tree Pose ~ *Vrkshasana*
Level 1

 Find a focal point while standing in Mountain Pose.

- Transfer weight to the left leg, and place your right heel on your left ankle with toes still on the floor.
- As you gain more balance, you can lift your toes off the floor like a kickstand.
- Hold your hands at the heart in Namaste.
- You will acquire strength and poise in short 5-10 second increments.
- Stand near a chair, wall or countertop for additional support.

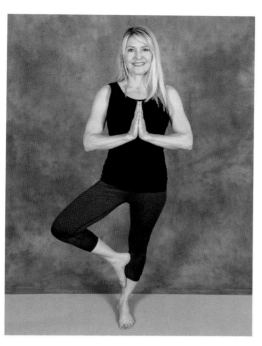

Level 2

- Move the right arch to your left calf. Toes facing floor.
- Don't turn the standing foot outward, as this will misalign the knee & hip.
- The left knee should be unencumbered. No compression on the standing knee.
- Continue externally rotating the right hip, drop the tailbone & elongate the spine.
- Ground deeper into the earth with standing leg and don't lock the knee.
- Hand to chair, hips or heart.

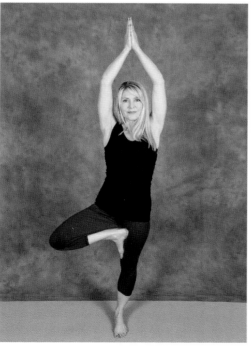

Level 3

- In the classical position, place the right heel at the top of the left thigh.
- Feel the four points of the foot on the floor.
- Inhale and reach your hands over your head.
- Elongate through side body.
- Drop the tailbone and lift the sternum.
- Feel the strength in the standing leg.
- Breathe comfortably for 5-10 breaths.

Benefits

- These poses develop core strength and tone your tummy.
- Increase balance and poise.
- Improve concentration and equilibrium to the mind.
- Strengthen legs, knees and ankles.

Contraindicated if you had knee surgery. I recommend practicing at Level 2 if you have delicate knees. Those with vertigo should avoid balancing postures without support or an instructor.

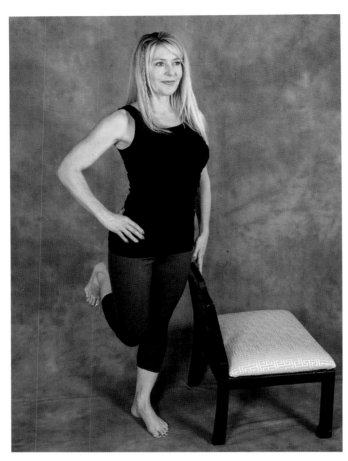

Quad Stretch ~ modified *Natarajasana*

- Stand tall on both legs equally.
- Transfer weight to your left foot and lift the right foot behind you.
- Lift your shin toward your buttocks lengthening the quadricep.
- Hold shin parallel to floor or higher up if possible.
- Increase the challenge by holding hand to ankle (Level 2).
- Stand tall and engage abs.

Benefits

- Releases tension in the quadricep, hip flexor and front of the leg.
- Improves leg and knee mobility.
- Increases range of motion.
- Keeps you walking upright. Keeps you independent.

Contraindicated for those with severe hip, knee or ankle injuries. If you get a cramp in hamstring then move to forward fold to lengthen back of leg.

Postures for Balance & Poise ~ Advanced

Remember, balancing postures should be fun. Acquire a little levity while practicing. It's just a game, a fitness game. Enjoy the postures and don't force yourself into something your body isn't ready to do. Consider the support of a chair or kitchen countertop.

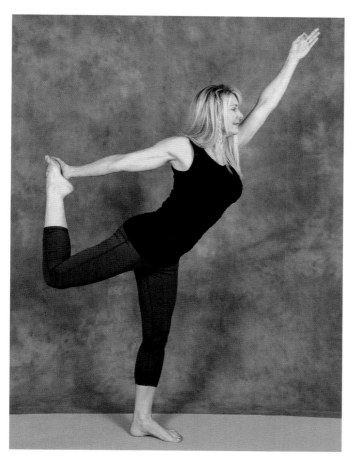

Dancer Pose ~ *Natarajasana*

- From Mountain, find your focal point.
- Externally rotate the right arm so the thumb lifts to the ceiling.
- Transfer weight to left leg and bend your right knee behind you.
- Exhale & bind right hand to right foot with palm to arch, thumb to big toe.
- Lift right leg stretching the quadricep while reaching left arm vigorously to the sky.
- Elongate the torso while opening the chest and shoulder on the right side.
- Feel the strength in the left leg and hold your upward alignment.
- Keep the left knee soft, not locked and not bent.

Benefits

- Stretches the shoulders and chest.
- Strengthens and elongates the thighs, groins, and abdomen.
- Improves grace and poise.

Contraindicated for those with ankle injuries. Do not stand on one leg without support if you have sensitive knees or ankles. Arching the back can improve spinal health. Dancer Pose is a backbend in the sky.

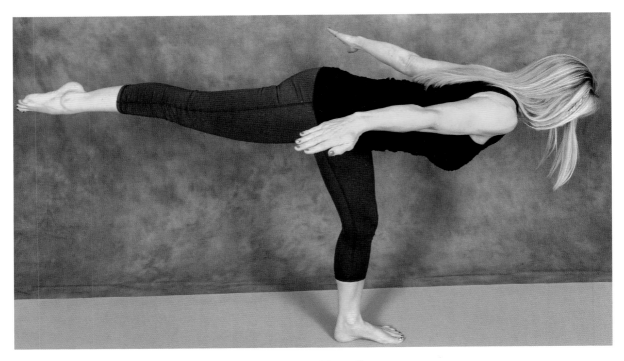

Airplane ~ *Dekasana*

- From Mountain Pose activate the arms down the ribcage & find your *dristi*, focal point.
- Feel the back body strong before transferring the weight to one leg.
- Lift one leg behind you as you tip the torso forward. Keep the neck long.
- Bend the standing knee softly & press on the four points of the standing foot.
- Tilt forward more, engage the abs, elongate the spine and neck.
- Reach the right leg behind, press through the toes, heel or ball of foot.
- Flex the calf and activate all the leg muscles in the lifted leg.
- Roll right hip down (in this photo) and reach the inside right thigh to the sky for a slight inward hip rotation.
- Extend through the fingertips like airplane wings.

Benefits

- Strengthens legs, hamstrings, knees and ankles.
- Tones lower back and abs.
- Improves balance.
- Increases concentration.
- Great challenge posture to build confidence quickly.

Contraindicated for those with leg, hip or ankle injuries. This is an advanced posture requiring significant strength and flexibility and should only be practiced if one has strong legs and lower back muscles. Avoid if you have high blood pressure.

ADVANCED YOGA ASANAS

Get your game on with these challenging yoga poses. These postures are only intended for seasoned students or athletes with a high level of mind-body awareness and noted strength, flexibility and balance. Consider locating a seasoned instructor to assist you with some of these advanced postures to confirm safe alignment. Remember, first you gain the neurological awareness then the muscular acuity will follow. Don't force yourself to achieve these postures the first time you try. Once you master the posture, then hold comfortably for 1-3 minutes. They are powerful postures requiring intense focus preferably in a quiet environment. I found advanced yoga postures took my confidence to a higher level and gave me a new sense of joy about being in a body. **Contraindicated** for anyone with any type of unmanaged injury.

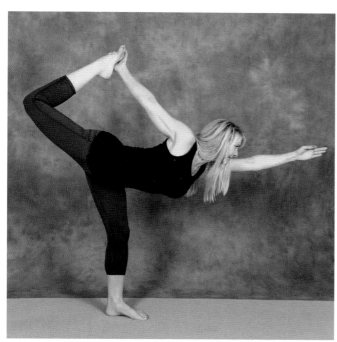

Bound Exalted Warrior ~ *Natarajasana*
- From Dancer Pose (shown previously) begin to tilt torso closer to the mat.
- Vigorously extend left arm away from the left hip.
- Lower torso and arm parallel to the mat.
- Feel the circular bind on the right side.
- Reach back foot over the head & hold the backbend in the sky.
- Push the right leg back opening the right chest and shoulder.
- Maintain the strength in the standing leg.
- Anchor through the four points of the foot.
- Soften your jaw and deepen your breath for 1-3 minutes.
- Slowly return torso upright as you release your leg to the floor and return to Mountain Pose.

Benefits
- Stretches the shoulders and chest.
- Strengthens and elongates the thighs, groins, and abdomen.
- Enhances flexibility.
- Improves grace and poise.
- Builds confidence quickly.

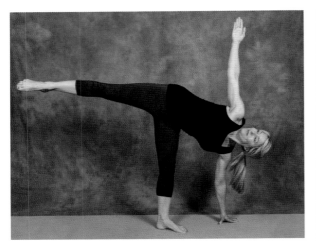
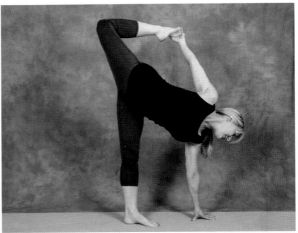

Half Moon ~ *Ardha Chandrasana*
- From Warrior II, inhale and push forward to balance on left leg.
- Lift back leg (right leg) parallel to the mat and breathe comfortably.
- Inhale, spin the lower ribcage (left) forward and top shoulder (right) backward.
- Lengthen through topside of body (right).
- Elongate neck and look forward or upward at right hand.
- Soften your jaw and deepen your breath and hold for 1-3 minutes.
- Slowly release leg, lift torso and return to Mountain Pose.

Bound Half Moon ~ *Baddha Ardha Chandrasana*
- From Half Moon, exhale & reach right hand to right ankle or foot.
- Hold this backbend in the sky for several breaths.
- Activate the standing leg without locking the knee.
- Maintain your focal point.
- For more intensity, take lower hand off the floor.
- Soften your jaw and deepen your breath and hold posture for 1-3 minutes.
- Slowly release binding, lower foot to floor while lifting torso.
- Return to standing upright in Mountain Pose.

Benefits
- Develops core muscles.
- Strengthens legs, knees and ankles.
- Stretches hamstrings.
- Opens chest and shoulder on bound side.
- Stretches abs, hip flexors, quadriceps on bound side.
- Calms the mind and builds confidence quickly.
- Increases stability and equilibrium.

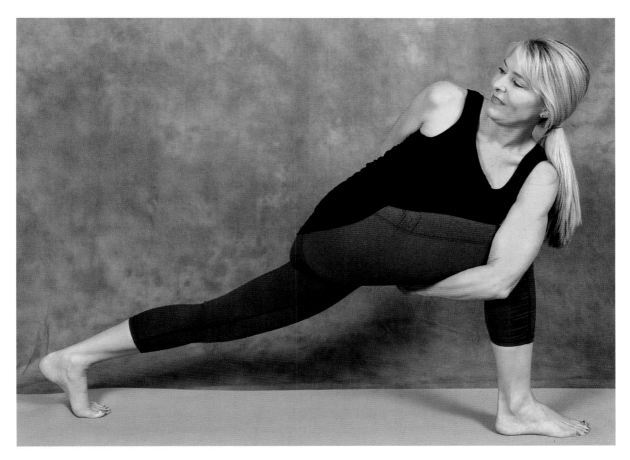

Prayer Twist ~ Bound Prayer Twist
Parivrtta Baddha Anjaneyasana

- From runner's lunge, elongate the torso and twist placing left elbow to the outside of the right knee. Namaste hands to the heart.
- Your feet should be about one leg's length apart.
- For those with flexible shoulders, reach right arm up and behind the torso for Bound Prayer Twist.
- Extend left arm below the right leg and bind hands underneath right leg (not at the crotch).
- Look over right shoulder.
- Soften your jaw and deepen your breath for 1-3 minutes.
- Slowly release binding, return to runners lunge facing forward, walk to forward fold and return to standing upright in Mountain Pose.

Benefits
- Requires intense flexibility and focus.
- Develops all major muscle groups
- Twists tone internal organs, kidneys and liver.
- Detoxifying.
- Stretches and realigns spine.

YOGA ON A PEG ~ A Yogi Recounts her Harrowing Motorcycle Adventure
Through the Andes

November 2018, my husband Tad and I decided to take an off-road motorcycle adventure tour through the beautiful wilderness of Chile, Argentina and the sparsely populated Patagonia. It was on Tad's bucket list, and I wanted to support him in his fantasy. My sister Laura, her husband Chris, and his son Dave, joined us on the tour. We affectionately call my husband GI Joe, Chris is Indiana Jones and Dave is MacGuyver. If you were ever going to do an adventure like this, these were the men to lead the way.

Dave joined as the fifth-wheel. We fondly called him Cinco (meaning five in Spanish). He owned it! He was so bold and confident on the bike and his youth gave us all a surge. I said to him, "Travel anytime you can. Even as a fifth-wheel, go anyway. Don't wait until you have someone to go with you or you may never get to go." I've been the third-wheel and fifth wheel more than once, and it can be awkward at times, but mostly it's not a problem. You do the main things together as a group, and when lovers want privacy, you explore independently or read a book. It's better than sitting at home bemoaning the fact that you don't have a date. Plus, you never know whom you're going to meet while on the road. Laura met Chris on an airplane to Peru 17 years ago!

The men made all the arrangements, decided on the self-guided tour and chose the bikes. We rented a 2017 GS 1200 black BMW with adventure sport suspension and knobby on/off-road tires. The traction control system made it safer when handling all-weather roads, with heated handgrips for the driver. It was a comfortable bike, but the engine guard crash bar was only 2" from Tad's shin. The touring company booked 3-5 star hotel accommodations and provided a basic map with very few roads indicated and a general itinerary. Tad charted the route on his GPS (which we used constantly). Laura & Chris had international calling plans and were on their cell phones daily to confirm reservations and handle business calls from America. MacGyver Dave brought a variety of tools and a can-do attitude. I was the spiritual warrior praying ceaselessly. Without the due diligence of the entire group, we would have been lost, injured or worse. Tad purchased the proper protective motorcycle gear including helmets, jackets, boots and gloves for full body coverage. Laura gave me a toasty onesie second skin, and that provided the much needed confidence knowing I wouldn't be cold or wet the entire expedition.

The two week adventure was planned well in advance, and I spent three months training almost daily. I continued my daily yoga and meditation practice, as well as teaching four times per week. Five times per week I ran on the elliptical for 30 minutes and lifted weights to increase my upper body strength. Once a week I visited a massage therapist with advanced nerve maneuvering certifications to assist with new and old injuries. I had a few injuries in the past that would have prevented me from this type of activity entirely. Sometimes sleeping on the wrong pillow, or even the right pillow wrongly, would ruin the next day rendering me almost debilitated (certainly without the ability to ride a motorcycle on a bumpy road for hours). My therapist manually manipulated the tissue and nerves once a week in an attempt to release pain in my hands and unlock my left thumb that was frozen. I didn't have full mobility of my hands when we committed to the voyage. I lost the ability to shuffle cards and pinch a chair to move it. Heck, I couldn't even flick a bic. I was seeing the results of the therapy; however, it was definitely an act of faith to embark on the idea of hanging onto a motorcycle for two weeks when I could barely open a jar. During my meditations, I continued to envision my hands and body with perfect health. I didn't watch the bike videos or even know the exact path we would ride. I knew my beliefs were generating feelings that would impact my outlook, so I continued to pray to God and the Andes Elders (the ones on the mountaintop and the ones in the sky) thanking them for a safe and successful tour.

 Excitement filled the air when we arrived in Santiago at 11am and we explored the capitol all day. The following morning we flew to Temuco, Chile, and shuttled to Enjoy Park Lake Hotel in Pucón, located in the Araucanía Region about 500 miles south of Santiago. Our stunning five star hotel rooms overlooked the pristine shore of Lake Villarrica with striking views of the Villarrica Volcano. Over the two week expedition the grueling 8 to10 hour rides were smoothed by the notion that a delicious meal and comfortable bed awaited us each night but that wasn't the case. Some of the hotels, like Alma del Lago in Baraloche, Argentina and Puyuhuapi Lodge in Chile, were absolutely breathtaking while others greeted us with little or no heat and small tepid showers.

The Andes are certainly a majestic sight to see, showcasing granite summits and enormous glaciers dotted with deep blue mountain lakes. Spires to the sky with spectacular views of the snow capped volcanoes and a plethora of fauna flourished the landscape. Chile, Argentina and Patagonia are a wild treasure. The volcano parks hosted 7-8 steeples, some even smoked, with a variety of microclimates throughout the terrain of glacially fed rivers and unmatched mountain peaks. It was the perfect photogenic backdrop Tad was seeking.

Each time I donned my helmet and began my ascension onto the bike I would say, "Thank you, God." Tad and I repeat that prayer every time we embark on a trip, whether by planes, autos or motorcycles. We use that simple prayer of protection to bless our path and bless our food. I also like to picture a four sided pyramid of protection shimmering with gold and indigo light all around me. I visualized a pyramid of protection surrounding each participant and one for the group many times throughout each day.

The footrest on a motorcycle is called a peg. It's a small 2" X 4" footrest that fits under your boot. We own a Harley Davidson Ultra Glide touring bike. We've clocked over 1000 hours together mostly through Central Texas. Our headliners up until this point were a 3300 mile excursion through Utah,

Arizona and New Mexico for two weeks. A few years later in 2015, we cruised the Great Smoky Mountains and Cherokee National Forest traversing the $100 Million Highway 129, Tail of the Dragon, with 318 curves in 11 miles. We continued the unforgettable ride "storm chasing" (or really being chased by a storm) for another 60 miles on the Cherohala Skyway. Exhilarating!

The peg was grated so that my boot didn't slide, and my boot had tread so I wouldn't slip; however, when getting on and off the passenger's seat you have to pivot on the left boot while swinging the right leg around to land on the opposite peg. With my hands on Tad's shoulders I tried to keep my foot slightly over the peg so I could pivot, roundhouse kick and slide down onto the passenger's pad praying I didn't bump my tailbone when I landed. The seat was a more than pee-pad but much smaller than our luxurious Harley. Two small handles on either side of my seat availed for hand gripping. My right fingers could hold the handle well with my thumb resting on the top, but my left hand was too large with the protective glove to hold the handle. I grabbed Tad's torso with all my might, and prayed to keep the rubber on the road. A prayer, two pegs, one handgrip and sheer physics kept me on that bike.

The microclimates shifted from lush and luxuriant to caramel colored dry and dusty, and unfortunately a deluge hit seven out of ten days. The bumpy dirt and wet roads were filled with 18-20" potholes. Our bike had off-road endurance suspension, and Tad handled it with precision. The treacherous roads demanded full attention, and the unpredictable weather made for slow long days. One day it was rainy, the next day windy and the next day both. While we were driving through the desolate and dry Patagonia dessert, every 15 minutes we needed to wipe the dusty film off our helmet shield so we could see.

Chris and Laura's bike had mechanical problems, and it took three days to resolve the issue. The battery cable wasn't secured tightly and would disconnect periodically. It was so frightening to watch Laura do the whiplash move when the bike would turn off for no apparent reason, and then fire up again with a blast. At one point, on a desolate road, their bike stalled, and the ride came to a screeching halt. No passing cars and no nearby gas stations, the guys donned their mechanic's caps. Waiting for them to fix the bike, I tried not to freak out in terror. I needed to busy my mind with positive thoughts or dread would set in. I began noticing the lovely terrain that surrounded me. I admired the glorious mountains and soaked up the sapphire sky. The rain hadn't set in yet, and 1000s of natural rocks contoured the road. Pink and blue stones lined the ditches, and I pocketed one of each color. They took my mind off the fact that my sister's bike wasn't working properly, they could end up with whiplash or worse, and we were in the middle of friggin nowhere. It was harrowing.

"Keep your head in the game" was my basic mindset. I continued my daily practice, adding a Virabhadrasana II (warrior II pose) or Trikoasana (triangle pose) here and there at the infrequent pit stops. I always had great success in unlocking my low back with Utthita Parsvakonasana (side angle lunge pose) and practiced those periodically in my bulky motorcycle gear. I clutched to my yoga sutra chants like a safety blanket and maintained my mantra ceaselessly. I couldn't help but sense that each day might be the last day of my life. I began offering very kind and gentle words to my body thanking it for the good life I led. I offered appreciation for the good and bad times with my body. Overall, I kept a sweet tone in these seemingly final hours periodically hearing Keith Urban's song Days Go By (2005). I offered gratitude to my family and friends and all the people I met along the path through 33 countries. I submitted a large gift of love to the planet and knew that if God wanted me to leave today that I would graciously vacate the body and return home. Occasionally, I saw myself dangling from the tree branches. I wondered if my sister would insist on yanking me out and shipping me back to America, or would they cremate me in South America and carry me home in an urn. Death offers a new adventure with the Superconsciousness; however, I wasn't quite prepared for that finality. As a tradition of renunciation, some High Tibetan Lamas leave their dead bodies on the mountaintop for the animals to feast. It's a final offering of detachment knowing that in the end the body returns to the Earth, ashes to ashes and dust to dust. I contemplated my offering.

My leather gloves never dried. After one to two hours of rain, my fingertips began to chill. I've heard of yogis melting the snow around them while meditating in the Himalayan Mountains. Native Americans have been known to ward off jaguars and snakes while on Vision Quests just through the power of their energy field. There is a way to strengthen your auric field so that your environment impacts you less. I thought I'd give it a try. I mean really, what did I have to lose? I was on the back of a bike, possibly about to die, silently singing my yoga sutra chants, enjoying the wet scenery. I knew I needed to think about what I wanted and not what I didn't want. I wanted to keep the rubber on the road, and I wanted warm fingers. At home, when my feet get cold, I give the command, "Heat Feet! Heat Feet!" and within one to two minutes my feet start to warm enough so that I stop noticing them. I've had much success with this simple method over the years and decided to try it in this challenging situation. I started with "Heat Hands! Heat Hands!" It required intense focus and worked for hours many times. When the cold grabbed my attention again, I slowly began Yoga Nidra from the crown down to my fingers. Yoga Nidra, mainly used for relaxation purposes and a highly successful method for insomniacs, is the practice of connecting deeply to the body through inward observation. Albeit, I knew I wasn't about to fall asleep but could I use this method to heat my hands? I focused intently on my fingers. Silently affirming, "the outside of my thumb is warm, the inside of my thumb is warm. The outside of my index finger is warm, the inside of my index finger is warm." And, so forth. I stated my intent to keep my fingers warm with proper circulation, and they began to heat automatically. The rain continued and my hands stayed wet and physically cold, yet I forgot about the discomfort for hours. When it would catch my attention again, I would repeat Yoga Nidra.

Hugging the mountain to the left and avoiding cliffs to our right, we traversed the treacherous wet lava rock gravel roads pocked with 18" potholes. Tad and I talked a time or two how it would be easier to go out (die) together. If God wants us, I'm good with that. May Thine Will Be Done! I resisted my morbid thoughts and kept thinking, "Train the brain!" I focused my attention on my sacred mantra that Dr. Deepak Chopra gave me. Think about what you want, not what you don't want.

Silently recite your mantra! Truly, there were many days I was surprised that I was so calm, vibrant, living in the leap, trusting God, Tad and the team with everything. Many times it was a sheer joy. I smiled and reveled at being Tad's dream girl. This was his fantasy, and I was part of it. I marveled at how we created this moment together. When I prayed for my Soulmate I included adventures with my Hunky Hubby but never as exciting as cruising through South America for a wild motorcycle adventure. I was thrilled to have this special bond with Tad, and we shared tender and dynamic sex each night. Thinking you're going to die the next day makes sex even better! However, everyday the rain kept coming and the roads got worse. At times it was hard to see and Tad lifted his shield to navigate the roads giving him rosy wind burnt cheeks.

One day we approached a construction team in the process of closing the road. Laura, fluent in Spanish, approached the lady engineer in charge who stood in a little booth the size of a port-o-potty. She came out into the rain to tell us the road was closed. Our men said, "We're going anyway. We must make that ferry." The female contractor said we could proceed, but we would be the last to pass, and they closed the road behind us. On that treacherous road, all of us drove through a puddle so big it splashed up over our heads. We drove 100 yards over the water-road (at least 1 foot deep with water, possibly more if you hit a pothole). We couldn't see the road at all. The 10 foot ditches brimmed over, and I prayed we stayed upright. Our helmet intercom communication system worked intermittently and this was a wonderful gift at this arduous pass. Dave, the trailblazer, gave clues regarding the upcoming terrain for the rest of us. Dave was heroic! We all were heroic! The men had to tow the line and stay vigilant. They all drove like experts. Little did we know at the time that if we had missed the ferry we would have to back track through gale force winds and rain for five additional days, but we didn't even have enough gas to return to the nearest gas station. If only I had prayed to the weather gods too.

Once on the ferry, we were spent. Our faces were filled with terror and delight. We hugged and patted each other on the back celebrating our amazing success. It was a huge relief to be in a safe dry environment. We had no idea how challenging this journey would be. Chris admitted that it was his most harrowing day over all the canyoneering, white water rafting and sailing that he had done around the world over decades. Laura and I nodded in complete agreement. We had a hot toddy and sandwiches and relaxed on the five hour ferry cruising just hours ahead of major hurricane-type weather while MacGuyver Dave fixed Chris' bike. We were so fortunate to only have a couple bruises by the end of the journey.

My daily meditation and yoga practice paid off BIG. I was met head on with sheer terror of loss of a loved one, injury or dying, yet didn't succumb to the fear. I experienced a divine conversation with my body and had a pseudo life review that revealed a spiritual maturity I'd not expected. And, Tad and I bonded in a deeper and more meaningful way. Now, when the final day comes, which could be tomorrow, I'm ready for the next adventure in the Afterlife!

Watch the 3-minute Patagonia Motorcycle Ride 360° video on YouTube at *GeorgetownMultiMedia.*

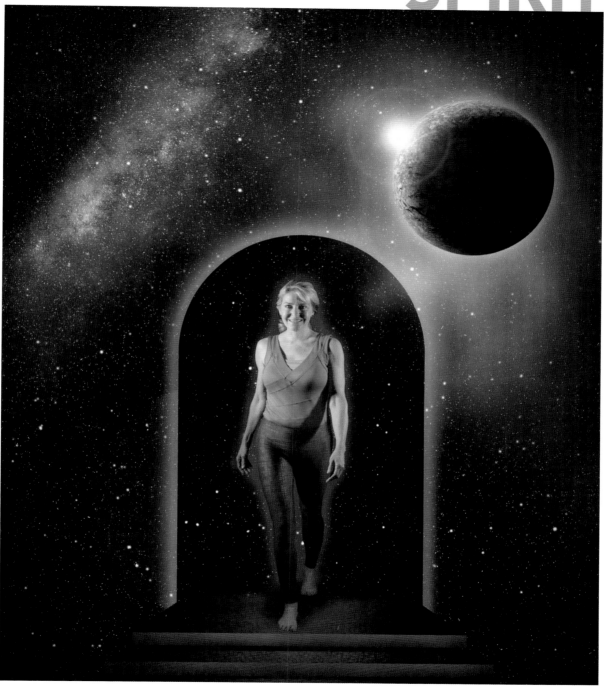

SPIRIT

WHAT IS SPIRITUAL WELLNESS?

Spirituality asks broad questions, like what is the meaning of life? How do I fit in? Why am I here? What is my purpose? Do things happen for a reason or is it random? What is the best use of my time and talent today? Without purpose and direction you can feel like you don't belong. When you ask these personal questions you tap into God. Spirituality respects all paths and offers a conduit to the Creative Forces through faith, belief and conviction. You can have faith in a certain savior or deity or even faith of the heart. You can believe in Spirit or a Higher Power or call yourself a member of a certain religion and still have your unique spiritual expression. Some people church-hop trying to find the right path. You may enjoy the message of your Minister and the connection to your church community, but many people don't know another path for spiritual development. They want a connection to the Divine and even invite miracles, but are perplexed by the church. Dogma, impending lawsuits and religious abuses in the past several decades (and centuries) confound many. This is particularly true with our modern understanding of geology, ancient archeology and the origins of humanity. It's difficult to believe some of the sacred texts, many heavily edited. For some people, even the word "God" can be a turn-off. Some are even mad at God and can't find a way back. Decreasing numbers in church attendance does not indicate a lack of faith, but a failure of the 'Traditional Church' to meet the needs of today's seekers. They are finding personal ways to connect to the Supreme Being. I've interchanged many different words for Omnipotence to be as inclusive as possible (indicated by a capitalization of the word).

Spirituality is individual whereas, religion is collective or communal. This difference explains why courses on comparative religions are offered in school but classes on comparative spirituality are not. When you identify with a specific religion and are ready to advance your consciousness, you may hold yourself back waiting for your whole tribe, or religion, to catch up to your advancing understanding. The tribe, religion or large groups in general do not transform as quickly as the individual. Through your unique spiritual expression you develop a personal path to make sense of life and invite a feeling of Inspiration into daily matters. Spiritual seekers are accountable to their own code of ethics and look for ways to express love and compassion as well as fulfill their Divine Life Purpose. They participate with the Universal Life Force by being kind and respectful without rigid behavioral expectations. Discernment is determining your best line of action; judgment is you deciding for others. Religion has a conventional code of conduct, dogma, rules, prejudices and states if you don't follow the code doing X, Y or Z, you will go to an unsavory place for eternity. Spirituality doesn't hold such pejorative proclamations. When those religious rules and codes don't mesh for you, how do you continue developing spiritually?

Spiritual seekers are free-thinkers, open to many ideas around the Great Mystery of Life and are not afraid to learn more about the many ways people worship around the globe. They accept other cultures and religions as a path to peace, wisdom and ultimate enlightenment. According to Wikipedia there are 4,200 religions worldwide, and quite possibly more, giving you plenty to investigate. For many, spending time in a park at the *Church of Mother Nature* brings them to a deep connection with Great Spirit. Time in nature connects you to your own organic nature. Walking through the park, appreciating the greenery, flowers and birds can lift your Spirit. Even playing Frisbee® at the park can awaken you to your own Inner Beauty. I invite you to spend a few minutes each week in nature (could be your own backyard) and find a favorite tree to sit under. The Buddha found enlightenment under the bodhi tree. Consider the many seasons, decades or even centuries for the tree's maturation. The strength and stability of an old large tree can ignite a sense of courage and potency. Simply resting under a tree can link you to your natural expression of gentleness, kindness and compassion. The Native Americans, Pagans and Wiccans honor the four seasons with a lovely celebration on the Equinoxes and Solstices. Uniting with nature on these significant days opens us to gratitude and manifestation. The Equinox is an indication that the day and night are equal (spring and fall) and the Solstice denotes when the sun is at its longest or shortest distance from the equator (summer and winter). The celestial voyage mirrors the inner spiritual journey.

Believing in a Power-Greater-Than-Yourself is a non-sectarian way to express spirituality. Having faith in something greater than yourself allows you to lean on the Supernatural to make life easier. Thinking you have to do it all can be quite overwhelming, but believing that your Guides, Angels and the Universal High Council are helping you strengthen tenacity. Asking for their direction and protection in small and large ways decreases fear and separation and increases trust and faith. Spending a few minutes each day in quiet contemplation improves your inner resolve, allowing you to act on those insights amplifying your Divine Intuition. The Small Still Voice resides in each of us. As you take time for mindful practices you increase the volume, if you will, to receive those pertinent answers to daily concerns. Spending time in some type of communion or ceremony developing a communication with your Wisest Self opens a world of possibility.

Mindful methods are numerous and varied. Meditation is a method that millions use daily, and you don't have to tie it to a Savior or Deity, although you can if that resonates for you. Quantum Physics expounds on the Unified Field of Oneness as our ultimate connection to life, each other and the Earth. Most religions say that we are all connected. You may not be able to relate to that statement, but you can't deny at a very basic level we are all connected through our feet touching the Earth simultaneously. Is there a way to connect to the loving vibration between us instead of fearing the competition for finite resources? Quantum Physicist Dr. John Hagelin presents the compelling "theoretical and experimental evidence that the Unified Field of Physics and the Unified Field of Consciousness are identical, and during the meditative state, human awareness directly experiences the Unified Field at the foundation of the universe." During meditation you can have moments that are ineffable. Ineffable occasions are indescribable, beyond expression and spiritually stupendous. Many meditators comment on a loss of time, space and words while achieving a deep connection to the Cosmos. Meditation improves the mind, body and spirit. It improves the immune system, reduces anxiety and opens the door to the Holy of Holies within you. When the rational mind (ego) relaxes, you can connect deeply with your Highest Council, and in that sense you become your own teacher. Jesus said at the Sermon on the Mount, "if thy eye be single, thy whole body shall be full of light" (KJV, Matthew 6:22). That is an exact corollary of the yoga teaching to focus on the point between the eyebrows as you relax into a meditative state during *savasana*, the final resting posture. You are then entering the Holy of Holies becoming illuminated by the Light. Christ was a Master of Masters, and you don't have to worship Him to benefit from His teachings; however, the more you meditate, the more ineffable and spiritually significant moments will transpire to strengthen your inner resolve.

Have you ever had an epiphany? An epiphany is a realization, a knowing, an awakening. After understanding the message an epiphany reverberates within you, you will never be the same. Your outlook is expanded and your pace is intentional toward a new heading for which the message directs. Some call it an "Oh Shit Moment!" It is a powerful realization in time that is hard to describe, but you are definitely talking about something unforgettable and life changing when you experience an epiphany. It is a spiritual message, and you are gifted with a higher perspective and the courage to take action on it.

Music can be a source of an epiphany. Some lyrics and rhythms can guide you into the heart for mending and healing emotionally. Have you ever heard a song that reflected exactly what you were thinking, maybe even answering the question on your mind? Many times I've been concerned about a relationship or career decision and right then the perfect song streams on the radio giving me the direction I'm seeking. It's uncanny, and it helps me spiritually move forward with conviction. There are no coincidences, some say. Belief that you will receive spiritual wisdom in mysterious ways, like from music, billboards or artwork is a method to develop your Mystical Union. Artists will frequently tell you that they experience artwork as a spiritual path. Whether creating it or enjoying it, artwork of any type or style can touch your heart. A visit to the museum or a musical ensemble might just awaken your spirit to an unexpected epiphany.

Synchronicity is another form of spirituality. Bumping into people in a timely fashion, thinking about someone right before they call, landing a job that ultimately leads you to your marital partner are a few synchronistic events that Spirit is sending your way. God is the ultimate friend and parent, and will bring someone to you at the perfect time to rectify uncertainty or restore love. The random smile received at the perfect time can shift your mood and reinstate your optimism. Calling out to the Parking Angels as you're leaving home for appointments can be proof that someone is indeed listening to you. When you expect synchronic events you learn to "manage the coincidences" in your life. Watching for these little gifts from the Universe can be the source of great pleasure.

Many connect to the Source just by being honorable people. For example, a Mensch is someone helpful and noble. A philanthropic spirit is one in service to humanity. You might not have millions for a charitable foundation, but you still enjoy serving humanity in small and even unseen ways. Altruism and volunteerism can be an expression of Love-in-Action. When I consider giving money to panhandlers at the stoplights, I access this direct communication with my Highest Council. I ask, "should I offer money or something else to this needy person?" Intuitively, I receive a message "yes or no." Some people are begging because they truly need help. Offering $5, $10 or $20 would really get them off the street but others are scammers. I don't want to enable someone to deceive, so I ask Spirit how can I help, and I receive direct guidance on the best line of action at that time. Spirituality allows you to decide how you can serve uniquely in each moment. You can call yourself Jewish, Christian, Hindu or another faith, follow those religious and cultural codes but not attend temple or church. You might have a personal relationship with Christ, Muhammad or Krishna and receive direct guidance instead of obtaining your answers through a Rabbi, Priest, Imam (Islamic Spiritual Leader) or Pujari (Hindu Minister). Many of you already believe you have direct communication to the Ultimate Supreme Being and receive insights personally. Spirituality opens that door for you to receive mystical experiences and express your personal convictions whether you go to a specific building on a certain corner one day a week or not. You can go straight to the Creative Power and know the best course of action for you on that day. The Temple of the Jedi Order believes that The Force is with them all the time. Chartered in Texas in 1980, this spiritual offshoot from the blockbuster film Star Wars offers a comprehensive guide to seeking The Force and uniting with a Supreme Being through acts of courageous service with a noble heart. There are countless ways to connect to God. Your Highest Consciousness wants to talk to you and participate in your life. Are you paying attention? Prayer is talking to the Creator. Meditation or intentional silence is listening to Omniscience.

Offering forgiveness is a significant part of spirituality. Forgive the trespasses of others as often as you can. You would be surprised how liberating it can be to release resentments. Negative feelings, anger or depression are signs that you're longing for some spiritual release from the bondage of fear, disgust and uncertainty. Silently stewing is a cry for love. The Creator knows your intent, and the intent of others. You don't have to know everything; you just have to trust that Spirit is on your side helping you even when you have a difficult ex-spouse. It is not a selfish act to strive for inner peace and happiness. For that is exactly what we need to do. When you are lost in perpetual feelings of hatred or revenge, you are part of the problem. Forgiveness, even in little increments, builds a bridge to the Universal Life Force that encourages you to turn the other cheek. The eye is directly above the cheek and by turning your cheek you turn your vision in another direction. Turn the other cheek to refocus your attention on more positive things. Your contentment is part of the Ultimate Divine Plan for the World. Seek higher ground.

Spiritual wellness allows you to move quickly into a compassionate state of being for self and others. You experience a sense of peace and purpose as you develop your ability to listen to your hunches and gut instincts. Instead of looking at the world judging this to hell and that to heaven, you spend more time on dismissing the negative and focusing on the Beauty of Life. Appreciate where you are today instead of bemoaning the trials of yesterday (or yester-year). Joy, Hope and Faith uplift your Spirit naturally when you shift negative thoughts into positive ones. You strengthen your Intuition when you release the litany of negative thinking or stewing. Intuition is a direct form of communication with the Divine. Your ultimate partnership is the spirit that transcends the union of the mind and body. Through mindfulness and intention, you can bring Heaven to Earth into your cellular structure.

Start by imagining what Paradise means to you and pretend that you're already living there. Acting as if you're already living in Paradise means offering and experiencing gentleness, compassion, forgiveness and truth today. You don't have to wait until you're dead to experience that heavenly feeling, and you don't have to go to a certain building once a week to connect to Spirit. Try not to limit the Supernatural; expand your awareness of what the Creative Forces may be, above and beyond the human mind. Having a spiritual practice will improve your relationships, increase your self-esteem, deepen your intuition and attract rich wholesome experiences to you. In my father's wise words, "We don't go to Heaven when we die, we grow into a Heavenly State of Consciousness."

 ZENERGY BOOST FOR SPIRITUAL AWAKENING
Write your spiritual autobiography. Create a timeline with 10-20 significant spiritual moments throughout your life. Even as an Atheist your outlook has been affected. What impacted your Spiritual Nature the most?

CONTACTING YOUR ANGELS & THE POWER OF PRAYER

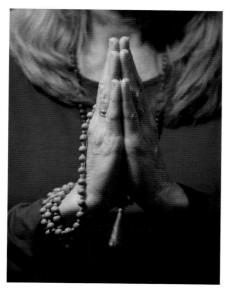

Do you believe in Angels? Studies show that about 55%-77% of Americans and one-third of Europeans believe in Angels (CBS News, Huffington Post and BBC). Many spiritual and religious people believe in Angels and the Power of Prayer. Religious scripture from the Sikhs, Judaism, Christianity and Islam promote that Angels are watching over us and protecting us. It is understood that Angels and Spirit Guides are committed to your Highest Good and are a part of every day life. Scholars, priests and pastors from many religions believe that Angels are celestial beings while Spirit Guides were once human, and now they are Helpers from Heaven. Many of you may believe that a deceased grandmother or uncle supports you from the other side. Even deceased pets make cameo appearances at times reminding us of their continued support. They would typically be considered a Spirit Guide not an Angel.

Angels seem not to interfere with our choices because we have free will. Most likely, however, they quietly prevent catastrophes that we enjoy unknowingly, like when someone walks away unscathed from a major auto collision or home fire. Angels can startle and awaken us. A startling dream or vision will awaken you to pay attention, discuss it with a friend and possibly interpret it. Dreams are a proven method of communication from your Angels and Spirit Guides, and the process has been documented numerous times in the *Bible* and other sacred scripture. Contemplating a potential prophecy opens your imagination to the miracle of spiritual communication through your dreams. Edgar Cayce and other spiritual leaders believed in the importance of dream interpretation as a gateway to the Unseen Forces.

Miracles are happening every day. In fact, there is something wrong if you don't experience miracles in your life. How do you define a miracle? Is it only the aberration of a burning bush, or could avoiding a wreck or a flat tire be a miracle? Restoring loving communication with a frenemy (former friend turned enemy) could be considered a miracle. Recognizing the flow in life opens you to the miracle of Synchronicity. Miracles are coming to you in countless ways. Are you paying attention? Expect miracles and accept miracles. They are contagious. When you receive one, be grateful. It opens the door for your best friend to get one too.

When you ask your Angels for guidance, their message may come to you in many different ways. Angels are thought to be Messengers trying to communicate with us. Sometimes our intuitive ability isn't refined enough, making it more of a monologue, with us alone at the microphone.

They may communicate with you during your meditations or you might see something in your peripheral vision. The message is rarely verbal although some people report hearing a voice loud and clear (but inside the mind). A message may consist of an aroma, a feeling of goose bumps or even a distant but relevant memory resurfacing. You may awaken singing a song or suddenly decide you need to visit a distant relative. Don't discard these magical messages. Enhance your intuitive ability by celebrating that contact is being attempted. A Leader in the Spiritual Community and dubbed *The Lady who Sees Angels*, Lorna Byrne confirms, "We all have a Guardian Angel who is watching over us." In her YouTube Videos (seen by millions), she indicates that Angels are always praying for us (2015). Her book, *Angels in My Hair* (2008) debuted as Number 1 on the UK Sunday Times Book Chart now translated into 30 languages, reveals a prophecy she received from her Guardian Angel at age 10 regarding her life story. The Angel showed her who she would marry and their love story, their children, her husband's ultimate poor health and their poverty, with perfect accuracy. Additionally, the Angel indicated that she would write books about the Angels and become very wealthy later in life (which again, is exactly what is happening to her now). These magnificent compassionate supernatural beings are helping us decode the symphony of life experiences, if only we would slow down to hear their messages.

Why can't most of us see Angels and Spirit Guides? Because they are in another dimension. Consider if we are in 3D then they are in 5D, 7D or higher. Quantum Physics tells us that 99% of the world is non-atomic, not measureable and presently not knowable. Angels are non-material, and we experience a knowing or a subtle conscious shift when we make contact. When you sit in silence and ask for guidance your prayer is heard. Be specific with your prayer and know the cogs are spinning to answer your request. The timing is not for you to determine. You only need to ask and patiently wait with an attitude of gratitude. Sometimes we don't like their answers or don't have the confidence to take action on their suggestions; however, they are guiding us away from dangerous choices, like a battered wife who needs to leave her abusive husband. Pray for the ability to act on the Angelic Wisdom you receive. Remember book knowledge, rationality, logic or intellect is not enough; you must act on what you know to do. Otherwise, you are remaining a victim. When you know to do something better but hesitate, you are wasting precious wisdom and energy. Prayers can manifest the greatest good for the maximum number of people.

Archangels are perhaps the most recognized in the ranking of the religious milieu. There is a hierarchy in the Angelic Kingdom and the four main Archangels Michael, Gabriel, Raphael and Uriel govern different arenas of life. Call upon Archangel Michael for protection and guidance, and to cut away old useless habits, bad relationships or karma. Reach for Archangel Gabriel for inspiration, opportunities and resources to finish assignments or pay the bills. Archangel Raphael is available for health and healing, and a prayer to Archangel Uriel will eliminate loneliness and reconnect you to the Power and Presence of the Creator. Remember, "all things work together for good to them that love God" (KJV, Romans 8:28).

Make your prayer requests specific. "I need help now" is too vague. "The mortgage needs to be paid in three days" is more specific without identifying yourself as the only one who can pay it. Set your intention and be specific. Intention is founded upon certain basic principles such as truth, tolerance, compassion, patience, humility, conscientiousness, joy and generosity. These qualities are voiced repeatedly throughout prayers. Praying with one or many Angels, Spirit Guides, Saints or Sages can ease your mind. Why limit yourself to just one Enlightened Being? Call them all to you! Your life can get easier when you access your Angels through the Power of Prayer.

ZENERGY BOOST FOR PRAYER
List seven things in different categories like health, money, career, communication, spouse, parenting, or relocating, that you need help with now. Set your intention and be specific. During and after your prayer hold an attitude of gratitude knowing your Angelic Protector is handling the details for you. Have Faith!

BECOMING ZEN

Many people think of Zen Buddhism when they hear the word Zen. Zen Buddhism is a mixture of meditation, dietary practices and regular exercise. Maintaining a serene state of being present, allowing your intuition to influence your actions rather than forcing an outcome on some type of methodology is being Zen. Permitting life to happen without all the judgments and worries, trusting Spirit and Self to accomplish your life goals successfully, is considered Zen. Deliberately focusing on a task at hand, without scatter chatter, whether mowing the lawn or cooking a meal is a Zen practice.

Some executives even have small Zen gardens on their desks now with the delicate assembly of natural elements like stones, gravel and sand that is raked. Raking the sand, whether in your office or in your backyard, can provide a moving meditation to keep you present. You become one with the garden, losing yourself to the task. Staying present is so important as many people are typically lost in the past or the future, and a Zen garden can bring you back to the precious present moment.

Trusting your intuition, not worrying about things you cannot change, opens the door for synchronicity. Synchronicity leads to spontaneity, not impulsiveness, and occurs naturally when you are in the flow. Being in the flow is another way of saying, "things fall into place," or "I didn't miss a beat," or "we hit all the green lights." Some people will say "dumb luck" or "it was a coincidence," but synchronicity acknowledges that you're in the Universal Flow. Things are not happening randomly, they are synchronized for your advantage, whether you recognize that or not. The structured mind can trap you into thinking that things are always a certain way, but being Zen relinquishes fixated ways of thinking so that you recognize the Universe is conspiring with you.

Being Zen opens the door for appreciating yourself exactly the way you are right now and continuously moving forward in authentic expression. As you become Zen you will experience more flow, energy, love, generosity of spirit and inner peace. Only you can stop the suffering and self-loathing in your mind. Your choices toward a healthier lifestyle allow you to enjoy simple things in life and stop wishing it were different. You make life different, or better, by focusing intently on what you love. Wishing is another way of pretending that you have no influence or control in your life and keeps you a victim of your circumstances. Being Zen is a way of stepping out of the old rut, and embracing a distinctive avenue of expression.

Sitting in quiet contemplation, or meditation, is a great way to awaken your Zen qualities. Reducing clutter, donating unused clothes and paring down elevates simplicity to an art form. Finding quiet time and creating a simple rock garden in your backyard embraces the Zen path. The minimalist philosophy reduces distractions prompting inner contentment known as Zen. You feel Zen after a soothing day at the spa, and a relaxing massage may just be your embarkation for enlightenment.

EQUINOXES & SOLSTICES

Honoring the four seasons on the Equinox and Solstice opens the door for connecting to nature with gratitude. The Equinox is an indication that the day and night are equal (spring and fall) and the Solstice denotes when the sun is at its longest or shortest distance from the equator (summer and winter). The stellar passage mirrors the inner mystical journey.

The year begins with the spring, attains the peak of life at the summer, matures at the autumn equinox and ends with the winter solstice. The Spring Equinox, typically around March 21, indicates the resurrection, an opportunity to tap into our Universal Consciousness, Christ Consciousness or Cosmic Consciousness. Jesus Christ's resurrection transpired during Jewish Passover, which is observed on the first full moon following the vernal equinox. The Spring Equinox is the return of the sun, the time to plant new seeds, and it marks the beginning of the astronomical year. It is an ideal time to set your intention, like a New Year's Resolution. Many of the great temples like the Mysterious Sphinx of Giza, the Temple of Angkor Wat in Cambodia and the Malta Mnajdra Temples on the Mediterranean Coast align with the rising of the Spring Equinox as a symbol of rebirth.

Summer Solstice, the longest day of the year, usually June 21, opens the day for festivities of the sun, ascension and enlightenment. It's a time to take a grander look at your life, stay the course toward the goals set at the Spring Equinox and adjust behaviors to achieve your mission. Refine your trajectory, like a pilot aiming toward a landing sight, to dynamically accomplish your goals. Like the farmer awaiting the seeds of spring to bare fruit, one must patiently anticipate the fulfillment of a dream. The Egyptian Temple of Karnak and the Ajunta Caves in India are the most revered salutes to the solstices erected thousands of years ago.

The Autumn Equinox, normally observed around September 21, marks a time for harvesting and conserving energy. Autumn indicates a ripeness or maturity as we embrace the evolving seasons. The colorful changing foliage mimics the ongoing transformation in all areas of life. Celebrate the day or the season by bundling your final herbal and vegetable picks and enjoying a pumpkin spiced tea at dawn or dusk. Acknowledge your efforts toward your annual goals here at harvest season and know the final quarter will bring ultimate fruition of your aspirations. The Pyramid of Chichen Itza on the Yucatan Peninsula offers the most intriguing view of the effects of the Equinox as the serpent-headed statue casts a shadow outlining the body of Kukulkan, the Mayan feathered-serpent god.

The Winter Solstice is for birth, rebirth, renewal and self-reflection. The shortest day of the year and typically celebrated on December 21, denotes endings and beginnings. It's the ideal time to reflect on the previous year and contemplate the upcoming one. Ireland's Newgrange Monument, Goseck Circle in Saxony-Anhalt, Germany, and the 5,000-year old monument Stonehenge in Wiltshire, England, are considered the most famous monuments dedicated to the Solstices.

Clearly, ancient cultures around the globe respected these significant days and erected permanent edifices to the sky. Spending some time in nature on these four auspicious days can reconnect you to Great Spirit. Celebrations, whether public or private, are a dynamic way to experience spiritual unfoldment independently.

 ZENERGY BOOST FOR THE EQUINOX & SOLSTICE

Imagine the Light illuminating your third eye. Feel the warmth moving down the spine to your toes. Appreciate your mind, body and spirit and allow that gratitude to expand around you to your home, family, neighbors, city and entire planet. Expand the Light. Acknowledge the four cardinal directions. Face East toward the rising sun and welcome new beginnings. Set a new goal or intention (either verbally or in writing). Pivot 90° right and look to the South for manifesting your goal. State your intended steps to fulfill your dream. Turn another 90° to the West for the setting sun and send your dreams into motion. Imagine your goal, vision or dream in a balloon, let it fly and see it traveling beyond the horizon toward the sunset. The final aspect of this simple ceremony is to face the North and invite strength and stability, direction and protection to manifest your Divine Life Purpose. Relax and trust that the Universe is conspiring to achieve your goals with you. Feel the warmth of the Light and rest for 5 minutes while incubating in your new vibration. Offer thanks and gratitude to the Great Spirit for bringing it in a timely manner.

SPIRIT ANIMALS

Some spiritual traditions, including the Native American customs, invite a rich connection with nature, seasons and solstices. Spirit Animals represent character, temperament or emotion. Those animals seen at birth often become the birth name of the newborn, like Standing Bear, Spotted Elk or Sitting Bull. A Totem Spirit Animal could be the clan symbol for a lifetime or for many generations. During life we can create a meaningful relationship with certain animals. They just seem to catch your eye here and there at auspicious moments. You might have periodic visitations from certain birds or dragonflies. These are messages that can assist you in developing your intuition and connection to the Mystery of Mother Nature.

If you're looking to develop your spiritual nature and are ready to receive messages from the Universe, look no further than your own backyard. When an animal or insect appears out of nowhere or continuously visits your mind, consider the symbolic significance of the animal. Spirit Animals are guides from nature, and they can appear out of the blue. For instance, you know there are spiders in your home and garage, yet rarely are they seen. You could see any insect or animal throughout the week or month, but when the emergence is recurring, obvious or startling, then ask, "What message can this Spirit Animal give me today?" When one appears it can be a deliberate message. Knowing the essence of certain creatures can open your mind to the messages the Universe is sending to make your life more manageable. Also called Medicine Animals, they can deliver a remedy for emotional health and healing in mysterious ways.

If you have a domesticated dog then you know the special communication between the two of you. No doubt, you probably receive useful messages from your pet almost daily. The Spirit Animal message would still be of loyalty or service but more in the sense that your dog is sharing the experience with you. Just as therapy dogs are in service to humans and heal us when in troubled times, we too are in service to our domesticated family. The rising popularity of canines is an indication of the powerful shift in consciousness toward respecting dogs, animals and nature in general. Dog may be your Spirit Animal that walks with you throughout your entire life, but this is different from owning a dog as a pet. Having Dog as a Medicine Animal means that you express a natural sense of loyalty and service to humanity, and nature mirrors your expression back to you by many dogs in a variety of circumstances being drawn to you. They seek you out with a friendly approach and want to befriend you. When Dog visits you (physically or metaphorically), interpret that to mean that you're reliable, dependable, approachable or loyal.

Completely different is when a spider makes a friendly pass on the floor. Spider Medicine is a message to awaken to the creative patterns in your life or that the winds of change are upon you.

Spider Medicine can indicate a windfall or financial gain coming your way soon. It's a fun game to consider the messages from nature when exploring your world a little deeper. Look for the clues all around by noticing the Spirit Animals in your life. You could walk into a spider web at any moment, why did it occur that day? Sometimes it could be completely random and have absolutely no auspicious meaning, but other times it's just too uncanny to dismiss as a coincidence (especially if it occurred four or five times in one day or one week). That's when we want to investigate the meaning of the Sprit Animal visitation.

The symbolic meaning of these Medicine Animals transfers to dreams also. Interpreting your dreams is a powerful tool for self-discovery. If you dream a certain animal then take a few minutes to contemplate the message being sent. For instance, if you dream of a hummingbird then it might be a good time to take action quickly, move fast, make a decision, and don't dilly-dally. Hummingbirds also represent resiliency and independence. It may be a message to move forward on a new path independently. Recognizing the messages of Spirit Animals can be a great source of wisdom and entertainment as you learn to navigate the spiritual world of symbology and cultivate your intuition.

SPIRIT ANIMAL DICTIONARY

Armadillo: Slow down, be in no hurry, self-preservation.
Badger: Aggression, independent, healing with herbs.
Bat: Seeing through ambiguity, changes for the better.
Bear: Strength, introspection, spiritual journey, healing.
Beaver: Power of working, achievement through cooperation, builder, team player.
Buffalo: Endurance to overcome, great emotional courage, provider to all.
Butterfly: Transformation, ability to know without evidence, change the mind, metamorphosis in life.
Cat: Independence, patience, curiosity, wisdom from dreamtime.
Cougar: Decisiveness, clairvoyance, clever, freedom from guilt.
Coyote: The master trickster, laughter, humor, foolishness, reveals truth behind chaos.
Crow: Manipulative, mischievous, audacious, adaptable.
Deer: Gentleness, sensitive, intuitive, graceful.
Dog: Loyalty, noble, protection, playfulness, in service, olfactory acuity.
Dolphin: Trust, loyalty, resurrection, cooperation, sexual.
Dragon: Inspiration, supernatural, invisibility, longevity, power.
Dragonfly: Lookout for deceitful people, adaptability, presence of fairy realm.
Eagle: Higher perspective, creator, teacher, spiritual connection to Divine Wisdom.
Elk: Stamina, very good luck, victory.
Fish: Purifier, quality character, ability to hide emotions, going with the flow.

Fox: Camouflage, melt into one's surrounding, be discerning and swift, tricky situations around you, caution.
Frog: Bringer of rain and abundance, fertility, camouflage, time to hide something.
Hawk: Messenger of the gods; keep a hawk eye, observe, laser focus, time to lead .
Horse: Swiftness, strength, enlightenment, possesses healing power, sexual energy, passionate desires, personal dominance.
Hummingbird: Act fast, respond quickly, resiliency, independence, stopper of time.
Lizard: Conversation, agility, self-care, dry, dehydrated, enjoy the harsh climate.
Lynx: The knower of secrets, clairvoyant ability.
Mole: Underworld, be inquisitive, use your feeling perception, be one with the Earth.
Moose: Headstrong, unstoppable, longevity.
Mountain Lion: Power of leadership, ability to lead without insisting others follow.
Mouse: Scrutiny, pay attention to the details, hide.
Otter: Laughter, curiosity, mischievous.
Owl: Can see what others cannot, true wisdom, recognize deception, a symbol for death.
Parrot: Celebration, recognize the good in your life, are you mimicking or being mimicked?
Porcupine: Meet challenge head-on & trust yourself, stick it to 'em, protection needed.
Rabbit: Virtue, serenity, sensuality, fertility, abundance.
Raccoon: Bandit, shy, hiding, resourceful, adaptability.
Ram: Sense of self worth, perseverance, virility, power.
Raven: Magic, a warning, auspicious message, a change in consciousness, watch out.
Seal: Family oriented, community minded, possesses power in numbers, imagination, creativity, vivaciousness, flowing with a group of people.
Sheep: Charity, purity, innocence, spiritual, following the herd.
Skunk: Very conspicuous, time to build your self-confidence, rely on yourself more, set healthy boundaries, refuse the offering and trust the best will occur.
Snail: Be gentle with yourself, focus on the details, slow down, isolation, loneliness.
Snake: Power of creation, transformation, life, death and rebirth, sexual, Kundalini.
Spider: Creative patterns of life, growth, winds of change, good luck, financial windfall.
Squirrel: Preserves for future, laugh & play more, get squirrelly, don't be so serious.
Turkey: Smart, fertility, elusive, festive, bounty, gratitude.
Turtle: Longevity, endurance, sure & steady pace, persistence.
Wolf: Teacher, pathfinder, sharing knowledge, strength, time for self-discovery.

ORACLE CARDS

Oracles, Prophets and Diviners have been the intermediaries with profound esoteric knowledge from the gods and goddesses since antiquity. Integrating information obtained from the Hebrew Kabbalah, Egyptian teachings and the Greeks, these Seers of the gods and goddesses would share interpretations of the symbols in temples or on mountaintops for whole communities through sacred rituals. Eventually these Seers became a part of the communities through religious practices of various types, and the prophecies were incorporated into the communities. Even the Apostle Paul considered prophecy to be the greatest gift from God. Gypsies incorporated the use of cards as entertainment and fortune telling in Italy, and the Tarot cards became popular there around 1840-1842 when Italian Artist Bonifacio Bembo painted a deck for the Duke of Milan. Like Nostradamus writing the Quatrains in code, the Oracle is chock full of symbols and hidden meaning to avoid persecution from the church.

Many believe viewing the card's symbols opens a door to the Akashic Records releasing sacred information about the Soul's journey through its many challenges. Metaphysical Pioneers Madam Helena Petrovna Blavatsky (1831-1891), Alice Bailey (1880-1949), Edgar Cayce (1877-1945) and others introduced the term "Akashic Records" in the 19th and 20th Century. They are the non-physical records of all time that some advanced spiritual seekers are able to tap into, melding the spiritual world with the physical one. With a regular meditation practice, listening to guidance from your Angels, and seeking answers from the Oracle, you can gain awareness from your Akashic Records.

Oracle cards are available now for the novice and can open the door to deeper meaning for just about anyone if used correctly. There are many decks to choose from. Angel, Psychology, Happiness, Osho Zen, the Original Rider-Waite Tarot, even Moon, Horse or Animal Spirit decks are available today. You can easily locate Mystical Shaman, Shamanic Healing or Goddess Cards at most bookstores. Seeking clarity on many topics like career, health, romance, money, relocation or family issues releases burdensome worry and reconnects you to your Spiritual Guidance. You don't have to know all the hidden symbols and special meanings. Each deck comes with a small booklet describing the cards' meaning and placing you in the driver's seat to start reading for yourself right away.

The beauty of having a session with a Professional Card Reader is that they intuitively feel the message of the cards and this allows a deeper meaning to be revealed. A Professional Reader is usually very skilled at understanding the significance of the cards you choose, and can offer objective messages to the recipient. Some expert Tarot Readers tie the cards into astrology for a more comprehensive discussion. You would be surprised how accurate these types of readings can be. A card reading won't necessarily tell you the future, since it is never set in stone, but you will learn more about the choices you have and what's on the horizon. You may receive insight about certain trajectories, but you have ultimate free will. **You** choose your path and response as the event comes to pass.

If you are ready to proceed on your own, then decide on a deck of your choosing. Hold the cards in your hands, shuffle a few times while you say a prayer of intention to receive guidance about ONE question and only ONE question. Phrase the question so that it remains open, stating a broader picture instead of getting lost in the minutia. Do not ask a yes/no question. Consider phrasing the question like, "what is working or what is missing in my marriage?" Instead of, "how can I get my spouse to help more with the kids?" By keeping the question open, you expand the range of information that can be revealed to you. In this example, you could ask two different questions and then draw the cards twice. Firstly ask, "How can I improve my marriage?" Secondly, "How can I improve my parenting skills?" Assuming that only your spouse's assistance with the kids would improve your family answers the question in advance. You want to come to the deck with an open mind and open heart seeking the best solution. Look for guidance, not a final answer. Your final answer will come from inside you when the event comes to pass, but a card reading can guide you on the next step. Hold your attention on receiving an answer to your ONE concern and then draw 1-3 cards. Many times one card will answer the question quite candidly.

ZENERGY BOOST FOR DEVELOPING YOUR INNER ORACLE
Draw one card a day and keep a journal of the events that happened that day. As you look at the card, expect to receive intuitive insight about the message. The card doesn't mean the same thing each time. The card is offering guidance and suggestions and your intuition gives you the ultimate answer. Learn two to three words for each card and let this knowledge build your sixth sense. Practice this for one to two months and find the correlation between the card and daily events.

While I was traveling the world alone I drew a few cards upon entering a new city. Then, on the train ride out of that city, I reviewed my notes and could see what the cards were trying to tell me. I did this daily and weekly over two years and gained a great understanding of symbolism while cultivating my intuition. Spiritual guidance offers relief from worry, even temporarily, and allows you to refocus on the important things at hand. The cards can give you insight into the unknown offering newfound confidence, and you definitely need to be self-assured to travel alone.

You don't want to ask questions when you're highly emotional as this limits your intuitive abilities. This is when a Professional Card Reader can support you. You want to be centered and calm while reading your cards. You may have a problem that needs healing, but you don't want to be frantic while looking for answers from the Oracle. We say the cards "speak" to us but really it's our intuition that has more volume when we see the images on the cards and hear the messages from our Spiritual Guidance. That voice can drastically reduce anxiety.

Some common questions to ask the Oracle:
• What should I focus on today?
• How can I improve my finances?
• What's going to happen tonight at the party?
• If I continue dating my current boyfriend/girlfriend what can I anticipate?
• What can I expect at my next interview?
• What is working with my current employment?
• What is missing from my current employment?
• What was the meaning of _____? Pull three cards and look for the storyline.
• What is my Divine Life Purpose? Pull three cards and look for a common theme.

Keep the card readings to important things, not petty gossip or insignificant topics. I found that the cards don't lie. You may not understand all the messages, particularly to something as important as your Life Purpose, but continuously searching will lead you to your answers. Seek and you shall find! You choose the card that you most need at that time. If you shuffle the cards right then and choose again, you will receive different insight, which may confound you. It's best to keep the question simple, direct and to the point. Take a deep breath and accept the card that arrives. You can ask for clarity with one more card, but don't keep choosing or you'll get confused.

One day I had writer's block for a couple hours. Painstakingly standing at my computer, I resisted my task at hand. I decided to choose a card to receive insight about my dilemma. Out of three decks, I chose the one card that had to do with "creative indolence" and specifically indicated writer's block. It was uncanny. I was forcing myself to be creative and really I needed to allow the ideas to percolate. With that information in hand, I shut down my computer without any guilt and headed for the gym joyfully. That day the cards gave me specific guidance and lifted a heavy weight off my shoulders instantly. You can also use this method with books. Hold one book in your hands. Say your prayer and ask ONE question. Then randomly open the book and read one page or one paragraph. Contemplate the meaning throughout the day. It's another way to quiet down the scatter chatter and reduce worry to make life easier. Your Guides, Angles and God are waiting for you to ask questions so they can assist you. As you develop your spirituality, you strengthen your inner resolve for taking action on your Divine Life Purpose.

NUMEROLOGY

Does the same number keep popping up in your life? Do you often look at the clock at the exact minute? Do you awaken at the same time during the night? Do you have a lucky number? The study of Numerology is a belief in mystical associations between numbers and corresponding events. Initially originated in the Kabbalah, every number has a frequency, and mathematics is the language of our Universe. Numbers are the letters of this mystical language. Those who use Numerology in their lives recognize the influence on personal and professional affiliations, finances, the mind-body-spirit connection and health status. Numerology is a science of numbers, and a fun approach to discovering strengths, weaknesses and the major events of a person's life. Expert Numerologists reveal layers of information regarding your background and life trajectory by investigating your numbers.

There are a variety of methods like Chinese Numerology, Chaldean and Kabbalah system. Pythagorean Numerology is the most common in the West and includes a few major numbers of most interest like Life Path Number, Personal Year and Destiny Number. Think in phases or cycles of 9s. 1 is the beginning, and 9 is the completion. Add the numbers together until you get to 9. Frequently people will say, "this is a 9 Year and therefore its time for me to wrap up projects." By calculating the annual numerology, you can use the momentum of the year to help you on your path. 2020 = 2 + 0 + 2 + 0 = 4. 2020 is a 4 Year. 2020 is a year for structure, stability and productivity. It's a good year for building and expanding. See details about the numbers below.

Examples:
To keep it simple we will use the first day of autumn, November 21, 1990 for these examples.

Life Path Number ~ Indicates your personality, divine life purpose, potential career and/or spiritual mission. It denotes how the world sees you and your karmic patterns. You calculate this number by your full birth date. Let's say you were born November 21, 1990. Calculate it by adding all the numbers together. 11 (for November) + 2 + 1 (day of month) + 1 + 9 + 9 + 0 (year) = 11 + 3 + 19 = 33 = 3 + 3 = 6. Your Life Path Number is 6. You most likely are family oriented, generous and find harmony between the material and spiritual worlds. See details below to know more about the number 6.

Personal Year ~ Glean a personal observation of what the year at hand has in store for you. This number allows you to anticipate the potential opportunities and pitfalls for the upcoming year. Calculate the year we're in (2020 = 4, as shown above) + your life path number (entire birthday and year) = add the two numbers together and arrive at your personal year number. In the examples provided, Life Path Number example above is 6 + 4 (for 2020) = 10 or 1. It would be a 1 Year in this example. A 1 Year is ideal for starting something new independently, stepping out as a visionary in your community or cultivating a creative talent. See details below to know more about the number 1.

Destiny Number ~ Describes your talents and attitudes. Your formal birth name gives the Destiny Number, and if you change your name you resonate with a new vibrational frequency. Many times children change their childhood names when they enter high school or college. This method is particularly useful for women considering a name change after marriage. Add the numbers according to the letters in your name. See the Pythagorean Numerology Chart below.

The name Susan Sample is 1 + 3 + 1 + 1 + 5 + 1 + 1 + 4 + 7 + 3 + 5 = 32 = 3 + 2 = 5. Based on Numerology, Susan may be a free spirit or adventurer; however, she may need to be careful of a restless nature and momentary pleasures. See details below to know more about the number 5.

When a number continues appearing virtually out of nowhere, consider the meaning from both the positive and shadow aspects. Occasionally, we receive a message from the Universe that something is unsuitable. Investigate the message intuitively. When a number repeatedly catches your eye then it most likely has the same meaning (positive or negative), but you haven't received the message yet. Is it a warning or a confirmation? When and where is the number appearing? Do you repeatedly awaken at the same minute each night? Do you see it only at work or only at home? Is it just when a particular person is nearby or anytime? We live in a polar opposite world so look at numbers from both aspects. Contemplate the potential message. This is a fun way to develop your intuition and strengthen your spirituality.

NUMEROLOGY DEFINITIONS

Number 1 (1, 10, 19): Leader, leadership, beginnings, innovative, creative, independent, visionary, inspired/inspirational. Great date to start a new project, go on first dates or present new ideas.
Shadow Side: Dependent on other's opinion or support, people pleaser, too detail oriented, need to delegate.
Number 2 (2, 20): Partnerships, romance, balance, cooperation, auspicious number for creating peace and partnerships ~ like signing a marital license or a divorce decree.
Shadow Side: Warning of danger, dealing with duality, feeling depleted or criticized.
Number 3 (3, 12, 21): Trinity, communication, socially magnetic, teamwork, optimism.
Shadow Side: Scattered energies, difficult to make commitments, shallow, discipline needed, overly/inappropriately optimistic.
Number 4 (4, 13): Structure, stability, foundations, strong will, building, good time for building, expansion, good time to expand.
Shadow Side: Restrictions, rigidity, lack spontaneity, overly-strict parenting.
Number 5 (5, 14): Change, adaptable, flexible, open-minded, free spirit, globe trotter, enjoy being single.
Shadow Side: Attracted to fleeting gratification, selfish, "don't fence me in" commitment concerns.

Number 6 (6, 15): Egalitarian, balance, family-oriented, generous, harmony.
Shadow Side: Willing to sacrifice too much without reward, missing the big picture, OCD (obsessive compulsive disorder).
Number 7 (7, 16): Spiritual, mysticism, 7 main chakras, 7 days of week, intuition, faith, uplifting others with inspirational words, wisdom.
Shadow Side: Hard to recognize the value of what you currently have in talent, material possessions or even spouse, ambiguous, aloof.
Number 8 (8, 17): Money, power, success, infinity, authority, attainment, organized.
Shadow Side: Stubborn, karma, egocentric, greed, lacks diplomacy.
Number 9 (9, 18): Completion, fulfillment, fund raising, good time for fund raising, time to create a non-profit, valor, genuinely love others.
Shadow Side: Judgment, overly focused on career or financial independence, give too much at your own expense, demanding, condescending.
11, 22 and 33 are considered Master Numbers.
You can add to make 2, 4 or 6, but typically you don't add these numbers together. They stand on their own. Consider both meanings.
Master Number 11: Spiritually aware, intuitive, much to offer others, sees the big picture, service-minded, psychics & prophets, fascinating.
Master Number 22: Great strength of inner power, balanced, service-minded, on a mission, old soul, wise, humble.
Master Number 33: Humanitarian, selfless, spiritual, fulfilling heart's desire, maturity, reaching full potential. Generally, we don't consider a shadow side to the Master Numbers. Usually, it is a High Five from the Universe to see these numbers consistently jump out at you; however, you could contemplate the following:
Shadow Side: Haughty, proud, meddling, let others do for themselves what they can, difficulty loving what you already have, not taking care of yourself.

PYTHAGOREAN NUMEROLOGY

1	2	3	4	5	6	7	8	9
A	B	C	D	E	F	G	H	I
J	K	L	M	N	O	P	Q	R
S	T	U	V	W	X	Y	Z	

ASTROLOGY

"When, exactly, were you born?" If it didn't matter, we wouldn't be able to get to know someone through his or her birth sign. The study of the stars had its beginning eons ago when our distant ancestors looked to the skies, noticed the heavenly bodies' movement coincided with the change of seasons and determined their lives through the rhythms they discovered. By knowing your connection to the stars and their influences at certain times of the year, you can reduce unexpected disappointments, strengthen self-confidence and increase your spiritual connection to the Universe.

Many people still use these ancient observations to plant and sow, weed and reap. The Old Farmer's Almanac, first published in the United States in 1792, is a testament to one facet of the Science and Art of Astrology. "Within the pages of The Old Farmer's Almanac, in addition to astronomical and meteorological reference material, you'll find an abundance of traditional astrological information, ranging from the dates of Mercury Retrograde (discussed later in this chapter) and the monthly 'Best Days to Garden by the Moon's Sign'" (*www.Almanac.com*). The patient observations of the natural world are an opportunity the study of Astrology gives to us all. Like the rhythm of a ceremonial drum, the movement of the moon and planets through the ecliptic remains constant and one can rely on its consistency in the midst of a chaotic world.

The planets make the journey around the Sun at independent speeds on a path called the ecliptic, and their placement coincides with the record of our birth. A Natal Chart, likened to a birth certificate that goes to the State as a record of the child's arrival, indicates the positions of the stars at birth. The time, date and location of birth comprises the Natal Chart or Birth Chart. The child is not imprinted with a permanent tattoo as to what the stars and signs signify in the child's life but the positions and angles suggest the attitude the child will commonly have with their experiences. The movements of stars and planets in our universe show patterns that have been recorded and studied for centuries. Planetary positions connect with our lives but do not control us. Ptolemy (100 CE – 170 CE), one of the world's great mathematicians and astrologers said, "The stars incline; they do not compel." Meaning, the celestial world doesn't control us, it influences. That being said, if you are a water sign (Pisces, Cancer, Scorpio) you will generally be more emotionally aware while a fire sign (Aries, Leo, Sagittarius) prefers to hide personal feelings. Of course, a water sign will still hide personal feelings at times but their basic nature is to be intimately expressive. A Natal Chart is a 2-dimensional capture of a moment in time in the Universe. It can be the birth of anything actually... a person, an idea, a company, or a nation. Upcoming events can be understood through the lens of Astrology by using a particular time plucked from the river of moments that pass you by.

Astrologers have been common advisors for centuries. Leaders employed Astrologers for major decisions such as travel dates, harvesting, upcoming events and even when to embark on a military campaign. Commonly used in India today, Vedic Astrological Readings determine marital partners and when to begin procreation for millions. Having an Astrologist read your Birth Chart can assist you with an in depth understanding of your basic nature and the general trajectory of your life expression, and your innate abilities and growth-opportunities along the way. A skilled Astrologer can be a guide to begin a new project, offer understanding if things are not falling into place, and advise on future stellar influences giving you peace of mind during the progress of certain endeavors.

Astrologist Kevin Burk states, "Astrology is the study of cycles. By observing the cyclical movements of the planets we gain a greater understanding of the cycles and patterns in our own lives. Astrology can be a powerful tool for healing and transformation, and it can be a key that unlocks a greater spiritual connection to the Universe. Although astrology is not fortune telling, when skillfully applied, astrology can be an extremely effective predictive tool. On a personal level, astrology can give insight into personal issues, patterns, fears and even dreams. Astrology is a tool that can help us understand and unlock our highest potential, and that can teach us how to live in harmony with the Universe."

We each have three illuminating factors: the Sun Sign (your sense of self) is most dominate of core values, the Moon Sign (your emotional nature and how you relate in intimate relationships) and the Rising Sign. The sign on the horizon at the time of the birth is called the Rising Sign or Ascendant and is located in the first house. The Rising Sign is like a window a person chooses to observe the world through, filtering the person's overall vision looking out at the world, and also the impression that person leaves on the world looking back. Basically, we are not just one sign, we are a combination of several.

The soul of the newly born baby is marked for life by the pattern of the stars at the moment it comes into the world.

Johannesburg Kepler (1571-1630)
German Astronomer & Leader of the Scientific Revolution
Kepler Space Telescope is named after him

The Astrological New Year begins on March 21st in the sign of Aries, the child of the Zodiac. There are 12-astrological sun signs and your birthday determines your sign moving between the 21st (+/-) of each month (i.e. January 21st to February 20th is Aquarius). Each sun sign has dynamic characteristics and general shortcomings. The *quality* of a sign shows how the energy is used. *Quality* means cardinal, fixed or mutable. Cardinal energy leads, fixed energy persists and mutable energy adapts. Cardinal signs (leading) are Aries, Cancer, Libra and Capricorn. Fixed signs (persistent) are Taurus, Leo, Scorpio and Aquarius. And, Mutable signs (adaptable) are Gemini, Virgo, Sagittarius and Pisces.

Astrological Signs

Month/Sign	Element	Positive Strength	Shortcoming
April/Aries	Fire/Leads	Pioneering/Adventurous	Impulsive/Selfish
May/Taurus	Earth/Persists	Steadfast/Loyal	Stubborn/Argumentative
June/Gemini	Air/Adapts	Thoughtful/Quick-Witted	Changing/Unreliable
July/Cancer	Water/Leads	Family-Oriented/Nurturing	Moody/Reclusive
August/Leo	Fire/Persists	Optimistic/Resourceful	Dramatic/Overbearing
September/Virgo	Earth/Adapts	Industrious/Efficient	Critical/Obsessive
October/Libra	Air/Leads	Balanced/Artistic	Indecisive/Gullible
November/Scorpio	Water/Persists	Healer/Dedicated	Secretive/Jealous
December/Sagittarius	Fire/Adapts	Travelers/Philosophers	Restless/Sexual
January/Capricorn	Earth/Leads	Prudent/Patient	Miserly/Stuffy
February/Aquarius	Air/Persists	Inventive/Humanitarian	Unpredictable/Detach
March/Pisces	Water/Adapts	Compassionate/Imaginative	Escapist/Weak-Willed

Your moon sign is determined individually by the date, time and location of your birth. The moon travels over a 27-day monthly cycle orbiting Earth counterclockwise. The moon's anticlockwise rotation on its axis also takes approximately 27 days leaving a near side and far side (or dark side) of the moon, which observers from Earth never see. The moon governs the oceans and tides, covering approximately 71% of the planet. Some tidal locations at certain times can rise and fall up to 40-feet in one day (near Anchorage, Alaska). We, too, are mostly water (approximately 60-75% depending on age), and are also impacted by the changing moon cycles. Albeit sometimes unavoidable, it is not recommended to have surgery during a full moon phase as you can retain additional fluids increasing recovery time. During the waxing, or beginning of the moon phase, is the best time to decide on goals, dreams and ambitions for the cycle. Review your progress during the movement through the signs and acknowledge and recognize your achievements at the full moon. Use the waning moon time to finish projects and plan for the coming cycle. Then, begin again the following period.

The Element's Influence on the Zodiac

Fire Signs (Aries, Leo, Sagittarius) spark action for new beginnings and a vision of what could be. Excellent at pouncing on opportunities, generally they see the big picture quickly and encourage the best in those around them. Fire signs are good leaders, passionate and optimistic, but can be impatient, impulsive and hide their emotions behind acts of strength. The element of Fire initiates.

Earth Signs (Capricorn, Taurus, Virgo) govern stability and substance, business and currency. Typically, Earth signs are said to be down-to-earth, dependable, trustworthy, productive and enjoy tangible results. This element embraces structure and cellular foundation (the bones of our bodies). People who have an abundance or prominence of Earth signs prefer to move carefully, taking time to evaluate the value of choices presented. This abundance of care can lead to procrastination or stagnancy. The element of Earth supports.

Air Signs (Aquarius, Gemini, Libra) represent thought, creativity, inventiveness, dreams and the power of mind. Musical compositions, dance, entertainment, written expression and data collection are related to the Air Signs. Over-thinking, analysis-paralysis, and talking too much are indications of an imbalance. The element of Air designs.

If **Water** is your ruling element (Pisces, Cancer, Scorpio), your natural tendency is to be emotionally aware, quite possibly your best and worst quality. Your emotional acumen may offer insight into your motivations as well as those of friends and family, but your sensitivity can also lead to moodiness and irritability. The effects of erosion demonstrate the potency and patience of this element. Water signs are fluid and may address concerns from an oblique perspective, or even sideways (as in the way a crab moves forward by shifting side-to-side). The element of Water feels.

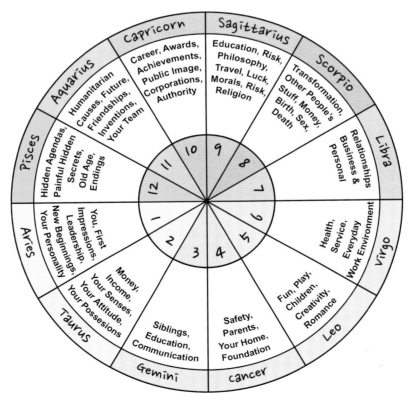

The Houses

The zodiac is divided into 12-sections (like a wheel or a clock), called houses, and your birth time, date and location determine the placement of the signs and planets. Astrologers read the chart beginning with the 1st house and proceed counterclockwise. These 12-sections are linked with a set of qualities for the self and extend to society and beyond. Each planet was in a specific sun sign and house at the time of your birth. When an Astrologer decodes your Natal Chart, she merges the meaning of each planet, the house it's in, and the corresponding sign to indicate the advantages and challenges you'll address in this lifetime. See wheel diagram on previous page.

When planets visit a house on their transit through the elliptic, they illuminate that portion of your chart with their unique flavor, and strengthen that House's attributes. The planets travel through the celestial bodies at their individual pace. Some proceed slowly, like Jupiter, and others move quickly, like Mercury. Jupiter influences us in almost 12-year cycles. As you can see from the preceding chart Jupiter represents luck and wisdom; however, Mar's 2-year cycle suggests desire and courage. Astrologers identify which area of your life will take the spotlight and best course of action based on the houses. The first six houses are "personal houses" about you and internal happenings. The last six houses are known as "interpersonal houses" corresponding with relationship and society.

The chart for the Astrological Houses is for teaching purposes so that you can learn what each house represents. The chart splits twice, from left to right (horizontally), and from top to bottom (vertically), like the four cardinal directions. The sun starts on the left or in the east at sunrise, and travels clockwise to set in the west on the right side of the chart. The top of the chart represents the midheaven or high noon, and the bottom indicates the nadir or midnight. Midheaven represents the exposed self, your highest aspirations and public expression. At the opposite end, the nadir indicates the deeply hidden part of self, your private, vulnerable and intimate space. Crossing over the top of the chart represents the daytime and underneath is the evening. If you were born in daytime you most likely are more outgoing or extraverted unless other factors dominate; if you were born at night you might find yourself more internal or introverted. The 1st House represents new beginnings, first impressions and leadership. This is the location for the Ascendant or Rising Sign.

The wheel in this basic example indicates the person was born in Aries. Let's say Maria was born on April 3 at 6am. Therefore, the chart would read correctly with her 2nd House governed by Taurus and 3rd House by Gemini and so forth; however, if Maria were born on April 3 at noon, the chart would rotate putting Aries at the top of the chart in the 10th House. Maria, with her Aries qualities (a natural pioneer who confidently leads, possibly even leaping before thinking) would manifest her skills in the 10th House. The 10th House represents corporations, authority and career. For instance, Maria may enjoy using her leadership skills to form new corporations, or being a spokesperson creating a public image for corporations, or exploring remote locations for National Geographic documentaries. Then, with Aries in the 10th House, Taurus moves to the 11th and Gemini to the 12th and so forth. Her Ascendant would be Cancer.

If Maria were born at midnight with her Sun in the 4th House of Cancer, she may have more challenges because that combo creates steam (Aries is fire and Cancer is water). Aries folks like a lot of activity, transformation and seeing the world, but being born in the 4th House of Cancer generally means staying home, focused on family's transformation, going slower and having roots. She might not feel as satisfied, or even flat out frustrated, because her natural Arian abilities would be thwarted unless she chose to get involved in the community making big changes, like being Mayor of a small town. Her Rising Sign would be Capricorn.

Understanding Astrological formulas you can somewhat predict what is on the horizon regarding certain upcoming astronomical events and their potential effects. Astrologically speaking, identifying your best qualities and knowing your weaknesses in advance can help you make decisions regarding your choices, therefore reducing stress. Knowing the zodiac's influence can aid you in choosing appropriate partners in business and romance. And, you can increase your spiritual wisdom and lessen fear and uncertainty in our chaotic world by knowing what is over the next hill.

Mercury Retrograde
The planet, Mercury, is situated closest to the Sun. Earth's orbit is longer than Mercury's. It speeds past Earth about three or four times per year. This position is what Astrologists call "Mercury Retrograde." Cycles last about three weeks each annual quarter. Once you begin to pay attention to how events in your life change during Mercury Retrograde phases, you will soon see how important it is to take note of them throughout the year. Keeping track of Mercury Retrograde periods can allow you to increase your productivity and avoid some of the frustration they can generate.

The biggest issue with Mercury Retrograde is communication malfunctions. I cannot tell you how many people say they had a computer or cell phone crash during Mercury Retrograde. It's annoying but even potentially devastating. If you're in Information Technology or you have a cell phone or a computer, it would behoove you to know these annual cycles. It's a bit like a police officer or emergency room doctor knowing when it's a full moon. Strange things are more prone to happen during that time.

The confusion and interference coinciding with Mercury's motion when it retrogrades affects our everyday lives. For example, if you and a friend were skating and your friend passed you, you would notice she was going faster than you. But if she slowed down and you passed her, it would appear that that she was going backward (retrograde). Then when she speeds up and passes you again, her trail kicks up dust and rocks in the road. As Mercury speeds by, it is like a car zooming past Earth, creating a potent, chaotic flurry in its wake. Wouldn't you benefit from knowing when potential chaos is headed your way?

Communication, scheduling, transportation and judgment calls may become cloudy or error-prone when Mercury is retrograde. It's interesting to know that Mercury Retrograde frequently occurs during the winter holidays and can explain for some of the dissatisfaction of that season. You can't do much with the behavior of others but by being aware and prepared, you can handle potential postponements and blunders more gracefully. One good measure is to always repeat numbers to avoid any potential transpositions. If there are miscommunications with several people in one week then check the Mercury Retrograde dates online. You might need to take additional measures to stay calm, confident and centered during the phase. (Staying calm is discussed in the Meditation Chapter.) On the other hand, introspection, contemplation and inner healing work are especially supported by the phase. Take advantage of those three weeks by organizing your closets, reducing clutter in the attic and finishing projects. It is not the time to sign any type of agreement or contract, launch a new website or have surgery, but if you must, then dot your I's and cross your T's, go slow and read the fine print twice.

The fractal relationship between the orbits in the heavens and human activity here on Earth pervades all of Astrology. Employing astrological knowledge once a year or throughout the year can connect you to a higher source of knowledge, amplifying your mystical awareness. Experiencing a connection to the planet, the stars and the cycles of life strengthens your spiritual understanding, reduces feelings of isolation and alights a sense of courage to take action. Astrology is one of many ways to develop a connection to the unseen influences of the cosmos.

Things to Avoid During Mercury's Retrograde
• Signing contracts and agreements – read the fine print year round
• Buying a house or leasing an apartment
• Launching a website or new endeavor
• Starting a new job or hiring a new employee
• Know that decisions may likely be modified during these four periods annually

THE POWER OF YOUR DREAMS

Wouldn't it be wonderful if you could grow mentally, emotionally and spiritually while you sleep? Well, you can and you are, whether you take advantage of it or not. We spend one-third of our life asleep. The body needs rest and rejuvenation, and while sleeping a fun video clip is left behind, a dream. Exploring the message is a powerful tool for understanding daily activities, physical health, relationships and spiritual progress. Dreams are a gateway for spiritual development. Today, psychologists, researchers, scientists and sleep doctors embrace the resurgence of sleep time investigation. The subconscious mind is like a computer and the dreamtime is an occasion for updating, reprogramming and defragging. Many times we just dream about daily events, possibly even becoming a character from a recently watched movie. Streaming through the day's activities, the subconscious mind catalogs and archives data for future use, and these visual images can leave us with information on nutrition, romance, career and even finances.

Recorded evidence of the power of dreams is found numerous times in the *Bible* and other sacred manuscripts. If dreams were powerful and potent enough for citation in the *Bible* over 20 times, then clearly we should be documenting and investigating our personal dreams today. One of the best known Biblical dreams, recorded in Matthew 2:13-14, is an Angelic warning for Joseph to flee into Egypt with Mary and Jesus to avoid the wrath of Herod. Joan of Arc, the most famous historical feminist, dreamed God instructed her to save France from England. Musical Legends like Richard Wagner, Billy Joel, John Lennon, Paul McCartney, Keith Richards, Jimi Hendrix, and many more admitted receiving some of their greatest music from their dreamtime. 1937 Nobel Prize Winner Albert Gyorgi stated, "My work is not finished when I leave my workbench in the afternoon. I go on thinking about my problems all the time and my brain must continue to think about them while I sleep because I awaken with answers to questions that have been puzzling me." Edgar Cayce, America's Sleeping Prophet, recommended watching dreams to glean insight about yourself and your life path. Cayce said, "Visions and dreams are given for the benefit of the individual, would they but interpret them correctly." He further stated that guidance only comes to "those who are doing something with their lives" (Reading 294-15). Clearly, we are given direction to watch our dreams from many different authorities.

In a normal sleep pattern you naturally flow from the beta brainwave, down to alpha and theta and onward to deep rest in the delta brainwave. During the middle of the night, repeatedly the brainwaves gently flow upward to theta and alpha and return back to theta and delta, naturally shifting between the three relaxed states of consciousness. The physical body rests while the consciousness accesses the inner plains for understanding and problem solving. Sleep drugs leave you in delta for the entire night, which is great if you haven't slept properly for awhile; however, it is natural to flow between the three phases (alpha → delta → alpha) throughout the night. Stopping this natural rhythm reduces or eliminates a very important aspect of sleeping. Without dreaming, and without the brainwaves flowing down and up through the night, one reduces the benefits of spiritual information from the dreamtime.

Asking for solutions to everyday problems opens the door to a plethora of guidance. *Edgar Cayce on Dreams* (1968) states, "Dreams work to solve the problems of the dreamer's conscious, waking life, and they work to quicken in the dreamer new potentials that are his to claim." If you're new to this type of investigation, consider leaving a journal with pen on your nightstand tonight. Write down a question for which you seek answers. Memorize your question and repeat it as you drift off to sleep at night. Each morning log everything you remember, even if only one symbol, word or feeling comes to you. We must train ourselves to awaken and remember the dream, as it is easily forgotten, and this type of dream incubation can aid systemically in dream recall. Even the slightest movement or opening the eyes can lose the images quickly because it is a different state of consciousness. It may take a week or a month, but soon you will develop the muscle for contacting your Superconsciousness, remembering your dreams and interpreting the messages accurately. Voice recording your dreams is an easy way to recall and retain the night's visions. If you receive a dream that you do not understand, ask for clarity on those symbols. Continue asking for a message until you receive your answer. Read your journal at the end of each month like a storyline regarding your questions, and eventually you will recognize the substantial information revealed to you almost daily regarding the bigger picture.

Dreams can help you with attitudes, habits, money, career and, of course, the unseen, as in a prophecy. Prophetic dreams are hard to recognize initially, because generally speaking, all the people in your dreams are different aspects of you. It would be difficult to understand the many sides to your personality if you showed up ten different times in the same dream; however, by presenting a businessman, the grocer or your neighbor, you can interpret that the message is about your career, your nutrition or your neighborhood. When you dream of someone you know, consider three words to describe that person. How do you relate to those qualities? Do you need to enhance those skills or tone them down within yourself? If you see no correlation between yourself, those potential attributes and the message of the dream, then possibly it is a prophecy. It is beneficial to log and maintain a list of how many times the insight came to pass, giving you validation of your ability to be a prophetic dreamer. If you dream a neighbor has a car wreck, you might say to her, "drive safely," and not disclose details of the dream because sometimes the meaning can be convoluted. Another interpretation of the dream may indicate that your upcoming project is about to end in a wreck. So, dreams can have oblique messages, but once you know your symbols you can interpret them quickly. My parents received many prophetic dreams throughout their lives, and I, too, have been given insight into the future through an occasional dream. They are the superhighway to clarity and spiritual development.

I reflect on a friend who owned a convenience store as a good example of receiving much-needed guidance from dreams. She knew she was losing money and inventory but couldn't catch the culprit. She double checked with vendors to confirm the delivery of certain products but couldn't find the supplies. She trusted her employees and couldn't imagine one stealing, but still the inventory was disappearing. She prayed a simple prayer, did the dream incubation mentioned above, and set the intention to receive guidance from the dreamtime. After a few weeks a very obvious dream was delivered. *Looking through a security safe with steel gray sides, she saw one employee sweeping the warehouse.* Sweeping the profits right out the backdoor. Within a few days she was able to physically confirm that employee was the culprit and appropriately discharge him. In another example while writing this book, I had technology issues. I was devastated thinking that I had lost three-quarters of the digital book. I prayed earnestly that night, "I've come so far in writing this book. Is it for the greater good that I finish it? I need an answer tonight." In the dream, I was driving, which is a good sign. You want to be in the driver's seat in your life. *Driving through the woods, I could not see out the front windshield.* I did feel blind at times in writing this book. So the symbol was accurate and understandable. *I could sense the blue sky above me, but I was driving blind in the Texas woods. Driving through the least-resistant area, I could hear the tree branches scratching on the sides of the car. Then, I felt a "plunk" as my tires hit the pavement, and the veil on the windshield lifted. I turned left, and I drove through a new neighborhood development. The paved streets provided a solid foundation, but the houses were not yet erected.* The people/audience were coming but not just yet. Apparently, I was ahead of schedule. You have to be ahead of the wave to catch the crest of the wave. Otherwise, you're in the crash on the seashore. To my relief in the morning, I learned one port was broken, but I didn't lose any data from the thumb drive, and the dream fueled my inspiration to finish this book. I've had many impressive dreams over the years that guided me out of troublesome times and lifted feelings of uncertainty instantly.

Interpretation of your dreams offers valuable insight. Have you ever asked, "How did I get into this situation?" Dreams can give insight into manipulations or karma. Watch for clever clues that someone may have the upper hand. Employers, parents, siblings, spouses, even children can find ways to manipulate, leaving you feeling obligated to perform or participate in an event that has no interest and no benefit to you. The message may come in the form of someone driving your car or you in the back seat. Shifty eyes or a hidden handshake also indicate foul play. On the other hand when dealing with karma, a boomerang may fly through the air indicating what goes around, comes around. You may be receiving what you've been dealing, and dream communication can gently indicate a need for personal responsibility and rectification. Symbols of water, large pools or the ocean indicate emotional wellbeing. If the water is calm and clear then so are you; however, turbulent and murky tides reflect a tumultuous time. One evening, I dreamt *I was walking on the bottom of the ocean breathing just fine. Above me were lots of sharks, but my father and I leisurely strolled along the bottom of the pristine translucent ocean.* At that time in my life, a few business propositions were presented and the dream was telling me to watch out.

Some dreams are in Technicolor while others are in black and white. The variety of images, experiences and context are completely unlimited. In the dreamtime, one-third of your life, you are supernatural. In a dream, you walk into a room and see a bouquet of flowers. If you think you would like to smell those flowers you don't have to walk across the room, you instantly whiff the bouquet. Whatever you want in the dreamtime happens instantaneously with no time restrictions.

There are many books to assist with understanding dream symbology. Even entering a word online will provide a few definitions to get you started on the path for dream interpretation. Although there is a general consensus on symbol definitions, there is still a wide berth for specific designations. Ultimately, you choose the meaning that accurately reflects the answer to your specific inquiry. For instance, if you see yourself running, are you running toward something or away from it? What is your mood? Are you frightened or elated? Noticing your gear, the terrain, weather and so forth give rise to the intended message. Understanding the mystical meaning of your dreams and milking these experiences, opens the door to greater spiritual development.

**Consider the following aromatherapies for a better night's sleep ~
bergamot, chamomile, lavender, sandalwood, clary sage or ylang-ylang.**

ABBREVIATED DREAM DICTIONARY

Anxiety: Insecurities, roadblocks, frustrations, warning, emotional fatigue.

Arguing/Fighting: A hasty decision; who are you fighting with or what do they represent? Sexuality, passion, frustration, explosive emotions.

Army: Discipline and obedience; A marching army is a sign of a long haul on its way; lots of protection needed. Collective group or community working together.

Baby: New ideas, new projects, starting anew, baby on the way.

Balloon: Rise above the crowd, create a new perspective, fly away, travel, lighten up.

Baptism: A blessing for you or someone nearby; good project is underway, spiritual renewal.

Being Injured: You may be neglecting that part of your body. Usually a diet dream.

Death/Dying: Letting go mentally, emotionally, spiritually or physically; change of employment; transformation, like the caterpillar, potential rebirth. Could be prophecy.

Desert: Not fertile, abandon project, wasteland, uncharted territory, diet dream indicating dehydration.

Disaster: Misfortune, choose a different course of action, watch out.

Driving: You are driving your circumstances, moving forward on the path; as passenger, you may be the manipulated or don't have all the answers. Whose car? Where are you going?

Exercise: Could be a literal message to exercise more. A new journey, path or work is on its way to you. Exercising at work could mean to articulate your point of view at work, or encouraging you to exercise on lunchbreak.

Falling: Out of control, lack of support, unsafe, potential out-of-body experience.

Female: Yin, internal, feminine qualities, collaboration, intuition, gentleness, maternal, multitasking.

Field: Get back to nature; learn more about your field of expertise, playing the field.

Finding: Learning or discovering something new, embracing a new quality. Look around more, pay attention, new opportunities.

Fire: Entering a phase of renewal or painful reflection, burning away that which does not serve you, letting go, time to pare down, sexuality, passion.

Fish: Christianity, spirituality, financial gain, about to catch something, big win, success, go with the flow, don't be rigid.

Flying: Longing for freedom, spiritual growth, out-of-body experience.

Head: Heads Up! Pay attention, mental condition, egotistical, head over heels, thoughts, state of mind, a crown rests on the head.

Heart: Love, emotions, stamina, main point; does or doesn't have heart for the person or project; heart condition, take heart, big decision.

Home: Private life and emotions; how you feel at home in dream indicates how you feel in life, safety, security, comfort. Kitchen: diet dream; bedroom: sleep or sex; bathroom: elimination; guest room: a stranger in your own home; closet: secrets, privacy.

Ice Cream: Seeking pleasures and the sweetness in life, may indicate what you need to stop eating, cream on the top.

King, Queen, Judge: Authority to give advice. Are you listening or ignoring? Justified or judgmental? A ruling presence in your life.

Left: Associated with feminine, yin energy, past, receptivity, unconscious self.

Lips: Sensuality, giving lip service, notice what you're saying on a regular basis; watch what food is crossing your lips.

Male: Yang, external, masculine qualities, action, courage, manifesting, single minded.

Mine/Mining: Work, repetitious work, salt mine fatigue, going within, mining for gold indicates your higher value is within reach.

Mirror: Looking into the unconscious or unknown, vanity, discover your true nature. Mirrors facing each other appear to expand into infinity. Is something being mirrored back to you karmically?

Money: Energy, security, choices, opportunity, things we value in life, possessions, moneymaking proposition, sexuality, power, success, tool for manipulation or persuasion or to provide and protect.

Naked in public: Open, exposed, unabashed, free, unprepared, taking a risk.

Orgy: Release pent-up energy, may indicate OCD or the need to masturbate.

Ostrich: Unwilling to see situation, head in sand, avoiding, neglecting self.

Paralysis: Unable to take action or protect self, feeling helpless.

Pyramid: Solid structure, afterlife, spiritual, sacred geometric shape; even though the pyramids have been proven to not be tombs many still perceive them as a crypt and therefore death may be another meaning for this symbol.

Rain: Troubled times ahead, washing away the stress & pain, releasing stagnant energy. Rainy day may indicate a need to relax.

Right: Associated with masculine, yang energy, future, conscious self, giving.

Sex: Connection, bonding, balanced yin-yang, exploited, examine your personal attitudes toward sex. May be time to hit the reset button and masturbate.

Swimming/Drowning: The quality of the water matters (see water); getting swept downstream indicates a bad situation at hand. Head above water indicates success & confidence. Treading water/barely staying alive. Emotional dream. What are your feelings upon awakening?

Terror: Extreme anxiety, apprehension, fear, uncontrollable circumstances. Beware.

Thorns: Dangerous situation, difficulties, obstacles, poking at you or you poking at another. You may be sticking your nose where it doesn't belong.

Vehicle: Progress through life; new vehicle/new ideas, next journey; jalopy/time to revamp project or improve nutrition; emergency vehicle/time for healing or need for rest; police car/order, discipline, protection, criminal activity.

Waltz: Rhythmical movement, precisions, dance of life, work together harmoniously.

Watchdog: Look Out! Warning sign. Be on guard.

Water: Spiritual or emotional wellbeing, wisdom, understanding. Quality of water indicates emotional awareness. Clear clean water/emotionally balanced; choppy water/turbulent emotions; dark stagnant water/stuck in life circumstances; flowing water/go with the flow; clam sparkling water indicates stability, spirituality and/or and contentment.

Wedding: Union, partnership, promise, integration of self, balanced yin-yang.

WHAT'S YOUR SUPERPOWER?

Have you ever had a strong feeling about something, but didn't follow it and regretted it later? We've all had those moments. Even though you know you should listen to your gut instincts and intuition, sometimes you don't trust the guidance received through feelings or extrasensory perceptions. Psychic and perceptive abilities are common but many people don't talk about it for fear of ridicule. The word "psychic" even has a bad connotation in some regions. Being psychic is no more mystical than learning computer code or programming which can seem quite cryptic to those of us who are not Techies. Some children have a natural knack for pulling wisdom out of thin air. It is human nature to be intuitive. You might not believe or trust in your innate abilities, either because you were told, "it's all in your head" or "where's your evidence" or you've never taken the time to actually pay attention. Many categorize psychic phenomenon as superstition unless you talk to people who share it. Many will dispute this topic entirely because they know with certainty that it has no value yet the scientific research on these types of skills and phenomena is growing.

The rise in popularity for movies like *Harry Potter, the Avengers and X-Men* indicate an increasing attraction to Superpowers. Thankfully, today there are a growing number of researchers and citizen scientists who are willing to investigate human supernatural tendencies with an open and discerning eye. According to the Pew Research Center, "Though the U.S. is an overwhelmingly Christian country, significant minorities profess belief in a variety of Eastern or New Age beliefs. For instance, 24% of the public overall and 22% of Christians say they believe in reincarnation — that people will be reborn in this world again and again. And similar numbers (25% of the public overall, 23% of Christians) believe in astrology. Nearly three-in-ten Americans say they have felt in touch with someone who has already died, almost one-in-five say they have seen or been in the presence of ghosts, and 15% have consulted a fortuneteller or a psychic." Some critics feel the need to oppose almost anything, but I invite you to keep an open mind during this conversation. Think of this topic like mind-candy and digest it in small bits. When you develop and strengthen your multisensory abilities, life gets easier and more exciting because you deeply align with your Higher Power. Connecting with your Higher Power gives you Superpowers.

Have you ever walked into a room and seen a couple looking at each other, and they stop talking as you enter? You can sense the unfortunate timing of your arrival and you politely excuse yourself. How did you know? What did you know? You sensed something. Was it a fight or a love affair or gossip about you? How did you sense it? Was it an odor? Did you feel something? Was it the expression on their faces? Registered or not, another form of communication is always at play. Stress levels surge giving us indications of social nuances. We might feel tension or the need to silence the moment or even leave that location to protect ourselves. The flight or fight cues are ignited, and we respond accordingly. Your senses are always evaluating your environment and informing you what's occurring beneath the cognitive chatter. Author of *Seat of the Soul* Gary Zukav asserts, "A multisensory human can learn more rapidly than a five-sensory human. With the help that is available to it, the multisensory personality can understand more quickly the meaning of its experiences, how they come into being, what they represent, and its role in creating them. It does not need to experience twelve or twenty or two hundred painful experiences to learn a major lesson of trust, responsibility or humbleness." You can reduce your stress, suffering and anxiety by developing multisensory perception.

Below is a partial list of psychic abilities from Wikipedia:
Astral projection, mental projection or out-of-body experience: The ability to voluntarily separate the astral body (or consciousness) from the physical body. Usually associated with the dreamtime but not required.
Aura Reading: The ability to perceive "energy fields" surrounding people, places and things.
Automatic Writing: The ability to draw or write without conscious intent.
Chronokinesis: The ability to alter ones own perception of time causing their sense of time to appear to slow down or speed up.
Clairaudience: The ability to acquire information by paranormal auditory means.
Claircognizance: The ability to acquire psychic knowledge by means of intrinsic knowledge. You just know it.
Clairgustance: The ability to taste without physical contact.
Clairolfactance: The ability to access spiritual or mediumistic knowledge through smell.
Clairsentience: The ability to psychically feel and to receive messages from emotions and feelings.

Clairvoyance: The ability to perceive people, objects, locations, or physical events via extrasensory vision.

Energy Work: The ability to manipulate physical or non-physical energy with one's mind. Reiki falls under this header.

Energy Medicine: The ability to heal with one's own empathic etheric, astral, mental or spiritual energy.

Levitation: The ability to float or fly by mystical means. Automatic or unintentional lifting of arms or legs without conscious intent.

Mediumship or Channeling: The ability to communicate with the dead.

Precognition or Premonition: The ability to perceive future events.

Prophecy or Prophetic Dreams: The ability to predict the future.

Psionics: The study of paranormal phenomena in relation to the application of electronics.

Psychic Surgery: The ability to remove disease or disorder within the body tissue via an "energetic" incision that heals immediately afterwards.

Psychokinesis or Telekinesis: The ability to manipulate objects with the mind.

Psychometry: The ability to obtain information about a person or an object through touch, like touching a ring or watch to learn more about the person.

Remote Viewing: The ability to see a distant or unseen target using extrasensory perception. Some Past Life Regression Therapists use remote viewing during sessions to understand and aid the client's recollection.

Postcognition: The ability to supernaturally perceive past events. This skill is particularly useful in solving crimes for the police force.

Second Sight: The ability to see future and past events or to perceive information that is not present to the physical senses, in the form of a vision (also see precognition, remote viewing, or seer).

Seer: Being able to view past or future events in the form of a vision.

Speaking in Tongues: The ability to speak a foreign language without conscious intent. When a believer prays in an unknown tongue, the Holy Spirit supernaturally directs the believer's prayer.

Telepathy: The ability to transmit or receive thoughts supernaturally, without words.

Thoughtography: The ability to imprint images from one's mind onto physical surfaces—such as photographic film—by psychic means.

It's amazing all the different ways we can receive information or manipulate the physical world. Where does a *vision, premonition or déjà vu* come from? Utilizing your Sixth Sense is another way to tap into your spirituality and experience the unfoldment of the Unseen Forces. When you have mystical experiences, your faith will be strengthened, and you will know that you are connected to something greater than yourself. Intuitive abilities, sensitivity, empathy or prophetic dreams allow you to channel your spiritual knowledge for insight, healing and guidance to move forward with confidence and inner peace.

Mental Telepathy

Human telepathy is quite a controversial topic. Telepathy means distanced feeling ("tele" means at a distance like a telephone or television and "pathy" is a feeling like empathy or sympathy). Thoughts are things. Your thoughts have a vibration and that changes your brain chemistry and consequently even your body odor (which mostly goes unnoticed by humans). That vibration carries weight, and energy follows thought. Don't think your thoughts stay in your cranium. Stop pretending that people don't know what you're thinking. Look at the people in your life; you know what they're thinking. You might not know every little detail but you get the gist of how your friends and family weigh-in on certain topics. You know who to call to get the response you want. If you want to whine, you talk to one person. If you want motivation, you call a different person. If you want to bitch about an objectionable politician, you know who will agree with you. As we get to know each other, we become connected energetically. How many times have you been thinking about someone and they called? Over time, developing your Superpowers allows you to communicate beyond the telephone. Being telepathic means that you have awareness beyond the obvious. It gives you an upper hand in dealing with relationships and the ability to resolve conflict sooner. When you know what someone is thinking you can communicate to that end instead of focusing solely on your own agenda.

ZENERGY BOOST FOR DEVELOPING MENTAL TELEPATHY
Find a friend or spouse who you can text whenever you think about them. Each time you think of each other text a word or emoticon. Do this for one to two weeks to understand their style. The second week or month, don't text, just write down each time you think of each other and the reason that stimulated the intent to text. Exchange notes at the end of the week or one month. Mental telepathy is a skill and a gift.

Currently, humans don't have a large vocabulary toward different ways of communicating (other than words) but animals do. Many pet owners will tell you that their pet knows more than just the commands of "No, Sit, Come, etc." What's that language called? Of course, pets communicate with each other, and it's not always a bark or meow. I like the motto, "if my dog doesn't like you, I don't like you." What is the dog noticing when it barks ferociously at a person? We are still learning about animal behavioral nuances and mental telepathy with pets; however, Cambridge Graduate Dr. Rupert Sheldrake spent the last two decades researching telepathy between dogs and their owners. In his fascinating research he was able to prove the line of communication with pets occurs on a mental level first. Many dog owners say their dog waits by the door knowing the owner's arrival is imminent. Critics of this experiment state that possibly the dog knows your routine, your vehicle motor noise, or hears the car door slam. Dr. Sheldrake did a double blind experiment wherein a computer called the owner at random times to invite the subject to go home. The subject would get into different taxis each time so that no familiar vehicle noise would be noted upon arrival. They set up a basic camera at the door or window where the dog would wait. What he found was that as soon as the owner decided to go home (even before getting into the taxi) the dog would walk to the door and wait approximately 85% of the time. Many skeptics, including more than 5,000 researchers and citizen scientists, repeated these experiments and documented their observations. The repetitive pattern of animals proves their significant mental communication with humans. Dr. Sheldrake's notable research continues to grow increasing his internationally based database. If you would like to participate, visit his website at www.Sheldrake. org. Due to his research and my own consciousness-raising experiences I view telepathy as a natural form of communication and not paranormal.

Learning more about telepathy with your pets may open your mind to telepathy with your loved ones. Many of you already practice this form of communication but may not document how often you actually make the mental connection. Many parents or grandparents comment on how they knew when a child was conceived, ill or injured. Twins show a remarkable ability to communicate beyond words. Occasionally, there is just a *knowing* about someone. You don't know how you know, you just *know*. Claircognizance is ineffable. You know but there are no words for that knowledge, and you trust following that internal wisdom even without evidence. You rely on your Higher Power when you are claircognizant.

A final plug for animals, we know how helpful working dogs are when they support the blind, aid those with PTSD and visit nursing homes. It's even becoming more common to trust dogs when they sniff for cancer. More than ever before trained therapy dogs can detect a physical or emotional imbalance before your doctor. And, let's not forget the multitude of animals that abandoned the Indian coastline two to three days prior to the deadliest earthquake-tsunami that hit the City of Banda Ache in 2004. Don't dismiss the connection you may already have with animals that gives you an automatic Sixth Sense with humans.

Empathy

Empathic ability means you feel what other people feel. You can feel their emotional intention, and it can provide clarity to a situation. Many parents have this natural Superpower with their children, and with a little effort could expand the awareness to others. If you see someone cry, you too might cry. You feel their pain. Some of that is sympathy but compassionate people hurt when they see human suffering, bullying or animal cruelty. Some very sensitive or empathic people can feel others' emotions, and it can be quite challenging at times to resolve this knowledge. You might not intend to know what others' feel but you have a Sixth Sense about it.

Feeling others' feelings can be very confusing if you don't know what's occurring. It's awkward when you're taking action on someone else's fantasy. I've had clients come into my office and say, "I don't know why I slept with that person. I just ended up in the wrong arms." Yes, that could be a cop-out and it could be the empathic one picking up on the pursuer's intention. A little bit of flirting or a common interest takes you into another dimension of the relationship, but you never intended it to go that far. You may very well feel someone fantasizing about you constantly, and that can impact your actions if you're not protecting yourself properly. (See Chakra Chapter to "Zip Up" for protection.)

One time while in college, I was listening to my science professor. I'll have to admit it was a little dull as that isn't my forté, but I wanted to graduate. While listening, suddenly I saw myself in a sexy rock video. Imaginatively, I hopped up on the lab desk naked and began strumming my electric guitar. I laughed, as I didn't think these types of things. I didn't play the guitar, nor had I watched a music video in years. (While in college, I sold my TV and many other possessions to reduce distractions. It definitely wasn't coming from my mind.) Initially, I laughed about the absurdity and just dismissed it, but the images didn't go away. Then, I realized I was seeing someone else's sexy rock video of me. I quieted my mental chatter and asked God, "Whose fantasy is this?" I opened my eyes and looked around the room and instantly saw a young man (18 or 19 years old) staring at me. He was so startled when I "caught" him. He never looked at me again for the remainder of the semester, and I never saw those images again either. It was quite interesting to notice the telepathy. My Sixth Sense kept me safe. As I walked around campus and in other locations, I realized that if I wanted to know more about my environment, all I needed to do was quiet my mind. The less television I watched the easier it was to develop that skill. While in school I learned to meditate and that helped me develop my Superpowers.

Have you ever had a sense of being stared at and then turned around to "catch" the person? Dr. Sheldrake wrote a book on this topic about his findings since the 1990s. Between 70-97% of Europeans and North Americans surveyed experienced this phenomenon. Even skeptics obtained significant positive results when duplicating the experiment. Albeit, the awareness that someone is watching you is more apparent with siblings and family members and especially amongst twins, anyone can develop the skill. If you would like be a citizen scientist and take part in Dr. Sheldrake's experiments, please see his website listed above. It's intriguing to know that many subjects in the experiment improved with practice.

Mediums Talk to Dead People
Mediums use different types of sensory skills to communicate with the deceased. Clairvoyance is seeing through the veil; clairaudience is hearing their words or whispers; clairsentience is feeling their presence. The most widely recognized form of mediumship is knowing that another entity is present in the room, and this is called claircognizance.

Mental Mediumship employs the use of telepathy, and some Mediums go into a trance allowing the spirit to transmit a communication to the bereaved client. Occasionally, the message could even be in another language unknown to the Medium. While receiving a communication from a Medium in trance, the client may experience the voice of the deceased or even an appearance of the deceased's face overlaying the Medium's face validating the experience. Taps, knocks or other noises may be heard or even random lights or orbs may be seen in the room during the experience. It's a fascinating and inexplicable phenomenon. Interacting with a Medium quite likely could save you from years of grief and bereavement, especially if your loved one died unexpectedly. Having some type of communication with the deceased could help you move onward instead of clinging to the past that no longer exists. Of course, loss of a loved one is challenging and the grieving process is different for everyone, but you can save yourself all kinds of bewilderment, confusion and anger if you could communicate with the dead, AND you can.

John Edwards on *Crossing Over* is probably one of the most famous modern day Mediums. Average Mum Teresa Caputo is on her third season with her own TV show justly named *The Long Island Medium* on TLC TV sharing her wonderful experiences with the dead. A&E Television Special on *Mediums: We See Dead People*, showcased John Holland's and other Medium's unique abilities. Rebecca Rosen seen on Oprah May 26, 2010, says, "Mediums rely on the presence of non-physical energy outside of themselves for the information relevant to the person being read." New Yorker James Van Praagh hosted many lectures with Hay House Publishing and other organizations to share his wisdom and teach mediumship skills. You could learn to be a Medium. There are many schools like the Los Angeles School for Spiritual Arts, and the most famous modern day Harry Potter School, Arthur Findlay College in United Kingdom which opened in 1923. You might be surprised to know that there are people in your hometown who communicate with the deceased. Some people are naturals at interdimensional communication and don't need any schooling at all, while others are formally trained. Regardless of their path, Mediums generally have one foot in each world with the intent to heal both.

It was documented in 1968 in the American Psychological Association Manuals and the American Medical Association Manuals that approximately 68% of widows and widowers frequently "talk" to their deceased spouses. We don't think of this as Mediumship, but it is a form of communicating with the dead. If your spouse died and you hear the voice of the deceased or feel the presence of the deceased, then you should feel normal. An article written by Simon McCarthy-Jones entitled "Sensing the Dead is Perfectly Normal and Often Helpful" (July 2017) shows that "A study of elderly widows and widowers in Wales found that 13% heard their dead loved one's voice, 14% had seen them and 3% had felt their touch. By far the greatest number, 39%, said they continued to feel the presence of loved ones." This is not a new phenomenon, but if you relay this information to your local psychiatrist or medical doctor, they should not prescribe any medication and/or label you as crazy because this is a natural phenomenon. Doctors frequently will prescribe something, sleeping pills or otherwise, since their main trade is to sell pharmaceuticals. Can you imagine how many people are talking to the dead and think they are crazy when it's actually normal? Spouses are the control group because the deceased do not talk to everyone in the family. They reach out to those family members or friends who are open enough to listen with their Sixth Sense, clairaudience. What does that mean for humanity? It means, that death does not part us. Just because you die doesn't mean that you're gone.

Some of you, like myself, may have been born with some of these gifts, or possibly you've developed multisensory skills throughout your life. Initially, I was very empathic as a child, but it lay dormant until I was older. I struggled with my emotions as a young person and young adult because I didn't realize that I was sensing my family and friend's feelings. I was under the impression that all those thoughts and feelings were mine, and it was very confusing at times. Once I learned that they were not all mine with the simple technique of saying "mine" or "not mine" then I knew how to protect myself. It helped me in the moment to recognize when I was sensing others' thoughts and feelings. In the example above, I didn't own a TV and wasn't watching rock videos so it was easy for me to say, "not mine." When you have certain thoughts of hatred, racism or judgment just ask, "Is this my thought?" Sometimes it is a habit to hate or judge someone or you may be sensing others' opinions. Knowing to "Zip Up" the chakras provides energetic protection (see Chakra Chapter).

If you get a feeling or a knowing that you should call a friend or get home right away or not take a flight, then listen to your hunch. We've all had an intuition and didn't act upon it, and the situation was a flop. Identify the nuances of your bodily sensations. Many people automatically label feelings as anxiety or anger instead of as a premonition. Just because you have sweaty palms, your breathing changes or your heart palpitates, it doesn't always mean you are worrying. You may be receiving insight about an upcoming event. Getting angry sometimes is a sign that your boundary has been crossed or you agreed to participate in something that is inappropriate. You may need to reevaluate a relationship or re-establish boundaries for a win/win situation. Quiet down so you can feel your own energy and learn what is "mine" and "not mine." You can save yourself a heap of heartache by developing your Superpowers.

 ZENERGY BOOST FOR CONNECTING WITH YOUR PARKING SPACE ANGELS
Next time you're headed out the door say a quick statement, "Thank you for giving me a free parking space near the front door." Notice what happens.

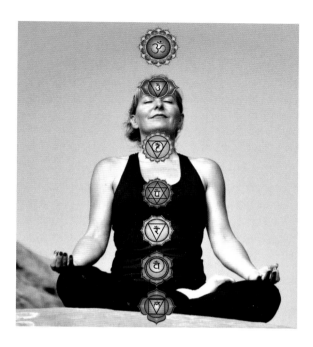

CHAKRAS & THEIR INFLUENCE

The term *chakra* is becoming more of a household word these days due to the New Age Movement; however, there is nothing new about the New Age Movement or chakras. The Movement is rooted in ancient wisdom dating back Before the Common Era (BCE). There is some mention of the chakras as psychic centers of consciousness in the Yoga Upanishads (circa 1200-900 BCE) and later in the *Yoga Sutras of Patanjali* (circa 200 BCE). However, the Vedas are the oldest written tradition in India, (1,500–500 BCE) recorded from oral tradition by upper caste Brahmans for thousands of years prior to written form (*Ancient History Encyclopedia*, 2013).

The chakra is an energy wheel that cannot be seen by the naked eye. You wouldn't find it if you cut someone open and looked into their body or spine. The chakra is a part of the ethereal body, the glow around you or your aura. It surrounds you and responds to your emotional-mental state. The etheric body or halo is around all plants and animals. We have a physical body and a light body, and the main chakras relate to specific areas of life.

There are seven main chakras overlaying the physical body along the spinal column, from the crown of the head to the tailbone where the root chakra sits. Through modern physiology, Ayurvedic Doctors and Doctors of Oriental Medicine, it is noted that the seven chakras correspond exactly to the seven main nerve ganglia that emanate from the spinal column to all of the bodily organs. Your chakras can become blocked or imbalanced due to a variety of issues that we will be reviewing in this chapter, and that blockage can lead to lack of focus, inability to manifest your desires, fear of self-expression, sleep apnea or even illness. Recognizing blocked chakras not only raises your consciousness beyond just the physical, but also can stabilize your physique, psyche and spiritual connection.

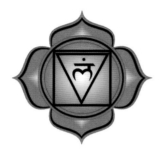

First Chakra ~ *Muladhara Chakra* ~ "I Am"

Sanskrit *mula* means "root" and *adhara* means "support." The first chakra is located at the perineum (near the base of the spine), and is generally translated as your physical foundation, need for food, shelter and survival. The root chakra governs the skeleton, bones, rectum, colon, and arterial blood that flows through the heart, transporting oxygen and nutrients to bodily tissues. The personality and ego reside in the first chakra, and it connects you to Mother Earth.

Energetically, the first chakra anchors your sense of safety, stability and security. It represents your first seven years. It's your identity, autobiography and connection to family. You anchor the ability to perform your life purpose (or walk your life path) by grounding your feet to the Earth. You either feel connected and at peace with yourself or flighty and fearful. The human ego is needed as it allows you to recognize yourself in the mirror and houses your memories. You need your ego to live on Earth, but you don't want your ego leading you. When the first chakra is imbalanced it can point to selfishness, addictions, predatory behavior or mindless violence.

The root chakra is the color red like blood or passion. Common colloquialisms like "don your red shoes" or "let's paint the town red" or "hop in my red sports car" traverse our language with an edge toward a passionate adventure, similar to a walk through the Red Light District. These references to a night of joyous expression are rooted in the first chakra. On the other hand, aberrant sexual behaviors indicate imbalances in the root chakra. I'm not rebuking hot and heavy sex or even classy nude photography, but you want your sexuality to take you to another dimension in your evolution not just get lost in getting-off. It's a team activity so make it wonderful for both parties. Find healthy ways to create sex-to-superconsciousness.

Generally speaking, addictions to cyberporn, prostitution or stripping are also symptoms of an imbalanced root chakra. Unhealthy sexuality can block or hinder progress along the life journey. Many adult entertainers and the "Johns" who visit the bars frequently have sex addictions. The performers find it difficult to quit stripping even when the financial goals are reached, and it remains an easy, albeit expensive, distraction from adult responsibilities for the "Johns." Sex and adult entertainment are needed but there are many facets to life that require the passion and energy of the root chakra. In fact, hobbies require passion and enthusiasm but rarely seduce like sex. Some people have venereal diseases like herpes, warts or pelvic inflammatory disease (PID) and not because of promiscuity but due to emotional angst in their primary relationship. When you don't feel supported and promoted by your significant other, you can contract yeast infections, hemorrhoids or similar irritations that prevent you from having sex. When you sublimate your sexuality (moving from the first chakra to the second chakra), you transform lust into desire for passionate connection. Lust is about wanting sex for a momentary pleasure, and passion is about sharing love.

Alcohol and drug addiction are also associated with an imbalanced root chakra. When someone is full of drugs, pharmaceuticals or recreational, they cannot listen to their intuition as well. Just because your doctor wrote you a prescription doesn't mean you can't get an addiction. Find the right dosage and monitor yourself. Continue your quest for higher and greater achievements, not perfection. Some people are arrogant because they don't drink or use drugs. Again, egotistical behavior is the culprit we're all looking to tame when harmonizing the chakras.

Egocentricity, depression, feeling like a victim and abandonment issues are indications of a blockage in the root chakra. Imbalances in the first chakra can lead to an overwhelming concern for security in relationship at the cost of one's autonomy. Conversely, feeling secure and comfortable in your own skin are signs of a stable first center.

Yoga Posture: Get grounded by standing tall in Mountain Pose, Tadasana.

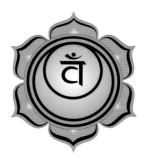

Second Chakra ~ *Swadhisthana Chakra* ~ "I Feel"
The Sanskrit word means "*vital force.*" The second chakra is located below the navel in the sacral-lumbar area. It is the seat of creativity, and the color is orange. When you sublimate your sexuality, you generate your passion into new creative endeavors. It could be a painting, musical composition, an entrepreneurial enterprise or even a child. The second center is considered the sexual center as it governs the reproductive organs. Balancing the creative center with your passion can generate a lot of satisfaction. Some people work almost 24/7 but never feel financially secure. Others have sex with pure abandon, but as Mick Jagger says, "just can't get no satisfaction." If you're tired of hollow victories, then create something remarkable with love, passion and enthusiasm. Works of art of any kind can offer a bounty of contentment.

Chakras correlate to the organs along the spinal column, and the digestive system is governed by the second center. When you're not expressing yourself authentically or you're uptight about life, you may experience constipation, diarrhea, IBS or other digestion disorders. Additionally, lumbar tension is a sign of an imbalanced second chakra. When the low back is out of alignment it can impact the proper functioning of the bladder, kidneys and adrenals. Although some overlap occurs within the lower three chakras, the second center governs the genitals and reproductive organs, adrenal glands, kidneys and intestines. The sacral chakra embodies our sensuality and sexual energy, intimacy, self-acceptance, personal relationships and our emotionality.

The intestines are governed by this center, and detoxifying the digestive track can rebalance the orange center creating a harmonizing effect throughout the entire parasympathetic system. (The sympathetic system manages the "flight or fight" response, and the parasympathetic system governs the "rest and digest" activities.) Softly massaging the second center in a clockwise direction encourages digestion. Colonics or enemas can improve and rebalance the lower GI track, and abstinence (even for a month or two) can purify the body and mind. Abstinence from sex, drugs, pornography, TV, even socializing for a month or two can be very healthy.

As a Mind-Body-Spirit Life Coach I'm always looking at life on all three levels. When there is an issue, say with the kidneys, then look first at what's occurring physically. Are you drinking enough water and reducing your caffeine intake? Do you need a chiropractic adjustment in the lower back to assist the organ's proper functioning? If you've handled what you can physically, then look at what's occurring mentally. Money worries, fear of poverty and family issues are stored in the second chakra and those issues can stop you from stepping up to your next level of achievement. It may be time to begin a new chapter in your life, invite new experiences, explore the world and invent something distinctive. An unfulfilled innovative endeavor might slow your creative flow and mental-emotional pain can become physical. Even developing a "poker face" to hide your discontent can become a permanent part of your self-expression. Resolving a kidney issue on a spiritual level may require reflection and forgiveness of a disappointment or criticism. Taking a more integrated approach to some of these common physical ailments and investigating them from all three areas can provide greater understanding and a deeper spiritual contentment.

Yoga Posture: Generate emotional stability and creativity with Sun Goddess, *Deviasana*.

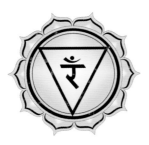

Third Chakra ~ Manipura Chakra ~ "I Will."
The Sanskrit meaning is *"navel,"* rightly positioned in that area, and it has a luminous energy of brilliant yellow. I call this the Manifestor. It hosts the part of us in business, money, materialism, maternity, paternity, parenthood and intellect, and the part that responsibly goes to work each day. Personal and professional agreements are governed by the Third Center. It's the part of you that remains professional even when you want to scream at someone. It's the side of you that feels dutiful, accountable and obligated.

This energetic center relates to the digestive system and includes the liver, gallbladder, spleen, stomach and pancreas. If there is a frustrating situation that you just can't "stomach" anymore, you might contract an ulcer. I've had several clients over the years who "blew out" their third center by staying too long in demoralizing marriages. They were giving, giving, giving and unfortunately, they were left with acid reflux, diverticulitis or other stomach disorders. Rebalancing the third center can dissolve tiresome situations to regain your personal power. It harnesses the influence of our drive and will.

When we receive an intuitive hit it is felt in the solar plexus, like a hunch or a gut instinct. Remember a time when you met someone that you didn't trust. You might have noticed that they gossip or were deceitful. If they are gossiping about someone TO you, then they are most likely gossiping ABOUT you. If they tell you how they cheated someone, guess what, you're probably next in line. So you must be mindful of these types of people. It is a human condition. Many people have those types of problems. You don't have to judge them or hate them for their shortcomings, just know the truth and the truth shall set you free. Free, that is, from getting into a professional contract with them, marrying them, loaning them money or sharing secrets with them. Avoid contractual agreements with untrustworthy people; however, sometimes you can't, and that's when you're thankful for our legal system. Remember you can abhor the behavior and remain compassionate toward the person. Don't expect people to be like you, but be thankful when you find the ones who are.

Greed is a sign that this center is imbalanced. It might be expressed when a CEO eliminates 30,000 jobs at the holidays or when politicians file another frivolous lawsuit against the federal government. The loss of our social connection in professional settings is an indication of an imbalanced third chakra across the nation. Conversely, acts of collaboration, cooperation and generosity express that you're not just on the right path but the Light Path.
The third chakra encompasses your ability to manifest a job, work in the world and express yourself professionally. Don't underestimate your intuitive ability while at work. Learn to listen to your Sixth Sense and set healthy boundaries as necessary. Even quiet power can be very useful at times. Be productive at manifesting something miraculous, enjoying your line of work and your contributions.

Yoga Posture: Foster personal power in Warrior I Pose, *Virabhadrasana I.*

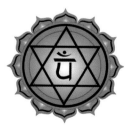

Fourth Chakra ~ *Anahata Chakra* ~ "I love"
The Sanskrit meaning is "unstruck note or unhurt." Notice the pace at which your heart beats. This emerald colored chakra resides at the center of the chest and includes the heart, cardiac plexus, thymus gland, lungs, lymphatic system and breasts. Taking a few minutes each day to feel your heart beating can restore kindness, affection and love. This simple exercise could be performed while driving, grocery shopping or even at a company meeting. Compassion will carry you on life's roller coaster ride with grace and understanding.

The heart can keep us connected to our loved ones. The fourth center provides a sense of devotion, connection, commitment and joy. Delight in the ways you enjoy life and all the meaningful relationships around you. Keeping an open heart is a huge source of pleasure. Conversely, hate also comes from the heart chakra and keeps us connected to our enemies. When you lament on a painful memory, you keep it alive in the present. The brain synapses fire and the stress hormones flow in the same way as if you were in that time and place still suffering through that unpleasant experience. Open heart surgeries and transplants are a huge indication of a congested heart chakra and with over 500,000 heart surgeries performed annually, we really need to look at how much love, or lack thereof, we are sharing (*TexasHeart.org*).

As I mentioned in the third chakra, you can abhor the behavior and remain kind to the person. Loving someone doesn't mean being at his or her mercy. Imagine if your child is a drug addict and (s)he keeps asking for money. It hurts your heart to not support your child, yet you know (s)he will spend the money on drugs. If you are acquiescing to the requests, it reduces the child's self-reliance and fuels addiction. Keep your heart open and your mind wise. You don't want to close your heart to set healthy boundaries. When you decline support to a child when you know the money or other gift will be squandered, you force the child to accept responsibility for their choices. You encourage the child to acquire new resources instead of turning to you when in a time of want. Listen to your intuition while deciding what is best for your heart intellectually. When you take care of yourself in a healthy way, you generate vitality for the entire family. Bridge the intelligence of your mind with the wisdom of your heart, and allow your children to mature in their unique way. Remember we are sensitive and vulnerable beings. If you let others take advantage of you willingly, ultimately you will pay the price with more karma.

Most of us have experienced a broken heart. It could be from the loss of a loved one, getting fired from a good job, having your car stolen or even miscommunicating with siblings. An unrequited heart can lead to disastrous behavior, and the shoulders may physically round to protect the wounded heart. Being guarded, angry, confrontive or rude is a way to hide how vulnerable you may feel. Self-sabotaging your accomplishments or undermining your family members is an indication of a blockage in the heart chakra. When the wounded child, or wounded adult, begins to intimidate others, that is a sure sign to pull back, sit down and reflect. We all make mistakes, and the quicker you forgive the better you will be. Forgiveness is a valuable skill worthy of consideration to restore leniency and humility. When the heart is open and loving, all things become possible.

Yoga Posture: Develop compassion for self and others through Camel Pose, *Ustrasana.*

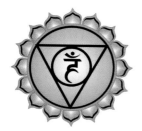

Fifth Chakra ~ *Vishuddha Chakra* ~ I Speak!
The Sanskrit meaning denotes, *"pure or purification."* The throat chakra is cobalt blue and governs our words or sounds. Music, prayers and inspiring affirmations are positive ways to keep this chakra balanced. Listening to ambient or uplifting music can generate a harmonic tone in your home or office.

Music is a divine art, to be used not only for pleasure, but as path to God-realization.
Paramahansa Yogananda

Enhance your communication and your thyroid gland through healing tones. Negative thoughts and emotions weaken the electromagnetic system of the body. Harmonic ambiance, rhythms and vibrations like chanting or humming can balance the throat chakra. Your voice chanting is the perfect sound for your body. Whether flat or sharp your tone is ideal for your spiritual development. Your sacred mantra can heal the physical body, balance the endocrine glands and align the spinal system.

Its important to remember that words can bring life or death to a situation or a relationship. Manipulative people will say something hurtful, and then say, "It's just a four letter word. Don't be so sensitive." Any word can hurt when the intention is to harm, and pretending that expressions and intonations don't have meaning can be a form of manipulation. Also, you can't un-hear something said, regardless of what the Judge's rule in the courtroom. Harming someone with your words can be an indication of an imbalance in the fifth center, and resolving conflict, even a decade later, could reduce countless future problems. You don't necessarily have to apologize but acknowledge that your words caused them to experience ill feelings (anger, sadness, resentment, low self-esteem). When you forgive a friend for misspoken words, it opens the door in your spiritual escrow account for someone else to forgive you. (e.g. Jane forgives Bill; Amy forgives Jane.) When you forget others' shortcomings it allows others to forget yours. Frequently, we associate forgiveness with the heart chakra, but it is certainly connected to the throat chakra as well.

Additionally, the Throat Chakra governs the neck. Restoring flexibility through gentle neck rotations can assist you in gaining 360° clarity on a topic. Seeing the world from another's perspective offers greater understanding and that can dissolve neck or throat tension.

Yoga Posture: Cultivate a healthy authentic voice with chanting while in Easy Pose, *Sukhasana,* or sitting in a chair.

Sixth Chakra ~ Ajna Chakra ~ I See!

The Sanskrit meaning is "*to perceive or to command.*" The third eye is probably the most known chakra. Our third eye points upward, and the color is indigo. It is vertical not horizontal like our other two eyes. Proper brain functioning and healthy hormones positively impact the indigo center. Vision from the sixth chakra comes from our Higher Self.

Have you ever had an unforgettable dream or vision that came to pass? Intuitions, premonitions or precognitions arise in the sixth center and leave us with an unforgettable experience. Now, this is different from a memory with the prefrontal cortex, the area of the brain at the forehead. Let's explore the difference. A memory of the night's news occurs in the frontal lobe (stock market fluctuations, employment statistics, car wrecks or a new recipe). The memory is complimented with an analytical explanation and compartmentalized for future recall. A vision comes from somewhere else –your Higher Self, Soul or Superconsciousness, not your brain–and you can't explain it. Unique and rare wisdom accompanies a vision, and it's usually a perception you didn't previously have. These types of experiences are well documented in the *Bible* and other sacred texts. You, too, can have visions that benefit your life and those around you. Visions and dreams didn't only occur in ancient history, they are happening daily if you are awake enough to notice them.

Opening the vision center will transform your life forever. When the sixth center is balanced you will think more clearly, have foresight and insight, develop your imagination, understand the big picture quickly, expand your consciousness and influence your environment. Hindus wear a bindi, a red dot or dry paint on the third eye, honoring this sacred center. Meditation can harmonize, balance and stimulate your sixth center while preparing you for the next level of your spiritual evolution.

When the sixth center is blocked, judgment reigns. Harsh opinions, irritations and quibbles float through the head impeding the flow of energy through the mind's eye. Until you actually know what scatter chatter is filling your mind, you can't really stop it. When judgments are in a blind spot and you don't recognize your own unconscious behavior, they will control you. If you can't specifically identify why you don't like someone, someplace or something then you will continue to make unconscious decisions and will avoid certain people, places or things. Alight your blind spots, clarify a pejorative outlook and release judgments through simple mindful practices to reclaim your sixth chakra.

Yoga Posture: Calm your third eye and all that scatter chatter by lowering your head to the earth in Child Pose, *Balasana*. Ask for God's guidance on how you can best serve the Earth. Connect to the Earth to magnetize your steps easily and effortlessly.

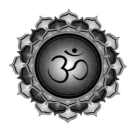

Seventh Chakra ~ Sahasrara Chakra ~ I Know!

The Sanskrit meaning signifies "one thousand petal lotus." Although growing in the swamp, the lotus strives to reveal its colorful petals and bountiful fragrance. As the outer edge of petals dies and disappears, the inner circle begins its journey through the flowering cycle. The Soul is likened to a thousand petal lotus and is so powerful that it couldn't possibly be contained entirely in a cellular form like the human body. It hovers overhead and animates the body. Imagine the wheel of a car wherein God is the center and the spokes reaching out are the individuals (you and me). The outside of the wheel (the rubber tire) is the Earthly experience, theater, relationship and individuality. The inside of the wheel is the Creator. The spokes don't touch, yet the inside wheel and outside tire unite it all. We are the individual spokes, and we are a part of the whole wheel. The human brain can't possibly imagine the power of a Soul and certainly not the Creator. We attempt to verbalize knowledge about the Soul, but words will never express all the details to one human existence, much less Universal Omnipotence.

When you are tired of feeling isolated or unhappy and relinquish the "know it all" stance to find peace of mind, that quest reconnects you deeply with your Soul. Being happy is one sign that you are connected to your Highest Consciousness and that your seventh center is balanced. The crown center is blocked when you are morose, pessimistic, scattered or cynical. Disturbances like epilepsy, migraines and brain tumors indicate a blocked seventh center.

Over intellectualizing, rigidity and feeling disconnected point to insufficient energy. Meditation, yoga and prayer are positive ways to rebalance the central nervous system, and stay connected with your Highest Council to receive counsel. Don't pretend that you, your ego, your prefrontal cortex, can do all the work that is required while on the Earth plane. Transcending Earthly problems of the lower self to attain wisdom from the higher self guides you to Superconsciousness.

Begin to see yourself as a soul with a body rather than a body with a soul.
Dr. Wayne Dyer

As you can see, the chakras function on multiple levels of the mind-body-spirit. Balance your chakras through pranayama (breathing exercises), meditation, mindfulness practices, nutrition, yoga and exercise. By working on one chakra, you also affect the entire chakra system.

Yoga Posture: Connect to your Highest Power through meditation. Sitting or lying in *savasana*, relaxation pose, touch the pallet to the roof of the mouth and lift the perineum (pelvic floor) while focusing on the pineal gland located at the center of the brain. Spend a few minutes in restful awareness practicing Kegels in five-second increments (with an inward eye on the pineal). Practicing Kegels periodically throughout the day is another way to incorporate a spiritual practice into daily lifestyle.

Connect the Centers ~

- The 7th Chakra connects to the 1st Chakra ~ Allowing the Soul to guide you on your path. Bring Heaven to Earth through your cellular structure. Feeling joyful and grounded are signs that you are on your Divine Life Path.
- The 6th Chakra connects to the 2nd Chakra ~ Your inner vision spurs your creative endeavors. Find your passion to create good works in the world. Consider reading *Do what you love and the money will follow* by Marsha Sinetar (1989) or other similar books. The feminine aspect of yourself (Yin) creates a Honey Do List, and the masculine aspect of yourself (Yang) manifests it into reality. Balanced Yin and Yang create harmony.
- The 5th Chakra connects to the 3rd Chakra ~ Speak your truth eloquently at work and at home. Bring life through your words to your relationships and notice how bountiful your world becomes.
- 4th Chakra ~ When we are balanced, the heart remains open and compassion reigns. Happiness is our natural state of being.

 ZENERGY BOOST ZIP UP!
Inhale and imagine the Light flowing from the crown chakra down the spine to the root chakra toward your feet. Exhale see and sense the Light moving back to the top of your head. Feel the warmth and see the Light flowing down and up the spine seven times for seven breaths balancing seven chakras. Expand the light all around you, above and below (approximately six feet in each direction). Each time you move your attention down and up the spine silently affirm, "I am balanced in all chakras, and they spin appropriately for my spiritual growth." On the seventh and final breath moving up the spine, imagine a zipper from your feet to your head, and zip up your energy field so that you are working from your Highest Center. This exercise reduces anxiety, fatigue, as well as feelings of isolation, and it can connect you deeply to your Highest Self. When you stop leaking your energy and giving it away unknowingly, you can recognize the best use of your time and talents. Many times people feel bad because a friend feels bad. Stop feeling others' emotions, thinking that they are your feelings. Feeling bad for others doesn't stop their suffering, it increases yours. Keep your good energy for your use so that you can focus on your Divine Life Purpose, and when it is time to help another, you will have enough energy do to so wisely. Zip up!

QUICK REFERENCE CHAKRA CHART

	MIND		BODY	
	Spiritual Direction & Transformation, Humility, Enlightenment, Wisdom, Bliss	**7**	Brain Stem & Spinal Cord, Pineal Gland, Regulates Biological Chemistry & Sleep Cycle	I KNOW
	Insight, Intuition, Vision, Dreams, Imagination, Expanded Consciousness, Life Purpose, Patience	**6**	Brain, Eyes, Hair, Ears, Sinus Glands, Petuitary Gland, Produces Hormones	I SEE
	Personal Expression, Speak your Truth, 360° Perspective, Communications	**5**	Neck, Mouth, Larynx, Vocal Chords, Thyroid, Regulates Respiratory System, Metabolism & Body Temperature	I SPEAK
	Compassion, Love, Connection, Joy, Grace, Devotion, Understanding, Acceptance, Commitment	**4**	Heart, Cardiac Plexus, Lungs, Breasts, Thymus Gland, Regulates Immune & Lymphatic Systems	I LOVE
	What I do with my energy for others. Business Chakra, Social, External, Manifesting, Self-worth, Making Money, Greed	**3**	Abdomen, Stomach, Liver, Gallbladder, Pancreas, Spleen, Digestion, Metabolism, Circulation	I WILL
	What I do with my energy for me. Creativity, Pleasure, Sexuality, Children, Fear of Poverty	**2**	Adrenal Glands, Kidneys, Intestines, Digestion, Bladder, Low Back, Ovaries, Testes, Reproductive Organs	I FEEL
	Self, Ego, Personality, Feeling Grounded, Securing Basic Needs, Home, Safety, Food, Addictions & Carnal Nature	**1**	Base of Spine, Pelvis, Digestion, Rectum, Reproductive Organs, Legs, Feet, Bones, Blood	I AM

287

REIKI HEALING ENERGY

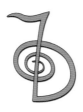

Cho Ku Rei

Reiki (pronounced "Ray Key") means Universal Life Energy. The word Reiki is made of two Japanese words – "Rei" which means "God's Wisdom or the Higher Power" and "Ki" which is "Life Force Energy." Reiki is an Asian healing art form devised by a Japanese Priest, Dr. Mikao Usui, in the early part of the 20th century. It is based on the principle that the Reiki Therapist can channel energy to the patient by means of prayer and light healing touch. This healing touch, which is now being offered in some hospitals, activates the natural healing process of the patient's body and restores physical and emotional wellbeing.

I am a Reiki Master, Teacher and Therapist, and I have given hundreds of treatments. I allow the Creative Forces to work through me to restore balance and reinforce the body's natural ability to heal by placing my hands gently on or over a patient. Although Practitioners do not diagnose injury, illness or disease, the patient can absorb the powerful Reiki energy like a sponge in the whole mind-body-spirit, restoring health and vitality. It's an intuitive and nurturing process like when a parent's hands quickly and naturally embrace a crying child. This act of giving love in a physical touch is a simplified way to explain Reiki. As the practitioner is giving Reiki, the hands feel like a heating pad. Once I left a pink handprint on a patient even though the patient was fully clothed and covered by a sheet.

The Father of Science, Sir Isaac Newton (1643-1727), used the term "ether" in the 1600s to describe the substance that comprised the universe, and it was linked with gravity and human sensations (The Method of Fluxions and Infinite Series with Its Application to the Geometry of Curve-Lines, 1736). The word ether describes the place by which electronic signals travel through the air broadcasting radio signals. A message is conveyed over or through this field. The Greeks also used the word ether to describe the material that fills the region of the universe above the terrestrial sphere, but we now know that this field is not just above the Earth, it is all around us like a matrix. Reiki travels through the matrix. 1902 Noble Prize Winner Hendrik Lorentz developed the equations that gave Einstein the tools to develop his Theory of Relativity. Lorentz stated, "I cannot but regard the ether which can be the seat of an electromagnetic field with its energy and vibrations... however different it may be from all ordinary matter." Einstein also believed in the field when he stated, "Space without ether is unthinkable." The scientific community accepted the field in the past and in 2012, CERN identified the Higgs Boson Particle also known as the *God Particle*. CERN is the European Organization for Nuclear Research located 150 meters beneath Switzerland and France. For the Higgs Boson Particle to exist there must be a Higgs Field. Scientists have been searching for this field for three centuries (or longer). I only mention this scientific data provided by Gregg Braden in *The Divine Matrix* (2006) because when thinking about Reiki one must also understand this field within which we live. *The field* is the container for all things we know. It is the bridge between the inner and outer world. Our prayers find their recipients whether nearby or on the other side of the planet through this energy field.

Although touching is not required, a treatment is likened to the "laying on of hands" as found in many faiths. It is non-sectarian yet an effective way to pray for people. Reiki lowers stress, reduces pain, promotes relaxation, and stimulates personal and spiritual growth. It's as if the patient is a battery that needs recharging, and the Reiki Therapist is a conduit for Universal Life Energy to flow to the patient through the matrix. You have a circulating central nervous system that flows through your bloodstream. Reiki healing energy uses this natural rhythm in the body together with the Soul. God, Guides and Angels heal the body and Reiki smooths the auric field. When people are troubled, ill or injured their vitality is weakened. Their energy field seems like static and not smooth like someone who is stable and in a good place in their life. I feel like an antenna reaching out for the greatest loving vibration to bless the patient. During this connection between us we can acquire messages for health and healing that alone the patient cannot do. Each of us is an antenna and Reiki attunes you to your best frequency stabilizing the emotional edges.

The Practitioner attains a calm meditative state and becomes like a generator sending healing light and love while the patient reclines fully clothed face up on a massage table. Reiki sessions are unique because the patient plays a major role in the session's success. A patient supports the Reiki process by mentally clearing their thoughts and setting their intention prior to the session. Focused intent and receptivity of the patient allows Reiki to clear obstacles from the human energy field and achieve a state of equilibrium. The more relaxed the patient feels and the more expectant of a remedy the patient is, the more beneficial the treatment.

The concept of Reiki is that the Practitioner is never in the position to dominate or dictate the channel of energy. The Therapist remains always at the service of divine healing; they are actually "Reiki Servants." Reiki Masters describe the process as one that links them with a Cosmic Radiant Energy. It involves the transfer of a harmonic luminous energy through the Reiki Practitioner to the patient. All the patient has to do is receive the energy fully. Unfortunately, some new Reiki Practitioners may be more like a sponge absorbing the patient's imbalances, leaving the Practitioner depleted after the treatment. A seasoned Therapist learns to be a conduit to channel the healing energy and not absorb others' pain out of empathy.

During a 15-60 minute session, the recipient relaxes or even falls asleep while the Reiki Practitioner holds a meditative mind focusing solely on the patient. Practitioners, frequently empathetic, will feel or notice imbalances in the patient's body and are intuitively guided to direct energy to certain areas. The Reiki Therapist and patient's mind become linked which enables an expansive connection, reducing pain, illness and symptoms of disease. The entire Reiki ritual, the soothing room environment, the calming music, the gentle hand positions, the skilled practitioner's attitude and confidence, and the length of the session, work harmoniously to support the patient's relief from physical pain and emotional discord. Following the treatment, some patients have vivid dreams or visions with the exact information they need to move forward in life.

Some hospitals and clinics provide a Reiki Practitioner as a cost-effective way to accelerate recuperation after surgery, reduce pain and anxiety, and decrease the negative side effects of medications and other medical procedures. "One 2013 study at UCLA confirmed with an electromyography (EMG) lab that studies electrical activity in the body found that 10-minutes of energy healing was as effective as physical therapy in improving the range of motion in people with mobility problems" (*NY Daily News,* 2014). Typically, a Reiki Practitioner would be in the recovery room to assist with rejuvenation and revitalization. I assisted one patient after a botched surgery. Being available to reduce pain, chills and nausea made a significant improvement in his recovery. Due to severe sepsis, near pneumonia and other considerable concerns while at the hospital, the patient and the family assured me that without these Reiki treatments he would not be alive. Furthermore, when he returned nine-months later for another operation, the doctors were amazed to see no excessive scar tissue, as is common after complicated surgeries. This is a huge success on an extreme case.

Many patients see vibrant colors or other visual images clarifying concerns. Some experience a *knowing* of what is the next path for them reconciling unresolved issues. Others encounter their Angels or Spirit Guides and receive direct guidance. It's an intuitive exercise, not an analytical one, using your imagination in connection with your divine spiritual intelligence. While relaxing in a tranquil meditative state, new solutions to old problems may be presented. Providing grief relief after the loss of a loved one can be very therapeutic. The patient can invite the deceased with whom they have unfinished business. Possibly a final expression or exchange needs to occur for the patient to move forward in their life. Reiki Practitioners do not call Spirits back from the dead although this can happen spontaneously. The patient's heartfelt desire and the deceased's ability to reconnect determine ancestral visitations. Although results vary, a Reiki session can transform your spiritual outlook profoundly, and radically reduce the time needed for the bereavement process.

After a session many patients look with astonishment and say, "I've never been that relaxed before." I frequently hear, "that's the closest to Christ that I've ever felt." While on the massage table I've had several patients receive bone adjustments. My hands were just lightly touching the skin when we heard the bones adjust. I didn't manipulate the bones or muscles in any way; they relocated on their own accord while I was focusing Reiki energy to the body. The patient got off the table and moved in ways previously unable. Reiki energy allows the body to heal itself and patients report feelings of relaxation, happiness, empowerment and relief from pain.

Long distance healing through the matrix is also common. Reiki, prayer and love are not bound by the time-space continuum. Sitting in Texas, I can easily pray and send Reiki to a patient in Australia, and the patient feels the soothing energy simultaneously. Think of it like making a phone call. Phones use electromagnetic radio waves to connect with other phones. Practitioners and recipients do not need to be near each other, we just need to be on the same wavelength. Long distance Reiki works according to the Universal Law of Oneness and Higgs Field, which hold that we are all connected through the divine matrix.

Sometimes the Soul needs to heal emotionally before a physical healing can be experienced. The Practitioner does not decide how the energy should be used. Reiki Practitioners are only instruments in the healing process, and the patient's Divine Mind makes adjustments as additional energy becomes available. The power of prayer has been well documented for eons. When two or more are gathered in the spirit of God, we create miracles. If you could patent God, then this information would hit the front page of every newspaper daily; however, since you can't patent God, the media doesn't give much attention to every day miracles.

Benefits of Reiki
• Improves stress reduction
• Offers deep relaxation
• Aids better sleep
• Reduces blood pressure
• Helps relieve pain
• Removes energy blockages
• Supports the immune system
• Raises the vibrational frequency of body & mind
• Aids spiritual growth
• Improves and maintains health

NEAR DEATH EXPERIENCES

The term Near Death Experiences (or NDEs) was coined by Dr. Raymond Moody in 1975 in his bestselling book *Life After Life*. As a trained surgeon it took him decades hearing numerous stories about patients who died and came back while on the operating table. Although, most would never utter a single whisper of the experience, there were a few who came forward with a remarkable experience of "Heaven." During the interview process Dr. Moody learned that many people have quite similar experiences and frequently return feeling connected to Universal Wisdom, which many call God. Summarized below are some of Dr. Moody's elements of an NDE.

Some experience a strange sound like a buzzing or ringing noise while others experience just a sense of peace and painlessness. More common is the "out-of-body experience" with a sensation of rising up or floating above the medical team and watching the event from the ceiling. Many admit to fearlessly traveling through a tunnel of light at high speed until they reached a radiant light or the Presence of God. Occasionally, Ancestors, Spirit Guides, Friends or Angels greet them while approaching or traveling through the tunnel of light. Some have an off-world experience, like what an astronaut would see, or the individual may go directly to a life review. During a life review the individual relives every act from a panoramic view. Even though there were painful situations experienced and/or mistakes made and/or regrets had because Earth can be challenging , they still return with a greater feeling of love and understanding. Overall, the less the individual judged while alive, the less they judge during the life review. The individual reluctantly returns to Earth mostly because they do not want to leave loved ones behind, and the reluctance to return to Earth stems from a desire to stay with the love experienced on the other side.

Millions of people around the world experienced this remarkable phenomenon and more are sharing it through thousands of YouTube videos. These two significant stories may confound you. Anita Moorjani and Dr. Eben Alexander wrote their autobiographies disclosing their unique journeys into the afterlife. Moorjani's compelling story in *Dying to Be Me* (2011) describes her unforgettable encounter. She was medically diagnosed with terminal cancer and it was physically evident from her deteriorating condition. After four years of cancer treatment, slipping into a coma and dying on the medical table, she came back from the dead and no longer needed any type of medicine or chemotherapy. She admits that she repeatedly sacrificed herself so that other family members could excel, and it crushed her, but she couldn't stop sabotaging herself. Motivationally she writes, "When you choose to live from a place of love, you are free to be yourself, to connect with your desires, and to take action from a place of empowerment. When you choose to live from a place of fear, you are always trying to fit in, denying who you really are in order to satisfy the expectations of others. The latter not only deprives you of tremendous joy, but it also deprives the world of the real you; the you that is unique, gifted, and a pure facet of the Universe. You see, in every moment, you have a choice to either honor the part of you that craves something more, or to continue squeezing into a role that doesn't fill your cup." Her ultimate motto is, "Self sacrifice is not a virtue; self love is." She is currently an international speaker inspiring huge audiences toward full self-expression.

Academic Neurosurgeon and Harvard Professor for over 25-years Dr. Eben Alexander and his medical colleagues dismissed NDEs as a neurological chemical process. Medical teams frequently explain away all the lights, music and visitations that people report when they return from the *other side*. Previously an NDE skeptic, Dr. Alexander contracted the perfect strand of meningitis that shut down his faculties so that science could not explain away the phenomena as they had with every other patient before him. Upon his return he wrote an inspiring book entitled *Proof of Heaven* (2012) sharing his eloquent account of this extraordinary experience. The audio sequel *Seeking Heaven* (2013) provides a guided musical meditation enabling the listener to tap into the inspiring sounds Dr. Alexander heard while on the other side. *Seeking Heaven* invites the listener to experience firsthand the power of the NDE experience through a sacred journey. I listened to it twice a week for a year and it's quite profound.

Discussions of the Near Death Experience reduce fear of death and dying. Dr. Elisabeth Kübler Ross (1926-2004), American-Swiss Psychiatrist and Pioneer in NDE studies, wrote more than 20 books on death and related subjects, including *To Live Until We Say Goodbye* (1978), *Living with Death and Dying* (1981), and *The Tunnel and the Light* (1999). Her extensive research and lectures in the 1970s opened the door for candid public conversations with those dying, and she spearheaded the hospice program. She identified the Five Stages of Death (denial, anger, bargaining, depression, acceptance), which is still taught in collegiate psychology programs today. Her mystical approach to the dying process removes the stigma of the final stages of life. She states, "I've told my children that when I die, to release balloons in the sky to celebrate that I graduated. For me, death is a graduation." In 2007, she was inducted into the National Women's Hall of Fame and was the recipient of 20-honory degrees. We learn from her and others in the field that life is meant to be lived not feared. Many people are petrified of death (as if being fearful of death changes the fact that it will arrive for each of us one day). The fear of dying provokes a fear of living. Not knowing what's on the other side of the veil can be debilitating for some, particularly the ones who are knocking on death's door; however, there are numerous YouTube videos of individual accounts of those who met the other side successfully and claim it is a loving compassionate place.

Paradise, or Heaven, is an individual creation. You imagine a place that you will visit when the body dies. Who is this "You" we're talking about now? You have a body, and you also have a Consciousness. When the body expires or dies, the Consciousness will move upward, onward, outward and expand beyond this limited existence. If you can only think of two places to go (Heaven or Hell) then that's a very limited imagination. As a parent, can you imagine damning your child to a fiery oven for eternity because of a common mistake? Seems very limited for a human, not to mention for an off-world Omnipotent Presence. The wisdom of the Near Death Experience expressed by millions indicates that a loving place awaits all of us at the end of this journey. Love yourself, your naivety, your mistakes and the opportunity to begin again. Be Born Again! Make today the first day of the rest of your life.

REINCARNATION

"Almost half of the world, about three billion people, including 26% of American adults, believes in reincarnation" (*Stastica.com*, 2016). Most religions that believe in reincarnation consider it the path to purity and salvation. Many cultures incorporate the belief in "cause and effect" or "what you sow, you reap" which can be considered an abbreviated form of reincarnation. Hinduism, Jainism, Buddhism, Sikhism, Taoism and 1st Century Christianity, now called the New Age Movement, incorporate reincarnation as a founding principal to gain inner peace and deep connection to the Creative Forces. (New Age is not new at all. It's Ancient Wisdom reintroduced in modern language.) The Dalai Lama said that you don't have to stop your religion to implement Buddhist practices into your life, like meditation or the belief in reincarnation. I invite you to see this section as mind-candy and ingest it in small doses.

Gary Zukav writes in *Seat of the Soul* (1989), "In the creation of a personality [and body], the soul calibrates parts of itself, reduces parts of itself, to take on the human experience. Your higher self is that aspect of your soul that is in you, but it is not the fullness of your soul. It is a smaller soul self. Therefore, 'higher self' is another term for 'soul', yet the soul is more than the higher self." Intuition is the communication between the self, higher self and greater soul. "The reincarnation conviction is that an imperishable principle (soul or consciousness) exists in every human being and returns to Earth after death in a new form. The fate of every person in this life and in future lives is determined by the consequences of good or bad actions in the past or present (karma)" (*AmericanMagazine.org*, October 2015). Karma means the cycle of cause and effect. What is happening to you now is because of something you did or didn't do in the past. Karma balances the past with the present. Dharma means "cosmic law and order" and directs our Divine Life Purpose. Dharma would be your virtues and blessings, and your way to contribute into your community via your career or talent.

You might think...
- If I ever had a past life, then it was probably with that person (name). We are so connected; we have so much in common. Or the opposite, we fight like cats and dogs.
- If I ever had a past life, it must have been in that country. I feel so passionate and alive when I'm there. I love that culture.
- I must have been really good in a past life because things often fall into place for me.
- I must have been really bad in another lifetime because I can't keep a good job or a good relationship.

If we knew that we lived before and that this life was the next episode of an ongoing series from a previous time, a bit like a Netflix Series, who would we be as a species? Would we be kinder to each other? Would we honor our parents and children more? Would war disappear? Today is a carryover from another time. Just like a movie, characters' faces and names change, but the actor is still the same. This time you're the mommy next time you're the son. One time you're the employee, next time you're the boss, another time you're partners. Varying levels of IQ, talents, gifts and opportunities arise in each lifetime.

Dr. Ian Stevenson (1918-2007) was a Reincarnation Pioneer as the Department Head of Psychiatry and the Director of the Division of Personality Studies at the University of Virginia. He began thoroughly investigating paranormal activities in the 1960s after Chester Carlson, inventor of Xerox copy machines, donated one million dollars to Dr. Stevenson's research. He dedicated decades of his life to researching and meticulously documenting more than 3000 cases of children's past life memories that gave undeniable evidence for the truth of reincarnation, and Dr. Jim Tucker resumed the research while Stevenson was still alive. They worked together extensively. Dr. Tucker continues his research at the Department of Psychiatry & Neurobehavioral Sciences, Division of Perceptual Studies at the University of Virginia Health System. All researchers in the field, myself included, are indebted to Dr. Stevenson and Dr. Tucker for their groundbreaking work.

Children from the ages of two to six are more likely to recall being someone else. They don't need hypnosis or to be in any type of trance to remember. A few simple questions get the ball rolling so that the child feels comfortable talking about past memories. After age 6, we all begin to forget or lose interest as the veil thickens between the two worlds. Dr. Stevenson's most notable documented case study was a young boy, age 2, who showed all the traits of post-traumatic stress disorder. Young James Leininger recollected images and feelings of a plane crash that were not pertinent to his current life and his parents confirmed the facts. The boy's physiological signs indicated the trauma ~ pupils dilated, muscles tensed, and respiration increased as the body braced for fight or flight ~ and this led the parents to Dr. Stevenson's research.

"James Leininger began having intense nightmares of a plane crash. He then described being an American pilot who was killed when his plane was shot down by the Japanese. He gave details that included the name of an American aircraft carrier, the first and last name of a friend who was on the ship with him, and a location and other specifics about the fatal crash. His parents eventually discovered a close correspondence between James' statements and the death of a World War II pilot named James Huston. Documentation of Boy James' statements was made before Huston was identified on a television interview with his parents that never aired but which Dr. Stevenson was able to review."

The extent to which Leininger and other children show heightened emotion in recounting apparent past life memories is an indication that something truly significant is occurring. The case studies reveal that some children become sensitive or distraught about the prior life circumstance and want to return home to finish business. Some children can be troubled by flashbacks and nightmares of the past life leaving them with unexplained debilitating phobias. Other children who recall good times can be blessed with inexplicable talent and skill or a level of comfort in typically uncomfortable situations, like being on stage. Child Prodigy Wolfgang Amadeus Mozart

(1756-1791) isn't particularly one we think of when discussing reincarnation; however, it is worthy of consideration to reflect on his biography and learn that by age 3 he knew piano basics and by age 6 he was a budding composer. Where does superior talent come from? You might find that you are or your child is a natural at music, dance, computers or engineering. You or your child might have an innate ability for gardening, architecture or design. These skills are carried forward from other lifetimes.

Helping a Child deal with the Impact of a Spontaneous Recall
1. Validate their feelings, memories and invisible friends.
2. Listen to their story.
3. Write it down and make sure you get all the details correct. Make it vivid and colorful.
4. Gets names, dates, street names, ages, terrain of location, occupation, etc.
5. Review it many more times. Daily or once a week for a few months.
6. Encourage the child to swim (in a pool, lake or ocean, even bathing) to recall more images and memories. Water stimulates the emotional body and feelings while allowing the analytical mind to relax.
7. Research the story. Look for historical information to validate the recollection.

To me, "Original Sin" makes sense when you tie it into reincarnation. Sin is an archery term from ancient times. It means to "miss the mark." You had a mission, a target, and you didn't hit it. To look at a sweet innocent child and say, "you're a sinner" sounds cruel to me; however, if in a previous life you missed the target or you didn't complete the mission, then you're fortunate enough to have another opportunity to try again today. So, you arrive on Earth with your densely materialistic Earthly vessel to help you "Hit the Target." Don't miss it this time. Remember your purpose! A past life regression could remind you what you did and didn't do in the past and awaken you to your Divine Life Purpose today.

When you repeat your actions, you upgrade your performance the second time. For instance, think about the first time you repaired a vehicle or changed a tire. The second time you performed the task weren't you a little better at it? By the time you changed the 10th tire, you were probably good and fast at it. Think about balancing your checkbook, wrapping a present or cooking a recipe. We improve with each successive try. Apply that understanding to the philosophical view of reincarnation. Each time we incarnate we are a little better, smarter, wiser, healthier and more conscious. We have a lifetime with a certain mission, tasks and experiences. Some things we don't complete or we try but were not successful so we ask God for another chance.

Think about a Rock Star, Ballerina or Surgeon. Highly successful and celebrated skilled professions require a level of awareness far beyond the common human. It might be easy for the talented, but how does one really get talented. Just dumb luck? Great genes? Fabulous parenting? It's many,

many lifetimes, hundreds maybe thousands of lifetimes at one profession to become a notable success. Sometimes professionals squander their success with excessive drug and alcohol abuse ultimately leading to depression and even suicide. "Next time I'll share my talent and enjoy the fame, not being afraid of it or squandering it," the Soul cries on its way out. Hence, another lifetime is born. Your unfulfilled desires create more lifetimes.

From Buddhism, we learn that the consciousness reincarnates generally between 49 days and two years after death. From New Age Christianity, we learn that the soul can reincarnate at anytime after a death. It is believed that the Soul in its ethereal form lingers about its household, near family and customary locations for ten days following the death of the body in the form of a ghost. Many religions believe that the Soul can take about ten days to two years to reach the final journey to judgment. Those Souls who return to Earth choose their next host body and parents depending on their karma from previous lifetimes. Your Soul chose your parents, siblings, birth order, demographics, socio-economic status, culture, IQ, hometown, health and medical condition, etc. prior to returning. You had a mission and only these people could help you achieve it. Your karma (unfinished business) and your dharma (virtues and blessings) determine the next host body and experience based on the quality of life your Soul led in the past and desires to live now. Being born with amnesia gives the personality an opportunity to try new approaches to similar problems with the same soul group instead of attempting to avenge the past.

The body and ego are considered the Earth vehicle of which the Soul oversees. God governs the Soul. Souls jockey for position and choose which womb would be most suited for them. A few days before or after birth, the Soul bonds with the brain and body of the baby. Improper connection can lead to mental illness or early death. Things like miscarriage and stillbirths are completely out of the ego's control. Upon arrival, a Soul might decide that it won't be able to fulfill its mission and therefore leaves Earth (as in death) quickly. Sudden Infant Death remains unexplained by the medical community, but the spiritual community sees this condition as a sign that the timing is not right. Frequently, that same Soul will return to those same parents but at a later more appropriate date.

Today many people long for their **Soulmate**, a lifelong companion and helpmate, and take great measures finding an appropriate partner. Online dating allows modern couples to find their lifemate virtually anywhere on the planet. Although not a requirement, many Soulmates talk of love at first sight or an instant connection. A natural feeling of comfort, anticipating behavior and sexual chemistry are part of recognizing a Past Life Lover. Soulmates generally have been together many previous lifetimes, and once the connection is made they rarely divorce or they separate amicably. When Past Life Lovers are together time seems to fly and passions ignite. The deep bond and ease in sharing almost anything poses no problems, and they naturally forgive each other quickly for shortcomings. Even though most lovers don't want to be apart, Soulmates feel connected regardless of distance. It feels like you're always together because the bond is so strong. The deep spiritual connection that Soulmates feel allows them to share authentically, dropping masks they may wear for the rest of the world. Soulmates encourage self-expression and exploring latent talents; the spark between them is vibrant and inspires those around them. This type of powerful union comes only after many lifetimes of being together and supporting each other successfully through many different trying situations.

Some questions the curious will ask are: Who have I been before? How would I know if a past life is impacting me now? Were any of my family members or spouse with me in the past? Curious people will look for answers in many different ways. Seek and you will find your truth.

Questions to Ask about a Past Life
- Are you beckoned to a certain area of the world, a culture, or a language that is uncommon for your family or region?
- Do you have exotic dreams of other worlds or other time periods?
- Do you have recurring dreams or nightmares?
- Have you met people to whom you were attracted instantly?
- Have you met people you disliked instantly?
- What keeps you together with certain family members and not others?
- How did you choose your profession? Are you "just a natural" at it?

These are a few questions which arise when one is considering a past life regression. I'm not a proponent of investigating a past life for entertainment purposes. Some people have so many problems right now that they have no need to delve into a past life. No need to look any further than the mirror and the last words you spoke to find something that needs improvement. That may be all the introspection that is appropriate right now; however, if you've tried other things and yet there is still something niggling at you, then a past life regression might be the perfect avenue for self-exploration.

Reincarnation is a useful tool in understanding that life is actually fair. It doesn't appear fair over 80-100 years, but it's fair over the course of 8-10 lifetimes. Each day, each year, each lifetime, you learn something new about yourself and your environment, and these experiences transform your outlook, providing spiritual maturity. Your transformed outlook gives you wisdom for the future. Unfulfilled desires draw us back into this Earth experience called samsara (the cycle of birth, life and death and rebirth).

According to Berkley Center in Georgetown, "Samsara is the continuous cycle of life, death, and reincarnation from which believers seek liberation. Samsara is a feature of a life based on illusion (maya). Illusion enables a person to think (s)he is an autonomous being instead of recognizing the connection between one's self and the rest of reality. Believing in the illusion of separateness that persists throughout *samsara* leads one to act in ways that generate karma and thus perpetuate the cycle of action and rebirth. By fully grasping the unity or oneness of all things, the believer has the potential to break the illusion upon which samsara is based and achieve moksha—liberation from reincarnation."

Your Soul has an agenda, a mission to awaken. There are certain people your Soul will engage, and certain experiences that your Soul will endure to balance the scales of samsara. Skills, talents and latent abilities surface in divine timing. We bring forward the good and the bad that needs to be healed each lifetime with the intention to awaken, become enlightened and liberated from samsara. You don't need to live a perfect life just move toward perfection each day and that will guide you to enlightenment, Moksha, Samadhi or Nirvana.

Examples of the samsara cycle include those who are 40, 50 or 100 pounds over weight. They typically attempt all the fad diets, try exercising and even therapy but those didn't work. Understanding the core issue to any problem can alleviate the conflict. A regression might just take you back to the Middle Ages when fat was beautiful and a sign of success. It might be that gluttony in a past life needs to be healed through a lifetime of disciplined nutrition and exercise. I find that people who are obese generally have a wounded heart. Ask the following questions and journal for a minute or two (or twenty). Come to learn more about the inner workings of your mind and heart. When did you start getting large? What was the pivotal point? Who was around at the time ~ parents, ministers, friends, a lover? Who contributed or didn't contribute to this habit of gorging? Past life regressions may point to a time when you ridiculed fat people and now you have to experience that in return (karma).

In the Spiritual Classic *Many Mansions, the Edgar Cayce Story on Reincarnation* (1999), Author Gina Cerminara reflects on numerous case studies showing how unfinished business in the last lifetime spillover to today. Take for instance digestive disorders. In one case study, a man currently had to limit his food intake due to digestive weakness. His sensitivity required constant precautions to digest properly and avoid social embarrassment. As it turned out, in a previous lifetime, he was a protector of King Louis XIII of France and had a weakness of gluttony. The pleasures of the table got the best of him in that lifetime and there was a spillover into the current life. Consequently, he had to monitor every thing he ate this time because last time he didn't have proper self-control. So, he is learning that now. It doesn't matter when you learn a lesson, just that you learn it. It could take 10 lifetimes or 300, but why would you want to stay in the 5th Grade when everyone else is going on to Middle School?

Many people are deeply unhappy or depressed and have absolutely no idea why. Just a general discontent, a low tone, undercurrent, which says, "I don't deserve to be _____ (you fill in the blank... happy, healthy, thin, married, independent). Basically, "I don't deserve to BE." Yet, God created you to BE a human BEing. Now you're here and a deep part of you doesn't want to be. Doesn't want to be here on Earth; doesn't want to be in your body; doesn't want to be in the family to which you were born. This emotional suffering could be a carry-over from another lifetime and medication is only going to mask the distress temporarily. Many feel forced to hide their feelings and this loss of self-expression can lead to a lifetime of inauthenticity. Inauthentic expression can be depressing and confusing and that can stir imbalances leading to bad habits, addictions and self-defeating behaviors.

In the Spiritual Community, we believe that to become more authentic a Soul chooses unique ways of self-expression with different customs and distinctive talents. The Soul is androgynous but generally resonates with one sex more than the other. It is imperative that you are both sexes numerous times as we have many different lessons and encounters which the other sex does not experience or understand. No man will understand what its like to transform the body and give birth to a 5-10 pound "bowling ball" from a small vaginal canal. And, no woman will understand how communicative a penis can be to its owner. So much that men name it. Even though asexual, the Soul expresses itself more as male or female. Possibly we have been that gender for 10 lives and now its time to cross over to the other sex. Gays and the LBGTQIA community fall into this section of the human experience. If you have been a man for 10-20 lifetimes and now it's time to be a woman, the man may incarnate gay. He's becoming more feminine but not entirely. It is a similar concept for lesbians who identify as masculine but are in a female body. Gays choose to experiment with a gender seldom used in previous lives. The Soul can choose to be gay or it can also be a part of a transition moving between male and female. Although society is gaining acceptance of gays and their important role in our community, today it is a difficult life path for the LBGTQIA population. Being gay may indicate a desire to accelerate personal understanding of the opposite sex with complex differences in gender identity. All three roles are equally important for human evolution.

Public understanding and acceptance is growing, but gays have been around for centuries. They contributed to society in countless positive ways. They are artists, painters, sculptors, photographers, dancers, cartoonists, usually sharp dressers, even trendsetters. Some of the most handsome men and women in the world are gay. Understanding that gay is a Soul choice takes the pressure off the person to try to alter it or hide it. Many gays are bullied for something they cannot change, and sometimes take their life in their own hands just to walk down the street. You can't pray gay away, just like you can't pray straight away. It's genetic. You either are or you are not which is usually recognized in puberty but sometimes as early as age 5. Western society is opening up more to gays and this gives rise to the entire LBGTQIA community allowing them to explore who they really are at any age. Gay neighborhoods in large cities offer a sanctuary for open authentic self-expression and that can only help the Soul to grow in love and honesty. To clarify, it is not a mistake for the soul to choose to be LBGTQIA. As Lady GaGa says, "Baby, I was born this way!"

Examples that a Past Life is Beckoning You
- If you suspect that a past life is impacting you today, your suspicion is usually correctly motivated.
- You feel trapped in the body of the opposite sex.
- You have a strong connection to a certain cuisine, region, city or country. Maybe you even married someone from that country.
- You have an unexplained feeling of anxiety, sadness and/or despair with no real trauma attached, just an underlying emotional wound.
- You have unexplained phobias.
- You have unexplained aches or illness for which there is no diagnosis.
- You experience extreme racial prejudice.
- You enjoy a thrilling love affair or infatuation to someone.
- You have a natural ability for a certain talent and/or way of thinking (i.e. engineering, mechanics, music, art) without any significant training.
- You sneak eat or you eat like it's the 1920s Depression and can't get enough.
- You starve yourself like you're in Ethiopia.
- You a "period actor," a Renaissance Festival Actor or Civil War Actor.
- You're a historian drawn to a specific era of time.

Why do we say some people are **Old Souls** regardless of their age? What is an Old or Young Soul? You've probably met a young accomplished and aware teenager and a 50-year old man-child. The Old Soul embodies a wealth of wisdom beyond her/his years, and prefers quality friendships and deep conversations typically with older people. Extremely inquisitive and intelligent they have an innate ability to appreciate the classics or blend the old with the new. Globally aware and service-oriented, Old Souls have a keen eye toward the big picture. Spiritually-minded and guided by their internal moral compass, Old Souls live differently from their peers or are the leader of their group. Generally they are very generous people who don't like to waste time, get lost in the latest fad or may even reject mainstream ideas. These are a few qualities gained in successful successive lives wherein the Soul brings-forward these gorgeous qualities and refined abilities. Generally speaking, Old Souls are usually on their final incarnation or nearing it.

The opposite is true for **Young Souls**. They may be 50-year olds with gray hair and wrinkles but still act like a child. Young Souls focus on prosperity, power and popularity. Seeking the spotlight, imposing their will on others, emotionally unstable or unavailable, selfish or even vengeful are common examples of a Young Soul. Over the course of many lifetimes we seek individual power and prestige but as time progresses the Soul matures giving rise to compassionate courageous character. Younger Souls typically end up with certain imbalances, disease or malformations while they are learning how to engage with the dense form of a human vessel. The refined energy of the Soul can get damaged as it bonds with the human body, and we learn to integrate properly with each passing life.

It must sound easier when you're in Spirit form than the reality of a three-dimensional body on Earth. A common joke I've heard in the spiritual community is that as Spirit you're sitting with your Angels, Highest Council and God deciding what you're going to do in your next lifetime. You choose your parents, siblings, birth order, profession, health, height, eye color, major lessons and opportunities, and then you decide to change something on the list. While looking at the spiritual computer you move to tap "delete" and inadvertently click "send." Whoosh! You fly through the earthly stargate, called the birth canal, to drink from the cup of forgetfulness and poof! Here you are! "Wait, wait, I meant to hit delete not send." If you're suffering and you've tried all types of remedies like nutrition, exercise, pharmaceuticals, acupuncture, chiropractic care, Reiki but nothing has resolved your issues, then you're likely a good candidate for a past life regression. Knowing that life is continuous really takes a lot of pressure off you to be Super Woman or Super Man. You really can have it all and do it all, just not on the same day and not in the same lifetime.

What You Can Do to Know more about Your Past Lives
• Keep a dream journal and earnestly ask for a dream confirming a past life.
• Sit in quiet contemplation for 30-60 minutes weekly or daily with the intent to receive knowledge about a past life.
• Expect hints and tips to arise in usual and uncommon ways in waking, sleeping and meditative states.
• Watch movies on reincarnation like *Ghost* (1990), *Defending Your Life* (1991), *Goundhog Day* (1993), *What Dreams May Come* (1998), *Cloud Atlas* (2012), and *Heaven is For Real* (2014).
• Read books on reincarnation like *20 Cases Suggestive of Reincarnation* by Dr. Ian Stevenson (1980), *Many Lives, Many Masters* by Dr. Brian Weiss (1988), *Life After Life* by Dr. Raymond Moody (1975), *Reincarnation in Christianity* by Geddes MacGreggor (1989), *Many Mansions, The Edgar Cayce Story on Reincarnation* by Gina Cerminara (1950), *Heaven is for Real* by Todd Burpo (2010), *Reincarnation: The Missing Link in Christianity* by Elizabeth Clare Prophet (1997), *Reincarnation: A New Horizon in Science, Religion and Society* by Sylvia Cranston (1993), *Journey of Souls* (1994) and *Destiny of Souls* (2000) by Dr. Michael Newton, and *Between Death and Life* by Dolores Cannon (1993).

PAST LIFE RECALL

Past Life Recall opens the door for understanding why your life is the way it is. A Past Life Regression could provide you with new insights never before considered, and take your personal wellness program into a new dimension. Past Life Regressions can clarify certain patterns, phobias, behaviors, addictions, trauma, illness and relationships and strengthen your spiritual understanding. It is especially useful if you divorced the same type of person more than once or cling to childhood issues in adulthood. We can awaken from the constrictions of past conditioning, release anxiety and fears through the use of Regression Therapy.

Past Life Regressions are not intended to supplant any clinical, cognitive or psychiatric therapy that resolving a serious emotional trauma may need. Some clients benefit greatly from weekly visits with a licensed trained professional over a prolonged period of time to heal major abuses. My clients are curious and seek understanding by recollecting a past life. Yes, they frequently experience substantial clarity around emotional traumas but still some patients need to see a local therapist on a regular basis.

Dr. Brian Weiss, the premier American Psychiatrist and Past Life Regression Therapist and Teacher states, "these experiences are all quite common. We change race and religions because we have to learn from all sides. Souls don't have those characteristics (like human personalities do). We're all connected. It's not about color or race. Sometimes we have to be nuns because we learn to live spiritual lifetimes. We've all been black, white, brown, yellow and red. We've been everything because we have to learn from all sides...that's part of our learning here on this planet." The way the last lifetime ended is how the next one begins. We roll out of one experience and into the next like a Netflix Series. Maybe you were born with an injury, illness or disease. You can reflect on the previous episode to acquire insight into this life's circumstances. Some people are aggressive while others are mild mannered. Many people are not interested in retaliation even though they've been abused and matching the hostility would be common, yet they do not harbor violence. For some reason, they have a calm disposition even though others have taken advantage of them or harmed them outright. Then there are others who get upset at the smallest things. They walk through each day expecting to be offended. This disposition of entitlement, as if the world should respond to your every mood, could have started in another time. Were you the Queen Bee in another tribe? Understanding the past, releasing resentments and restoring emotional wellbeing can transform the mind-body-spirit connection.

If you didn't complete the mission last time or you "failed" in your last lifetime, you may be dealing with repetitions of failure now, failing at love, finances or health. Find the origination of that "failed mission" and transform it. Then, you can have the success you earned in this lifetime. Just because you took a vow in a previous lifetime, like a vow of poverty, doesn't mean you have to fail at acquiring financial security today. That was then, this is now. How much of a previous life is influencing this lifetime? If you took a vow of poverty in the last lifetime you may find a fulfilling career but are still unable to meet your financial requirements. If you just can't provide for yourself, you may have taken a vow of poverty in a previous lifetime. Nuns, Priests, Monks and Yogis walk the monastic path without focus on finances for many lifetimes. These same groups frequently were required to take vows of celibacy (or at least attempt it), and this can carry forward with it sexual discomfort, uncertainty or inadequacy.

Sexual promiscuity or addiction could be a pendulum swing after a lifetime of religious repression. For many, those vows came/come easily with deep commitment, but for others a vow of celibacy could have left one feeling tormented sexually for a lifetime. That can lead to other types of deviant behavior in the current or future lifetime. Conventional psychiatrists and the prison system have vastly overlooked Past Life Regression Therapy. Why wouldn't you consider this therapeutic method when nothing else has worked?

Vows of obedience that most women are required to give can cause a rift in the Soul as it traverses the spiritual realms looking for equanimity. If a woman was locked away in an abusive marriage or culturally repressed for a lifetime or two, she may need to investigate the world in the next life. A life as a female is appreciably different all over the world. Being born an American woman offers significant independence and opportunity versus being born a woman in rural India. Today many Western women are choosing not to marry or to marry later in life, and that may be a strong inner commitment for worldly exploration after a lifetime of intense oppression.

Vows of piety and devotion are life path choices that can provide a Soul with discipline and order but can also lead to punishment and chastisement. Many religious people are hypercritical monitoring everyone's "sin ratio" and avoiding their own. This can be a carry-over from the *amen corner* to office water cooler. Do you hate a certain religion or culture or damn someone to hell? Have you ever contemplated how you might know the culture or the person from another time? Maybe life is presenting you an opportunity to resolve unfinished business. Remembering a previous life, taking responsibility for past mistakes or general ignorance can occur naturally, and that aids in moving forward with understanding today. Other times, tearing up the spiritual contract is the best resolution for releasing hate, revenge or severe criticism. A spiritual contract signed and secured in another time may be looming over you now. This type of contract could be with a person, group, region, religion, profession or even with a substance (addiction). Caroline Myss eloquently traverses this delicate topic in her book entitled *Sacred Contracts* (2001). Simply, when you're ready to end the conflict, think of the person or certain group with whom you have difficulties, imagine a contract between the two of you and tear it up. Burn the treaty and establish a spiritual truce between you. Respectfully affirm, "You go your way, and I'll go mine." It may be time for you to dissolve a previous vow or contract to move forward with your Divine Life Purpose now.

Were you born with an injury, illness or disease? Did you have asthma or colic as a child? These signs of disharmony indicate a tumultuous previous lifetime that you departed. The way the last influential lifetime ended is how the next one begins. Louise Hay's book *You Can Heal Your Life* (1984) indicates asthma is a sign of "fearing life and not wanting to be here." Colic indicates "mental irritation and impatience" at the environment. (See her book on the numerous ailments and potential meanings for a deeper understanding of how illness and disease are linked to emotions.) Knowing that you were born with weak lungs and the associative emotions, can allow you to uncover your hidden past and heal today.

Vows Can Carry over Lifetime to Lifetime
1. Vow of Poverty
2. Vow of Celibacy
3. Vow of Obedience–"love, honor and obey"
4. Vow of Piety/Devotion– to a particular religion or person. Long Live the Queen!

We are Human ~ *Hu* being the Light or Spirit, and *Man* being the physical part of us that will eventually die. The spiritual side, the Hu, will carry onward. There is a pattern of lessons throughout your life, and you might not recognize it until you're 40 or 50 years old. Reflecting on your life and recognizing the recurring theme is essential in finding meaning in life. (We call it a midlife review or midlife crisis depending on how the first half went.) The Soul is experiencing life, encouraging the maximum amount of encounters for greatest growth. It takes many lifetimes with similar themes to workout karma, release bad habits and habitual negative thinking, or create a star like talented quality. The Soul progresses each lifetime building character from good, bad or stressful events.

If you believe in reincarnation, then you know some portion of the past is influencing you now. What part of a previous life is unfinished? The disposition you have today is directly related to your most influential past lives. If you know you will live again then you definitely want to utilize your time wisely now to prevent future karma. The Soul chooses different experiences, and they're all valid, ultimately restoring love and understanding.

What's a Session Like?
The session starts with general hypnotic suggestions as you recline fully clothed on a massage table (face up) or sit in a chair. It's important that you are very comfortable and relaxed during the session so that your body or common daily thoughts don't distract you. This process must be performed with a safe person that you trust. Even if the Therapist has high credentials, if you don't feel relaxed with that person, you likely will not have a deep experience or recall. You could take a friend with you so that you feel more at ease, but that isn't necessary. Most people attend the sessions alone, but if they bring a friend it does change the dynamics of the regression. If you're regressing to learn more about your spouse it's best not to bring the spouse with you. You'll be more likely to have a breakthrough about someone who is not in the room. Some Therapists don't allow others in the room, as they can be a source of much distraction. This is a decision between the Therapist and client.

The Therapist watches the clock so you don't have to worry about the current timeline. Typically, sessions take two hours with an additional hour for a pre- and post-interview. The intention is for you to access your Higher Self and let the ego rest. Moving out of the beta-brain, the hypnotic suggestions take you deeply to the alpha-theta brainwave where you can have all types of profound experiences.

Regression work can take you to a past life or you can recall an earlier time in the current life where healing may be needed initially. If the client is anxious or fearful, then different types of healing modalities, like Reiki or creative visualization, are utilized to dissolve that fear first. We don't want to rush a past life remembrance. Many people want to have a past life recall immediately but this sacred information is only released according to soul development. If awareness is needed regarding the current lifetime it should be discovered first. For instance, a childhood trauma may need review prior to a full regression. In this instance, two or three sessions may be needed to resolve certain emotional blockages relevant to the present time. Go to the source of trauma and heal it there. Resolving distress can transform you and those who are closest to you, even though you don't share your insights with them, or they may seem unrelated. Awareness is a powerful tool that can offer insight and compassion to a painful situation, releasing you from the shackles of the past whether in this lifetime or a previous one.

In a regression, the Therapist visits the past with you, metaphorically holding your hand as you investigate another time that is relevant to today, which might be painful. Not all past lives are painful but there is intriguing information revealed during each session. It's best not to do a past life regression alone, although if it's too difficult most will just fall asleep and not recognize any discernible information. It would behoove you to have a Therapist especially if you think the regression will be tumultuous. In fact, the reason some people haven't resolved matters more quickly is because typically it is too sorrowful to do alone. Likened to Catholic Confession or the 6th Step (*making amends* in the 12-Step Recovery Program), admitting a painful wrong and experiencing your remorsefulness truly can transform you forever. Just recognizing your emotional vibrational signature in a previous life can heal today instantly. Can you take responsibility today for your shortcomings in a previous life? Personal responsibility offers the greatest benefits that can resolve karma immediately. The truth can set you free.

For instance, Mary came into my office to learn more about her husband, Bob. They were together for twenty years, but he still had a lot of stress associated with the War in Vietnam. Although they both did a lot of work resolving the depression associated with the conflict, he just couldn't get unstuck. She had been with him for 20-years and was really tired. She didn't particularly want to leave, but she didn't have anything else to offer, and the relationship wasn't fulfilling for her anymore. During her session, she recalled a previous time when they were hiking together in the mountains. In that lifetime, they were adventure seekers, very healthy and very much in love.

They enjoyed nature and all types of athletic sports. One time, they were rock climbing, and he fell to a premature death. She was devastated by the loss and spent the rest of that lifetime depressed. She eventually died old and lonely. In the follow-up interview, she realized how they both were depressed just in different lifetimes. I wasn't sure if her recognition and release would allow her the freedom to stay or leave her marriage, but she regained a sense of clarity and awareness about the relationship by the time she left my office. Due to her ability to resolve her own grief and depression in the previous lifetime, it mysteriously opened the door for Bob to start resolving his PTSD in this lifetime. After she did the regression and healed herself in the previous lifetime, Bob was able to heal himself today. They are still together five years later. Quite fascinating!

In another case study, the client recalled being a common male laborer in the 1800s who had an affair with a married female neighbor. She wanted to end the affair but couldn't make the suitor leave. The laborer forced himself on her but didn't perceive it as rape since prior to that time it had been consensual. Remorsefully, a humble apology was offered to all souls involved in that lifetime for overstepping a basic boundary. It was quite tearful and obvious that the client wasn't that type of person anymore. The release opened the client to recognizing a similar situation that occurred in this lifetime. During the post-session interview, unexpectedly the client remembered when a man pressured her into an affair that she refused. Even though it was a brief exchange and she wasn't raped, the boundary violation niggled at her that a "friend" would expect that. By offering spiritual reconciliation in the previous life for the laborer's shortcomings, the client could truly forgive the violation that happened to her decades prior in this lifetime.

Sessions vary from client to client and even if the same client had five Past Life Regressions, each would be completely different. Some clients discover untapped talents and gifts during their sessions. Some have visitations from their deceased relatives and ancestors, while others encounter a connection to the Divine. The experiences can be vivid, realistic and often deeply life affirming. After a few sessions, some clients who were depressed, filled with unfounded phobias, or stress from trauma, say the intensity of their feelings diminished significantly, and a new sense of purpose was restored. Many clients receive clarity on current situations, and it's common to resolve disruptive relationships in a couple hours.

After crossing through the death scene, the expert Hypnotherapist or Past Life Regression Specialist guides you on a unique journey to meet your Highest Council, Angels and Guides to learn about the past life you just recalled. You discover insight about yourself and your loved ones and embrace the wisdom of your life similar to those who had a Near Death Experience (NDE). Those who died on the operating table and were revived express with elation a newfound insight and understanding. They speak of a gentle guiding force embracing them with a loving vibrant feeling while in the Tunnel of Light. Of course, a Regression is less complicated since your body is not in shock or physical trauma; you are, in fact, reclining in a comfortable chair and safe environment. A regression is one way to access your personal wisdom and connect with your Highest Council without having a near fatal accident.

Once beyond the death scene (and I've seen people "die" in numerous ways), you enter the spirit world where you gain insight about the recent life recalled as well as the current life you're living. This in-between interlude is called the Life Between Lives. Dr. Michael Newton (1931-2016) coined the term Life Between Lives (LBL). He, his staff and trained therapists conducted over 30,000 case studies mapping the spiritual world. He trained many Regression Therapists who continue this work today. His groundbreaking research is available in his many books and YouTube videos and at *NewtonInstitute.org*. Typically, FDA approval of pharmaceutical drugs requires several hundred to 3,000 case studies in clinical trials. 3,000 vs. 30,000? Why wouldn't you investigate this type of therapy?

Dolores Cannon (1931-2014) generated and refined her own regression method called Quantum Healing Hypnosis Technique (QHHT) during her nearly 50 year career. "Dolores took one client back through 25 separate lives jumping backward in 100 year increments. Each personality the woman displayed in each life was distinctly different to the others, and it was a truly remarkable way for Dolores to explore history and life in different time periods. She wrote two books based on the work with this client. The first book was *A Soul Remembers Hiroshima* (1993), which reports the life of a man who describes his experiences as a Japanese man in Hiroshima in 1945 when the atomic bomb was dropped on the city in World War II. This shocking account of the dropping of an atomic bomb from the perspective of a person who was there provides a chilling lesson into the horrific effects of war and nuclear weapons. The second book was *Jesus and the Essenes* (1992), which describe the life of a young man who was an Essene teacher of Jesus. Many truths about Jesus himself, his personality, his background, his life and the times he lived in are revealed in this fascinating account of a teacher who describes her personal relationship with Jesus in loving detail" (*DoloresCannon.com*). The Cannon Method (QHHT) "enables direct contact and communication with the Subconscious of any individual for answers to any questions and can also provide the basis for instant healing."

When you are ready to explore the limitless boundaries of your mind and Soul, according to your spiritual maturity, more guidance and understanding is offered through a Regressive Journey. Where one travels during a session can be quite mystical and fascinating. Many people step off the table with a brand new pair of eyes to enjoy the rest of their life. By understanding that life does not end but it is continuous, we can heal our past, embrace our present and guide ourselves into a lovely future. We don't have to continuously repeat the past, allow others to take advantage of us, feel guilty for mistakes or harbor revenge. Past Life Recall can dissolve years, even centuries, of past transgressions. I assert if more people (specifically those 10-30 years old) would have a Past Life Regression we could transform society and evolve humanity within one decade.

Benefits of Past Life Recall
- Discover remarkable details about your past
- Release unfounded phobias
- Dissolve fears today from prior lifetimes
- Practice innovative visualizations and meditations
- Embrace love and understanding to transform your life
- Gain clarity on your relationships
- Discover new tools for intuitive and psychic development
- Become more emotionally-balanced
- Restore health and healing

HEAVENLY STARGATE ~ BIRTH, LIFE, DEATH AND BEYOND

When we are born there is a plan, Great Spirit's Plan. We arrive in a specific region of the world to parents of a particular race, faith and socioeconomic status. We intend to meet certain people at specific times, possibly marry and maybe have children. We explore the world, develop our careers, find ways to contribute and learn many lessons. Some people make lifelong decisions from something that happened in kindergarten or elementary school and live that notion for 80 years. Many will never question what was stated to them by an absentminded teacher or a distracted parent; they just believe one person's opinion and live into it. It becomes like a sentence ~ a noun/verb sentence and a judge, jury and trial sentence. Something happened, was said or heard, and the interpretation lasts for many years, even decades, regardless of how much suffering it causes or how limiting it may be. For instance, if a stressed parent doesn't have time for the child, the child might believe (s)he is unworthy of attention and begin self-sabotaging. Stressed parents love their children very much, they just don't have enough energy for all the adult responsibilities and parental duties. It takes two people to make a baby and a community to rear it. A sentence like "I'm not worthy" could lead to low self-esteem, addictions, workaholism, selfish acts or worse. These sentences are "delivered" when we are young because they are a part of an unfinished episode from a previous lifetime. We are here today to resolve that past and refine our Soul qualities. One whole lifetime can be surmised into that one sentence if you let it. Don't get stuck believing what you, as a child or teenager, assumed to be true. You can create a new sentence at any age and any stage. Periodically, try on a different pair of glasses and look at life through your sibling's eyes or an adversary's perspective or your mentor's vision. As we travel through life's colorful playground we continue to believe certain things about it, people and ourselves. Some of those notions are true and some just are not. Some things you can't change, like what others are doing or thinking, but many things you can change just by re-evaluating your perception. Don't waste the rest of your days in a daze. Consider creating an empowering, inspiring sentence with a joyous viewpoint and an exciting trajectory.

Nearing the end of life is a fitting time to gather your good memories, your childlike sense of humor and easy temperament. In the winter of life, the body slows down. Every wrinkle, gray hair, ache or pain is a sign that you are in God's Waiting Room nearing the Heavenly Stargate. We travel through the human birth canal and exit through the Tunnel of Light. We are born on an inhale and die on an exhale. All the fussing and fighting, impatience and frustration and then whoosh the Joy Train arrives, and you're whisked away to the next dimension. You're already in the Waiting Room. In fact, we're all in the Waiting Room together regardless of our age. Don't get damaged by cynicism and bitterness in the ever-changing stages of life.

I invite you to spend time letting go of this crazy world, its unrelenting demands and depressive human suffering. All that was happening way before you and I arrived, and it will continue way after you and I depart. Begin affirming, "good enough." It wasn't perfect but it was, you were, good enough. You gave your best shot. Instead of being mad that the world is so dysfunctional, begin to accept that some things in your life are sufficient. Authentically embracing the highs and lows of this planet will reduce the karmic chains. This type of acceptance offers spiritual maturity. It shifts the focus from others' shortcomings and failings to you, your joy and your inner fulfillment. When you approach the Tunnel of Light and review your life, it will be easier to say, "Not perfect, but good enough." As you reduce judgment now, you reduce samsara. If you judge yourself harshly you force yourself into another lifetime to correct that perceived karma. Consider releasing self-criticisms that stop you from feeling joy on a daily basis. "A child shall lead them," is a well known Biblical passage that invites innocence and enthusiasm to sparkle again (KJV, Isiah 11:6). You're approaching the successful completion of your life regardless of your age; feel joyous anticipation about that upcoming graduation.

What if you were going to die in one, two or three years? How would you live life differently today? Consider pretending that tomorrow is your last day so you don't miss today. Find activities that generate a joyful spirit. It's better to fulfill your life purpose sloppily than to fulfill someone else's purpose successfully. Get ready to hop on that Joy Train and take off into the Heavenly Stargate to the next dimension, the next reality. Death is the end and the beginning.

 ZENERGY MINUTE OF GRATITUDE
Spend one minute in gratitude at high noon. From 12:00-12:01pm think about someone, something, a pet, a hobby or anything that brings you joy. I assert if we had the maximum number of people in a state of gratitude at the exact same minute, we could evolve humanity. Be happy. Be thankful during One Zen Minute.

And, that is Zenergy!

GLOSSARY

Adverse Childhood Experience Study (ACES): Dr. David Clarke spearheaded the ACES program in the 1990s documenting psychophysiologic disorders in adulthood associated with negative psychosocial experiences in childhood. 1. Physical Abuse 2. Emotional Abuse 3. Sexual Abuse 4. Physical Neglect 5. Emotional Neglect 6. Substance Abuse 7. Parental Divorce 8. Mental Illness 9. Mother was Abused 10. Incarcerated Relative.

AHA: American Heart Association

Akashic Records: Records of all time found in the etheric higher realms of consciousness. Some psychics can read this non-physical information intuitively and reveal valuable information to the patient. Helena Petrovna Blavatsky (1831-1891), Alice Bailey (1880-1949), and Edgar Cayce (1877-1945) and others introduced the word and concept during the past recent centuries.

Alpha brainwave: Relaxed, somewhat alert, watching TV, zoning out, staring out into space.

Alpha-theta brainwave: Very relaxed. Restful awareness. Slow subtle forms of thinking, more mental imagery and less words. The ineffable place of meditation and/or deep hypnotherapy.

Antioxidants: Antioxidants are molecules that fight damage by free radicals, unstable molecules that can harm cellular structures. Antioxidants do this by giving electrons to the free radicals and neutralizing them.

Amygdale: One of two almond-shaped clusters located in the temporal lobe. Thought to be part of the limbic system within the brain, which is responsible for emotions, survival instincts, and memory. Prolonged stress can be experienced when the brain gets stuck on one side repeating traumatic event(s).

ARE: Association for Research and Enlightenment, Edgar Cayce Foundation, *www.EdgarCayce.org.*

Artificial Flavors: Are synthesized in laboratories and come from petroleum or other chemical substances and mimic a natural flavor.

Auric Field: The energy field that glows around the body as seen in pictures of antiquity. The "Hu" part of Human. The hue, light or aura around people, animals, plants and vortexes. Your personal iCloud.

Beta brainwave/beta brain: Common usage of the human brain in active problem-solving mental activity. Highest mental activity level.

Black Hole Machine Patent: A method for gravity distortion and time displacement. A method for employing sinusoidal oscillations of electrical bombardment on the surface of one Kerr type singularity in close proximity to a second Kerr type singularity in such a method to take advantage of the Lense-Thirring effect, to simulate the effect of two point masses on nearly radial orbits in a 2+1 dimensional anti-de Sitter space resulting in creation of circular timelike geodesics conforming to the van Stockum under the Van Den Broeck modification of the Alcubierre geometry (Van Den Broeck 1999) permitting topology change from one space-like boundary to the other in accordance with Geroch's theorem (Geroch 1967) which results in a method for the formation of G{umlaut over ( )}odel-type geodesically complete spacetime envelopes complete with closed timelike curves. US Patent 20060073976A1. Publication: 2006.

BPA/Bisphenol A: A chemical found in plastics, plastic bottles, straws and many cans for canned food items. Is known to be a neurological disrupter. Strongly recommended not to ingest BPA or other plastics is you have breast cancer, probably any cancer.

Carpal Tunnel Syndrome: Tension in the wrist that can start in the jaw, neck, shoulders, elbows or fingers. Nerve maneuvering massage therapy alleviates pressure in nerves that can cause tension.

CERN: The European Organization for Nuclear Research, known as CERN, is a European research organization that operates the largest particle physics laboratory in the world. A provisional body founded in 1952 with the mandate of establishing a world-class fundamental physics research organization in Europe discovered the "God Particle" in 2012. The organization is based in a northwest suburb of Geneva on the Franco–Swiss border and has 23 member states. The name CERN is derived from the acronym for the French Conseil Européen pour la Recherche Nucléaire.

Citizen Scientist: A person who individually participates in research and maintains rigorous records. Examples: Telepathy between pets and owners; Lady Bird Johnson's national documentation of birds and flowers; micro-dosing psilocybin.

Cloaking Device Patent: A method for cloaking an object from an observer is provided in the illustrative embodiments. A hardware device is affixed to the object such that the observer observes a presentation on the device when observing the object. The device is enabled to receive a signal, wherein the signal corresponds to a portion of an ambience obscured by the object from a view of the observer. The signal is processed, at the device and without using a data processing system, to generate a version of the signal. Using the device, the version of the signal is presented to the observer as the presentation, wherein the version of the signal cloaks the object from the ambience in the view of the observer. Patent US20150365642A1. Publication: 2019.

Contraindicated: Not recommended; do not use.

Delta brainwave: Sleep.

Detox: Cleaning the body through fasting, diet, exercise and pranayama (breathing techniques).

Earth Vehicle/Vessel: Body and ego to which the Soul oversees.

Edgar Cayce: Father of Holistic Medicine; America's most documented psychic. Over 14,000 readings cross-referenced on mind-body-spirit wellness methods stored at the Association for Research and Enlightenment (ARE) in Virginia Beach, Va. Visit *www.EdgarCayce.org*.

Ecliptic: An astronomy and astrology term indicating a great circle on the celestial sphere representing the sun's apparent path during the year, so called because lunar and solar eclipses can occur only when the moon crosses it.

EMDR: Eye Movement Desensitization Reprocessing. A phychotherapy treatment designed to alleviate the distress associated with trauma. Visit *www.EMDR.com*.

Endocrine/Endocrine System: Relating to or denoting glands which secrete hormones or other products directly into the blood; the glands that produce and secrete hormones, chemical substances produced in the body that regulate the activity of cells or organs. These hormones regulate the body's growth, metabolism (the physical and chemical processes of the body), and sexual development and function. The endocrine system, closely related to cortical and subcortical centers in the central nervous system, is one of the body's instruments to regulate and modulate its immune response.

Enema: Colonic irrigation; flushing water into the rectum to cleanse the large intestine. Enemas are typically self-administered but in the past the hospitals would help patients with this type of therapy. Colonic irrigation clinics have sanitary equipment that flushes water in and out of the bowel. Can be helpful with detoxifying and to alleviate constipation.

Energy Field: The auric glow that is seen around the body in pictures of antiguity The "Hu" part of Human. The Hue, light or aura around people, animals, plants and vortexes. Your personal iCloud.

Ether: A medium that in the Wave Theory of Light permeates all space and transmits transverse waves.

Etheric: The electro-magnetic field around humans, animals, plants and in the entire universe.

Femur: Thigh bone.

Force: May the Force be with you! A common term for Universal Life Energy, Omnipotence, that supports us in our life quest. Also, a term used in the blockbuster film Star Wars meaning "Good Luck and Good Will" (1977).

Free Radicals: Free radicals are a toxic byproduct causing significant damage to the cellular structure. Saturated fats, processed meats and alcohol are examples of some products that release free radicals into the body. The vitamins and minerals the body uses to counteract oxidative stress are called antioxidants.

Globetrotter: International traveler, usually solo.

Goose Bumps: When the hair stands up on your skin; usually around the neck and arms.

Homeostasis: The body's ability to maintain metabolic and hormonal balance and heal naturally.

Hybrid Aerospace-Underwater Craft Patent: Craft using an inertial mass reduction device. A craft using an inertial mass reduction device comprises of an inner resonant cavity wall, an outer resonant cavity, and microwave emitters. The electrically charged outer resonant cavity wall and the electrically insulated inner resonant cavity wall form a resonant cavity. The microwave emitters create high frequency electromagnet waves throughout the resonant cavity causing the resonant cavity to vibrate in an accelerated mode and create a local polarized vacuum outside the outer resonant cavity wall. US Patent # US1014453282. Publication: 2018.

Ineffable: No words can express or explain the feeling or experience. When we get into the gap while meditating, we can experience an ineffable moment in time that is indescribable and very enjoyable.

In the gap: The feeling in meditation that is indescribable, frequently associated with a loss of time and space. Feels fantastic!

Karma: The cycle of what goes around, comes around; the sum of one's previous actions and how they impact the present or future. Dharma is one's good deeds or life purpose being fulfilled currently.

LBGTQIA: The Gay Community. Lesbian, Bisexual, Gay, Transgenders, Questioning, Intersex or Asexual.

Lucid Dreams: Awakening in the dream and consciously altering it.

Micronutrients: Essential elements or substances required in trace amounts for the normal growth and development of living organisms.

Natural Flavors/Spices: Can refer to anything that comes from a spice, fruit or fruit juice, vegetable or vegetable juice, edible yeast, herb, bark, bud, root, leaf, meat, seafood, poultry, eggs, dairy products, or anything fermented from those foods, according to Food and Drug Administration.

NDE: Near Death Experience. Those who medically die and return to life.

Nocebo effect: Symptoms worsen when given a fake diagnosis because the subject thinks they have a disease. Worrying yourself sick when you don't know all the facts and find out by morning everything is fine after all.

NPDs Dieting Monitor: Consumer trends corporation. *Visit www.NPD.com.*

Parasympathetic Nervous System: Rest and relax. The part of the involuntary nervous system that serves to slow the heart rate, increase intestinal and glandular activity, and relax the sphincter muscles. The parasympathetic nervous system, together with the sympathetic nervous system, constitutes the autonomic nervous system.

Peristalsis: The involuntary constriction and relaxation of the intestinal muscles or another canal, creating wave-like movements that push the contents (fecal matter) in the canal toward elimination at the rectum.

Phytochemicals: Fresh, raw vegetables teeming with nutrients. A variety of biological active compounds found in plants and vegetables, important for humans to eat. Increases the body's immune system. Detoxifying.

Pineal Gland: A small, pea-shaped gland located in the midbrain. Researchers know that it produces and regulates some hormones, including melatonin and serotonin. Melatonin is best known for the role it plays in regulating sleep patterns. Serotonin is the happy hormone.

Placebo Effect: Symptoms improve when given a fake treatment, usually saline or sugar water.

Psoas Muscle: A long fusiform muscle located on the side of the lumbar region of the vertebral column and brim of the lesser pelvis. It joins the iliacus muscle to form the iliopsoas. The psoas is a general term, but most often refers to the combination of two muscles, the iliacus and the psoas major muscle. Together these two muscles are better known as the Iliopsoas muscle. They are linked together because of their common and combined attachment to the femur.

Pollyanna/Pollyannaish: Refers to seeing the best in all situations to a fault. When sadness or anger is appropriate a Pollyanna person will revert to optimism and miss the true message of the experience. For example, if your birthday cake falls on the floor it is only natural to feel disappointment even though you might laugh later. Derived from the 1913 children's book by Eleanor H. Porter, *Pollyanna*.

Prefrontal Cortex: The front region of the brain, located at the forehead, is responsible for cognitive reasoning, creating strategies, organizing social behavior and modulating emotions.

Psychosomatics: When the mind thinks something and the body responds with symptoms, like worrying yourself sick. Or when pre-med students read information about symptoms of diseases and begin to contract those symptoms/feelings for no apparent reason.

Reincarnation: To die and be born again in a different body. Unfortunately, amnesia is frequently associated in subsequent lives.

RnR: Rest and relaxation.

Self-loathing: Negative remarks made to self that make you feel bad like shame, blame or guilt.

Stay-cation: Instead of a vacation when you visit another city or country, a stay-cation is when you stay at home for a week and enjoy your own hometown without the daily grind of work.

Stenosis: The sciatic nerve is located in the low back and buttocks area, branches down each leg and delivers nerve signals to the feet. Compression is commonly caused by a herniated disc, protruding vertebrae in the low back, spinal tumors, spinal twist or injury. Some have a congenital effect in the spine with the narrowing of the nerve root passageway. It can be very painful. Nerve manipulation massage therapy can aid greatly with this type of tension.

Subluxation: When the spine is out of alignment, a chiropractor refers to it as a subluxation, and a spinal adjustment can correct it.

Sympathetic nervous system: Flight or fight; when the sympathetic nervous system is activated, your pupils dilate, your heart rate rises and you feel primed to run. If you're confronted with danger, such as the sudden appearance of a wild animal, the sympathetic nervous system controls how you react.

Synchronicity: Everything falling into place. Timely; in the flow; catching all the green lights.

Techi/Techis: Those who are technologically skilled and trained; computer savvy.

The Field: References the area around objects and people. It refers to the ether or energy around us all by which radio waves or thought waves transfer.

Theta brainwave: Very calm, almost asleep, hypnosis state of mind, suggestible. This state of consciousness is experienced right before falling asleep into the delta brainwave and upon awakening. Perfect brainwave for retraining the brain quickly.

Twelve-Step Program: A twelve-step program is a set of guiding principles outlining a course of action for recovery from addiction, compulsion, or other behavioral problems. Originally proposed by Alcoholics Anonymous (AA) as a method of recovery from alcoholism. The Twelve Steps were first published in the 1939 book *Alcoholics Anonymous: The Story of How More Than One Hundred Men Have Recovered from Alcoholism*. The method was adapted and became the foundation of other twelve-step programs.

Vibrational Signature: Addresses when people die they leave a vibration behind. Some people can sense a presence of another who cannot be seen. It's a frequency. Is this why you're required to disclose a death in a home prior to selling it? Also, relates to a notion of what you've done or would do, an expected response to something.

Weather Machine Patent: A sound device Patent Application was filed in 2003 to create a Hurricane and Tornado Control Device. "A method is disclosed for affecting the formation and/or direction of a low atmospheric weather system. Audio generators are positioned to project sound waves toward the peripheral area of the weather system. The sound waves are generated at a frequency to affect the formation of the weather system in a manner to disrupt, enhance or direct the formation. The sound waves can also be projected in a manner to cause the system to produce rain." US Patent 20030085296A1. Publication: 2003.

WHO: World Health Organization

SANSKRIT DICTIONARY

Acharya: Respected teacher(s) in India.

Agni: Strong digestive fire; digestive heat and energy are responsible for all transformative processes of the body and maintain vitality.

Ama: A product of improper nutrition, sluggish digestion, slow metabolism and negative emotions that lead to disease.

Anulomana: Timely elimination.

Asana/Asanas: Yoga postures, the physical part (exercise) of yoga.

Deepana: Strong digestive fire.

Dristi: A focal point to maintain balance and neutral expression during yoga practice, specifically balancing postures.

Kapha **Dosha:** Curvy frame, moves slowly and deliberately, usually more grounded or even community minded and compassionate. Governed by the earth and water elements.

Ojas: Vibrant health, not just absent of disease.

Panchana: Correct assimilation.

Pitta **Dosha:** Medium build, athletic, have a more intense personality, strong leaders, big picture type of people. Governed by fire and water.

Rishi/Rishis: Respected teacher(s) in India.

Samsara: Birth, life, death. Reincarnation. Recycling the Soul.

Vata **Dosha:** Thin, small frame; expends energy, enjoys change, constantly in motion. Governed by the space and air element.

Vippassana: Meditation technique of simply watching the breath.

Yoga Nidra: A sequence of yoga postures designed for deep relaxation and rejuvenation, ideal for insomniacs and those with anxiety.

BIBLIOGRAPHY

MIND SECTION

Anwar, Yasmin. "Some of Us May Be Born More Empathic, a University of California at Berkley Study." Proceedings of the National Academy of Sciences of the United States of America. 16 Nov 2009.

Art of Living Editors. "Pranayama: The Beginner's Guide to Yoga Breathing Exercises." Art of Living (US), www.ArtOfLiving.org/us-en/yoga/breathing-techniques/yoga-and-pranayama.

Brown, Brene. Daring Greatly. Penguin Random House, 2012.

Chodron, Pema. *Getting Unstuck.* Sounds True, 2005.

Cuddy, Amy. TED Talk "Fake It Till You Make It." YouTube, 7 July 2016. Contributor: Sarah Moore.

Dispenza, Joe. *Breaking the Habit of Being You.* Hay House, Inc., 2012.

Dispenza, Joe and Gregg Braden. *Becoming Supernatural: How Common People Are Doing the Uncommon.* Hay House, Inc., 2019.

Docter, P., Del, C.R., et. al. *Inside Out Movie.* Walt Disney Studios Motion Pictures, 2015.

Dubner, Stephen J. and Steven D. Levitt. *Think Like a Freak.* HarperCollins USA, 2015.

Emerman, Ed. "Business Group Press Release." *National Business Group on Health*, 18 Apr 2019. https://www.businessgrouphealth.org/news/nbgh-news/press-releases/press-release-details/?ID=355.

Gray, John. *Men Are from Mars, Women Are from Venus: the Classic Guide to Understanding the Opposite Sex*. Harper, 2012.

Hagelin, Dr. John. "*An Introduction to the Transcendental Meditaiton Techni ue.*" YouTube, 7 Apr 2012. www.YouTube.com/watch?v=ZjT831cjaUY.

Hendrie, Stephanie Widener. *Secrets for Exceptional Speaking: an Extraordinary Personal Communications Course That Gets Remarkable Results.* Hendrie Communications, 2000.

Japsen, Bruce. "*Employers Boost Wellness Spending 17 From Yoga to Risk Assessments.*" Forbes Magazine, March 27, 2015. www.Forbes.com/sites/brucejapsen/2015/03/26/employers-boost-wellness-spending-17-from-yoga-to-risk-assessments.

Kolakowski, Dr. Shannon. "*Emotional Wellness: Seven Daily Signs.*" PsychologyTomorrowMagazine, 19 Aug 2013. www.PsychologyTomorrowMagazine.com/dr-shannon-kolakowski-the-seven-signs-of-emotional-wellness.

Levine, Lange, et. al., "Meditation and Cardiovascular Risk Reduction." Journal of the American Heart Association, 2017, vol 6, no 10, www.ahajournals.org/doi/abs/10.1161/JAHA.117.002218.

McCraty, Rollin. Heart-Math Institute website. www.heartmath.com/science.

Mayo Clinic Editors. "A Beginner's Guide to Meditation." *Mayo Clinic,* Mayo Foundation for Medical Education and Research, 17 Oct 2017, www.mayoclinic.org/tests-procedures/meditation/in-depth/meditation/art-20045858.

MayoClinic Editors. "*Post-Traumatic Stress Disorder PTSD).*" Mayo Foundation for Medical Education and Research, 6 July 2018, www.mayoclinic.org/diseases-conditions/post-traumatic-stress-disorder/symptoms-causes/syc-20355967.

Ritberger, Carol, PhD. *Your Personality, Your Health.* Hay House, 1998.

Scientific American Editors. "*What is the Function of the Various Brainwaves?*" Scientific American, 22 Dec 1997, www.ScientificAmerican.com/article/what-is-the-function-of-t-1997-12-22.

Shell, Ellen Ruppel. "Artificial Sweeteners May Change Our Gut Bacteria in Dangerous Ways." *Scientific American*, Scientific American, 1 Apr. 2015, https://www.scientificamerican.com/article/artificial-sweeteners-may-change-our-gut-bacteria-in-dangerous-ways/.

Simon, David and Dr. Deepak Chopra. *The Wisdom of Healing: a Natural Mind Body Program for Optimal Wellness*. Harmony Books, 1997.

The Carol Ritberger Show. *Medical Intuition*. Hay House Publishing, May 2007.

Thorp, Tris. " *Meditations to Calm Your Mind and Help You Fall Asleep.*" The Chopra Center, 13 Feb 2017, www.Chopra.com/articles/3-meditations-to-calm-your-mind-and-help-you-fall-asleep.

Toastmasters Editors. "*Build a Better You Toastmasters International Can Help You Improve Your Communication and Build Leadership Skills.*" www.Toastmasters.org.

WikiHow Editors. "*How to Make Amends.*" WikiHow.

Yoga Journal Editors. "Beginner's Guide to Pranayama." *Yoga ournal,* 10 Oct 2014, www.yogajournal.com/practice/pranayama.

Zeidan, Fadel, et. al. "Brain Mechanisms Supporting the Modulation of Pain by Mindfulness Meditation." *The ournal of Neuroscience: the Official ournal of the Society for Neuroscience,* 6 Apr 2011. www.ncbi.nlm.nih.gov/pmc/articles/PMC3090218.

BODY SECTION

"45 Alarming Statistics on American's Sugar Consumption and the Effects of Sugar on Americans' Health." *TheDiabetesCouncil.com,* 10 July 2018. https://www.thediabetescouncil.com/45-alarming-statistics-on-americans-sugar-consumption-and-the-effects-of-sugar-on-americans-health/.

Axe, Josh. *8 Best Natural Supplements for Better Sex.* MSN:Muscle & Fitness, 10 Dec 2015, www.msn.com/en-us/health/nutrition/8-best-natural-supplements-for-better-sex/ss-AAgfVs7.

Balch, Phyllis A. *Prescription for Nutritional Healing.* Avery: Penguin, 2010.

Bello, Walden. "Twenty-Six Countries Ban GMOs-Why Won't the US?" *The Nation,* 29 June 2015, https://www.thenation.com/article/twenty-six-countries-ban-gmos-why-wont-us/.

Beyond Celiac Editors. *Celiac Disease: Fast Facts.* BeyondCeliac.org. www.beyondceliac.org/celiac-disease/facts-and-figures.

Bjarnadottir, Adda. "*How to Read Food Labels without Being Tricked.*" Healthline.com, 27 Feb. 2019, www.healthline.com/nutrition/how-to-read-food-labels.

Bolinger, Ty. "The Truth About Cancer: A Global Quest   Episode 1." YouTube, 15 Oct 2015, www.YouTube.com/watch?v=KqJAzQe7 0g.

Boseley, Sarah. "The Guardian: Epidemic of Untreatable Back and Neck Pain Costs Billions." University of Washington - Department of Global Health, 10 Feb 2017, www.GlobalHealth.Washington.edu/news/2017/02/10/guardian-epidemic-untreatable-back-and-neck-pain-costs-billions.

Brod, Ruth Hagy and Harold J. Riley. *Edgar Cayce Handbook for Health through Drugless Therapy*. Macmillan, 1988.

Byrne, Rhonda. *The Secret* Film. Prime Time Productions, 2006.

Carlson, Andrea. *Investigating Retail Price Premiums for Organic Foods.* United States Department of Agriculture, 24 May 2016, www.ers.usda.gov/amber-waves/2016/may/investigating-retail-price-premiums-for-organic-foods.

Carroll, Robert. *Bible-King ames Version.* Oxford University Press, USA, 2008.

Chaudhary, Kulreet. *The Prime: Prepare and Repair Your Body for Spontaneous Weight Loss.* Harmony, 2016.

Chikly, Bruno. *Silent Waves: Theory and Practice of Lymph Drainage Therapy: an Osteopathic Lymphatic Techni ue.* I.H.H. Publishing, 2004.

Chopra, Dr. Deepak. "*Microbiome 101: It's a Small World After All.*" The Chopra Center, 24 Feb 2017, www.Chopra.com/articles/microbiome-101-its-a-small-world-after-all#sm.0000dyizogwjlf9fbgn1fz2rd32m8.

Chopra, Dr. Deepak. *Perfect Health: The Complete Mind Body Guide.* Three Rivers Press, New York, 2000.

Chopra, Dr. Deepka and Rudolph E. Tanzi, PhD. *Super Genes: Unlock the Astonishing Power of Your DNA for Optimum Health and Well-Being.* Harmony Books: New York, 2015.

Clarke, David. *They Can't Find Anything Wrong: 7 Keys to Understanding, Treating, and Healing Stress Illness* and Author of ACEs. Sentient Publishers, 2007.

David, Lawrence A., Turnbaugh, Peter, et. al. "Diet Rapidly and Reproducibly Alters the Human Gut Microbiome." *Nature*, vol 505, no 7484, Nov 2013, pp 559-563, doi:10.1038/nature12820.

Dean, Amy, and Jennifer Armstrong. *"Genetically Modified Foods."* Academy of Environmental Medicine, 8 May 2009. www.aaemonline.org/gmo.php.

Desikachar, TKV and RH Cravens. *Health, Healing and Beyond: Yoga and the Living Tradition of Krishnamacharya.* North Point Press, 1998.

Dispenza, Joe. *You Are the Placebo: Making Your Mind Matter.* Hay House, 2014.

Dodson, Elaine, *Cooking for the Guru.* Sacred Journey Publishing, 2010.

EWG Editors. *EWG's 2019 Shopper's Guide to Pesticides and Produce.* Environmental Working Guide, 20 Mar 2019, www.ewg.org/foodnews/summary.

Ferrari, Nancy. *Is there a Link Between Diet Soda and Heart Disease?* Harvard Health Publishing, Harvard Medical School, 21 Feb 2012, www.health.harvard.edu/blog/is-there-a-link-between-diet-soda-and-heart-disease-201202214296.

Firger, Jessica. *"12 Million Americans Misdiagnosed Each Year."* CBS News, CBS Interactive, 17 Apr 2014, www.cbsnews.com/news/12-million-americans-misdiagnosed-each-year-study-says/.

Fischer-Rizzi, Susanne. *Complete Aromatherapy Handbook: Essential Oils for Radiant Health.* Sterling Publishing Co. Inc., New York, 1990.

Frawley, David and Vasant Lad. T*he Yoga of Herbs: an Ayurvedic Guide to Herbal Medicine.* Motilal Banarsidass, 2016.

Frazier, Karen. *Nutrition Facts: The Truth about Food.* Rockridge Press, 2016.

Gallinsky, Michael and Suki Hawley, et. al. *All the Rage, Saved by Sarno* Documentary Film, RumuR, Inc. Studios, 2016.

Gray, John. *Mars and Venus in the Bedroom: a Guide to Lasting Romance and Passion.* HarperTorch, 2001

Grbi , Milica Ljaljevi , et al. "Frankincense and Myrrh Essential Oils and Burn Incense Fume against Micro-Inhabitants of Sacral Ambients. Wisdom of the Ancients?" *ournal of Ethnopharmacology,* vol. 219, 2018, pp. 1 14, doi:10.1016/ j.jep.2018.03.003, 12 June 2018.

Griersonoct, Bruce. *What if Age is Nothing but a Mind-Set?* New York Times, Oct 2014.

Gursche, Siegfried, and Zoltan P. Rona. *Encyclopedia of Natural Healing: the Authoritative Reference to Alternative Health & Healing: a Practical Self Help Guide.* Alive Books, 2002.

Hartman Group Editors. *"Gluten-Free: What's Really Driving the Sales Boom."* Forbes Magazine, 20 May 2015, www.Forbes.com/sites/thehartmangroup/2015/05/20/gluten-free-whats-really-driving-the-sales-boom/ #14c241993ace.

Hay, Louise. *You Can Heal Your Life.* Hay House Publishing, 1999.

Hicks, Ester and Jerry Hicks. *Vortex: Where the Law of Attraction Assembles All Cooperative Relationships.* Hay House, 2009.

Hyman, Mark. *Food: What the Heck Should I Eat?* Little, Brown and Company, 2018.

Kirschmann, John D. *Nutrition Almanac.* McGraw-Hill Education, January 2007.

Iyengar, BKS. *Light on Yoga.* Schocken Books, 1966.

Johnson, Jon. *Does CBD Oil Work for Chronic Pain Management?* Medical News Today, 29 July 2018, www.medicalnewstoday.com/articles/319475.

Juntti, Melania and Andrea Meltzer. *"The Very Real Science Behind Sexual Afterglow.'"* Men's Journal, 4 Dec 2017. www.mensjournal.com/health-fitness/the-very-real-science-behind-sexual-afterglow-w47892/.

Kunal Ahuja, Shreya Deb, "Gluten Free Food Market Statistics 2026: Industry Forecasts 2019-2026." *Global Market Insights, Inc.,* Nov 2019, https://www.gminsights.com/industry-analysis/gluten-free-food-market.

Kaptchuk, Ted. *The Power of Nothing.* New Yorker, 12 Dec 2011.

Keating, Dan and Christina Rivero. *"A Florida Case Study in Surgical Necessity."* The Washington Post, WP Company, 27 Oct 2013, www.WashingtonPost.com/business/economy/a-florida-case-study-in-surgical-necessity/2013/10/27/5cb52864-3ce5-11e3-b6a9-da62c264f40e graphic.html.

Kubota, Taylor. "37 Sex Stats You Need to Know." *Men s ournal,* 4 Dec 2017, www.mensjournal.com/health-fitness/37-things-everyone-should-know-about-sex-20150327/.

Lang, Elizabeth. *22 Reasons to Stop Drinking Soda*. Killer Aces Media, 21 Dec 2011, www.wisebread.com/22-reasons-to-stop-drinking-soda.

Langer, Gary, et al. *"POLL: American Sex Survey."* ABC News Network, 21 Oct 2004, www.abcnews.go.com/Primetime/PollVault/story?id=156921&page=1.

Law, Sally. "The 10 Most Surprising Sex Statistics." *LiveScience*, Purch, 8 Apr 2009, www.livescience.com/11387-10-surprising-sex-statistics.html.

Levin, Neil E. *Who's Afriad of GMOs? Me Say No to GMOs,* June 2005. www.saynotogmos.org/ud2005/ujun05b.html

Lipton, Bruce H. *The Biology of Belief: Unleashing the Power of Consciousness, Matter & Miracles.* Hay House, Inc., 2012.

Lugo, Dianne. *U.S. Senate Passes GM Food Labeling Bill.* ScienceMag.org, 8 July 2016 www.sciencemag.org/news/2016/07/us-senate-passes-gm-food-labeling-bill

MacGill, Markus. *How Sodas Impact Diabetes Risk.* MedicalNewsToday.com, 18 Dec 2018.

McCall, Timothy. "*5 Ways to Practice Bhramari.*" Yoga International, 24 May 2013, www.YogaInternational.com/article/view/5-ways-to-practice-bhramari.

Marx, Natalie. "*Alternatively Speaking: Getting in the Mood.*" The Jerusalem Post, 18 Aug 2013, www.jpost.com/LifeStyle/Alternatively-Speaking-323468.

Mayo Clinic Editors. "*Lymphatic System.*" Mayo Foundation for Medical Education and Research. www.MayoClinic.org/diseases-conditions/swollen-lymph-nodes/multimedia/lymphatic-system/img-20007995.

Mohan, AG and Dr. Ganesh Mohan. *Hatha Yoga Pradipika: Translation with Notes from Krishnamacharya.* Svashtha Yoga Press, 2017.

Moss, Michael. *Salt Sugar Fat: How the Food Giants Hooked Us*. Random House, 2013.

Murray, Michael T. and Joseph E. Pizzorno. *The Encyclopedia of Natural Medicine.* Simon & Schuster, 2014.

National Kidney Foundation Editors. *Say No to that Diet Soda*. National Kidney Foundation. www.kidney.org/news/kidneyCare/spring10/DietSoda.

Ng, Chi-Fai, et al. "Effect of Niacin on Erectile Function in Men Suffering Erectile Dysfunction and Dyslipidemia." *The ournal of Sexual Medicine,* U.S. National Library of Medicine, Oct 2011, www.ncbi.nlm.nih.gov/pubmed/21810191.

Ni, Maoshing. *The Yellow Emperor's Classic of Internal Medicine: A New Translation of the Neijing Suwen with Commentary*. Penguin: Random House, Canada, 1995.

NID Editors. "*Digestive Diseases Statistics for the United States.*" National Institute of Diabetes and Digestive and Kidney Diseases, US Dept of Health and Human Services, 1 Nov 2014, www.niddk.nih.gov/health-information/health-statistics/digestive-diseases.

NID Editors. "*Preventing Type 2 Diabetes.*" National Institute of Diabetes, Digestive and Kidney Diseases, Dec 2016. www.niddk.nih.gov/health-information/diabetes/overview/preventing-type-2-diabetes.

NIH Editors. "*Endocrine Disruptors*". National Institute of Environmental Health Sciences, 10 May 2019. www.niehs.nih.gov/health/topics/agents/endocrine/index.cfm.

Noll, Meenakshi, and Fransisca Shepperdson. "Sugary Drinks and Artificial Sweeteners." *The Scrutinizer*, 27 Apr. 2019, https://thescrutinizer.org/sugary-drinks-and-artificial-sweeteners/.

NonGMOProject Editors. "GMO Facts." NonGMOProject.org. www.nongmoproject.org/gmo-facts.

NPD Group Editors. "*Percentage of US Adults Trying to Cut Down or Avoid Gluten.*" The NPD Group, 2013. www.npd.com/wps/portal/npd/us/news/press-releases/percentage-of-us-adults-trying-to-cut-down-or-avoid-gluten-in-their-diets-reaches-new-high-in-2013-reports-npd.

Ogle, Marguerite. "*Pelvic Floor Muscles Need to Be Strengthened with Exercises like Pilates.*" VeryWell Fit, 22 June 2018, www.VeryWellFit.com/the-pelvic-floor-muscles-2704828.

Perlmutter, David and Kristin Loberg. *Grain Brain: the Surprising Truth about Wheat, Carbs and Sugar-Your Brains Silent Killers.* Yellow Kite, 2019.

Petre, Alina. *"5 Benefits and Uses of Frankincense and 7 Myths."* Healthline.com, 19 Dec 2018. www.healthline.com/nutrition/frankincense

Chris Prentice and editor, Jonathan Oatis, "USDA Outlines First-Ever Rule for GMO Labeling, Sees Implementation in 2020." *Reuters,* Thomson Reuters, 20 Dec. 2018, https://www.reuters.com/article/us-usa-gmo-labeling/usda-outlines-first-ever-rule-for-gmo-labeling-sees-implementation-in-2020-idUSKCN1OJ2TF.

Sarno, John. *Healing Back Pain: the Mind-Body Connection.* Grand Central Life & Style, 2016.

Satchidananda, Sri Swami. *The Yoga Sutras of Patanjali: Translation and Commentary.* Integral Yoga Publications, 1978.

Scheer, Roddy, Doug Moss and EarthTalk Editors. "Should People Be Concerned about Parabens in Beauty Products?" Scientific American, 6 Oct 2014, www.ScientificAmerican.com/article/should-people-be-concerned-about-parabens-in-beauty-products/?redirect=1.

Schecter, Anna, et. al. "Farid Fata, Doctor Who Gave Chemo to Healthy Patients, Faces Sentencing." NBCNews.com, NBC Universal News Group, 17 Aug 2015, www.NBCnews.com/health/cancer/farid-fata-doctor-who-gave-chemo-healthy-patients-faces-sentencing-n385161.

Schlosser, Eric. *Fast Food Nation: The Dark Side of the All-American Meal.* Mariner Books/Houghton Mifflin Harcourt, 2012.

Scientific American Editors. *"Should People Be Concerned About Parabens in Beauty Products?"* Scientific American, 6 Oct 2014, www.scientificamerican.com/article/should-people-be-concerned-about-parabens-in-beauty-products.

Seifer, Darren. *"Is Gluten Free Eating a Trend Worth Noting?"* NPD's Industry Analyst Dieting Monitor, March 2013, www.npd.com/perspectives/food-for-thought/gluten-free-2012.

Simon, David and Chopra, Deepak, *The Chopra Center Herbal Handbook,* Three Rivers Press, New York, 2000.

Smith, Jeffrey. *"Doctors Warn: Avoid Genetically Modified Food."* Institute for Responsible Technology, www.responsibletechnology.org/doctors-warn.

Spritzler, Franziska. "8 Benefits of Nuts." Healthline, 17 Jan 2019. www.healthline.com/nutrition/8-benefits-of-nuts#section2.

Spurlock, Morgan. *Super Size Me* Documentary Film. Columbia TriStar Home Entertainment, 2004.

Stewart, James. *Hypnosis in Contemporary Medicine.* Mayo Clinic Proceedings, Apr 2005, vol 80, issue 4, www.mayoclinicproceedings.org/article/S0025-6196%2811%2963203-5/fulltext.

Sunhil, Joshi. *Ayurveda and Panchakarma: The Science of Healing and Rejuvenation.* Lotus Press, 1997.

The Essential Life: Doterra Essential Oils Reference Manual, 5th Edition. Total Wellness Publishing, 2018.

Thomas, Pat. *"Eat GMOs, Get Fat?"* Beyond GM. 30 Jan 2018. www.beyond-gm.org/eat-gmos-get-fat/.

TodayShow. *"6 Foods to Get You in the Mood."* Today.com, 30 July 2014, www.today.com/health/6-foods-get-you-mood-1D80246732.

Trudeau, Kevin. *Natural Cures "They" Don't Want You to Know About.* Alliance Pub Group, 2007.

Van Hare, Holly. *19 Facts About Diet Soda That Might Make Your Stop Drinking It.* The Daily Meal.com, February 2019, www.thedailymeal.com/healthy-eating/scary-facts-diet-soda-gallery.

Watchusgrow.org, https://www.watchusgrow.org/2019/01/08/everything-you-need-to-know-about-gmo-labeling-in-2019/.

WebMD Editors. *Natural Sex Boosters: Can You Rev Up Your Libido?* WebMD. www.WebMD.com/a-to-z-guides/prevention-15/vitamins/sex-drive-supplements?page=2.

Weil, Andrew. *Natural Skin Care.* DrWeil.com, 20 June 2019. www.DrWeil.com/health-wellness/body-mind-spirit/hair-skin-nails/8-natural-skin-care-tips.

Weis-Bohlen, Susan. *Ayurveda Beginners Guide: Essential Ayurvedic Principles & Practices to Balance & Heal Naturally.* Althea Press, 2018.

Wells, Katie. *Dry Brushing for Skin: 5 Benefits and How to Do it the Right Way.* WellnessMama.com, 30 July 2019. www.WellnessMama.com/26717/dry-brushing-skin.

Wired Magazine Staff. *"Placebos Are Getting More Effective: Drugmakers Are Desperate to Know Why."* Wired, Conde Nast, 4 June 2017. www.wired.com/2009/08/ff-placebo-effect/.

"What Is Gluten?" *Celiac Disease Foundation*, https://celiac.org/gluten-free-living/what-is-gluten/.

Zuardi, Antonio. *Should Cannabidiol CBD) Be a Medical Option?* Medical Marijuana Pro-Con.org, 12 July 2019. www.medicalmarijuana.procon.org/view.answers.php?questionID=001656.

SPIRIT SECTION

"6 Ancient Tributes to the Winter Solstice." *LiveScience*, Purch, www.livescience.com/42152-ancient-tributes-to-witner-solstice.html.

A Course in Miracles. Foundation for Inner Peace, 1976.

"A Heart Surgery Overview." *Texas Heart Institute*, www.texasheart.org/heart-health/heart-information-center/topics/a-heart-surgery-overview/.

Abadie, MJ. *The Everything Tarot Book.* Adams Publishing, 1999.

Alcoholics Anonymous: the Story of How Many Thousands of Men and Women Have Recovered from Alcoholism. San Bernardino, CA: Publisher not identified, 2018.

Alexander, Eben. *Proof of Heaven: a Neurosurgeons ourney into the Afterlife.* Large Print Press, 2013.

American Magazine Editors. "*25 Percent of US Christians Believe in Reincarnation. What s Wrong with This Picture?*" America Magazine, 22 Jan. 2017, www.americamagazine.org/faith/2015/10/21/25-percent-us-christians-believe-reincarnation-whats-wrong-picture.

Andrews, Ted. *Animal Speak: The Spiritual & Magical Powers of Creatures Great & Small.* Llewellyn Publications. 2002.

BBC Editors. *Post-Religion Poll finds Most Have Spiritual Beliefs.*' BBC.com, Oct 2013, www.bbc.com/news/uk-24576115.

Bagnall, Roger S. *The Encyclopedia of Ancient History.* Wiley-Blackwell, 2013.

Belsebuub, with Lara Atwood. *The Path of the Spiritual Sun.* Mystical Life Publications, 2017.

Bering, Jesse. "Ian Stevenson's Case for the Afterlife: Are We 'Skeptics' Really Just Cynics?" *Scientific American Blog Network*, 2 Nov. 2013, https://blogs.scientificamerican.com/bering-in-mind/ian-stevensone28099s-case-for-the-afterlife-are-we-e28098skepticse28099-really-just-cynics.

Berkley Center for Religion Editors, and Georgetown University. "*Samsara Hinduism)."* Berkley Center for Religion, Peace and World Affairs. www.berkleycenter.georgetown.edu/essays/samsara-hinduism/# english.

Braden, Gregg. *The Divine Matrix.* Hay House, 2006.

Bro, Harmon Hartzell. *Edgar Cayce on Dreams.* Warner, 1968.

Burke, Kevin, *Astrology: Understanding the Birth Chart.* Llewellyn Publishers, 2001.

Byrne, Lorna. *Angels in My Hair.* Century, 2011.

Byrne, Lorna. YouTube Video, 2015, www.youtube.com/watch?v=ssAmweLstLE.

Cannon, Dolores. *A Soul Remembers Hiroshima.* Ozark Mountain Publishers, 1993.

Cannon, Dolores. *esus and the Essenes.* Ozark Mountain Publishers, 2012.

Castelnovo, Anna, et al. "Post-Bereavement Hallucinatory Experiences: A Critical Overview of Population and Clinical Studies." *ournal of Affective Disorders,* vol 186, 2015, pp 266 274, doi:10.1016/j.jad.2015.07.032, www.ncbi.nlm.nih.gov/pubmed/26254619.

Cayce, Hugh Lynn. "*The Edgar Cayce Collection*" Wings Books, New York, 1968.

Edgar Cayce Readings . Edgar Cayce Foundation, 1971, 1993-2007, www.EdgarCayce.org.

Cerminara, Gina. *Many Mansions, The Edgar Cayce Story on Reincarnation.* Penguin Group Publishing, 1967.

Cheung, Theresa. *The Dream Dictionary from A to .* Harper Collins Publishers, 2008.

Colson, John. *The Method of Fluxions and Infinite Series with Its Application to the Geometry of Curve-Lines, 17 6 by Sir Issac Newton.* Printed by Henry Woodfall, London. https://archive.org/details/methodoffluxions00newt/page/n4.